CARDIOPULMONARY EMERGENCIES

CARDIOPULMONARY EMERGENCIES

Springhouse Corporation
Springhouse, Pennsylvania

Staff

Executive Director, Editorial
Stanley Loeb

Editorial Director
Helen Klusek Hamilton

Clinical Director
Barbara F. McVan, RN

Art Director
John Hubbard

Clinical Editors
Joanne Patzek DaCunha, RN, BS,
Diane Schweisguth, RN, BSN, CCRN,
CEN

Drug Information Editor
George J. Blake, RPh, MS

Editors
Stephanie Forbes, Carole Gan, Kathy
Goldberg, Peter Johnson, Brigid
Wallace, Mary Lou Webster

Copy Editor
Doris Weinstock

Editorial Assistants
Maree DeRosa, Beverly Lane

Designers
Stephanie Peters (associate art
director), Mary Stangl, Lesley
Weissman-Cook

Art Production
Robert Perry (manager), Anna
Brindisi, Donald Knauss, Catherine
Mace, Robert Wieder

Typography
David Kosten (director), Diane Paluba
(manager), Elizabeth Bergman, Joyce
Rossi Biletz, Phyllis Marron, Robin
Rantz, Valerie L. Rosenberger

Manufacturing
Deborah Meiris (manager), T.A.
Landis, Jennifer Suter

Production Coordination
Aline S. Miller (manager), Laurie J.
Sander

© 1991 by Springhouse Corporation, 1111
Bethlehem Pike, Springhouse, Pa., 19477.
All rights reserved. Reproduction in whole
or part by any means whatsoever without
written permission of the publisher is prohib-
ited by law. Authorization to photocopy any
items for internal or personal use, or the internal or personal use of specific clients, is
granted by Springhouse Corporation for
users registered with the Copyright Clearance Center (CCC) Transactional Reporting
Service, provided that the base fee of $.75
per page is paid directly to CCC, 27 Congress St., Salem, MA 01970. For those organizations that have been granted a
license by CCC, a separate system of pay-
ment has been arranged. The fee code for
users of the Transactional Reporting Service is 0874342694/91 $00.00 + $.75.
Printed in the United States of America.

CPE-010890

**Library of Congress
Cataloging-in-Publication Data**
Cardiopulmonary emergencies.
   p   cm.
   Includes bibliographical references.
   Includes index.
   1. Cardiopulmonary system—
Diseases—Nursing. 2. Intensive care
nursing. I. Springhouse Corporation.
   [DNLM: 1. Angina Pectoris—nursing.
2. Asthma—nursing. 3. Emergencies—
nursing. 4. Heart Arrest—nursing.
5. Heart Failure, Congestive—nursing.
6. Myocardial Infarction—nursing.
7. Respiration, Artificial—nursing.
8. Respiratory Distress Syndrome,
Adult—nursing. 9. Respiratory
Insufficiency—nursing. WY 154 C267]
RC702.C36 1991
610.73'691—dc20
DNLM/DLC   90-9760
ISBN 0-87434-269-4   CIP

Contents

Contributors and consultants

Contributors

CHAPTER 1: Cardiac arrest

Lynne Atkinson Rosenberg, RN, BSN, CEN
MSN Candidate, Gwynedd-Mercy
College
Gwynedd Valley, Pa.
Consultant in Emergency Nursing
Past President, Philadelphia Chapter
Emergency Nurses Association

Mark Rosenberg, DO
Director, Emergency Services
Roxborough Memorial Hospital
Philadelphia

CHAPTER 2: Angina

Dawn M. Angst, RN, BSN
Staff Nurse, Critical Care
Lehigh Valley Hospital Center
Allentown, Pa.

Dana A. Bensinger, RN, CCRN
Staff Nurse, Emergency Medicine
St. Luke's Hospital
Bethlehem, Pa.

CHAPTER 3: Myocardial infarction

Kathryn Dolter, RN, BSN, MA, CCRN, CPT/AN
Head Nurse, Neurosurgical Intensive
Care
Brooke Army Medical Center
Fort Sam Houston, Tex.

CHAPTER 4: Congestive heart failure

Deborah Panozzo Nelson, RN, MS,
CCRN
Cardiovascular Clinical Specialist
Consultant, Visiting Assistant
Professor, Staff Nurse
EMS Nursing Education
Purdue University–Calumet
LaGrange, Ill.

CHAPTER 5: Acute respiratory failure

Donald St. Onge, RN, MSN
Pulmonary Clinical Specialist
Allegheny General Hospital
Pittsburgh

CHAPTER 6: Adult respiratory distress syndrome

Phyllis Roach Sutton, RN, MA, CCRN
Clinical Assistant Director of Nursing
New York University Medical Center

CHAPTER 7: Acute asthma

Janet D'Agostino Taylor, RN, MSN
Pulmonary Clinical Specialist
St. Elizabeth's Hospital
Brighton, Mass.

CHAPTER 8: Mechanical ventilation

Karen Sudhoff Allard, RN, MSN, CCRN
Staff Development Educator, Critical
Care
University of Cincinnati Hospitals

Consultants

Linda S. Baas, RN, MSN, CCRN
Cardiac Clinical Nurse Specialist
Nursing Consultation Department
University of Cincinnati Hospitals

Sheila Glennon, RN, MA, CCRN
Critical Care Consultant
New York

Foreword

As changing systems of reimbursement have led to rising acuity levels among hospitalized patients, many patients once cared for in the intensive care unit are now in med/surg units, in outpatient rehabilitation centers, or in home care. As a result, nurses in all clinical settings must keep pace with accelerating technology and be prepared to provide patient care that's consistent with the latest approaches to treatment of major cardiac and respiratory disorders. For example, they must be ready to maintain adequate respiration in critically ill patients because respiratory failure can strike suddenly as a complication of many disease states. They must provide quick remedial interventions based on a thorough knowledge of cardiovascular and respiratory mechanisms and the effects of their dysfunction on interacting vital systems. They must know how to help patients recover by correctly using drug therapy, ventilation support, nursing diagnoses, care plans, and patient-teaching plans that enlist the patient's family in helping to manage acute cardiac and respiratory illness.

Cardiopulmonary Emergencies provides an updated and comprehensive guide to nursing care of acute cardiac and respiratory illness that can be applied to a wide range of practice settings—from critical care units to outpatient care. It provides this information in a unique format that encompasses the latest technical information within a holistic nursing approach.

Each of the first seven chapters in this volume focuses on a major cardiac or respiratory disorder: cardiac arrest, angina, myocardial infarction, congestive heart failure, acute respiratory failure, adult respiratory distress syndrome, and acute asthma. The final chapter, on mechanical ventilation, explains the mechanisms and uses of mechanical ventilation and offers specific recommendations for successfully managing nursing care of patients who require it.

Each chapter begins with an introduction that summarizes its importance to practicing nurses and offers a review of fundamentals related to pathophysiology, assessment, and diagnostic tests. Interwoven among major sections of the text, a complete case study illustrates the practical applications of the information contained in the text. By highlighting real nursing transactions during the treatment of a single patient, the case study personalizes the educational content and encourages the reader to relate specific content of this volume to her own patients.

Each chapter also provides current treatment options with emphasis on nursing management. For example, the chapter on cardiac arrest incorporates American Heart Association guidelines for Advanced Cardiac Life Support, including the use of external pacing and defibrillation; nursing measures to prevent or recognize clinical situations that may lead to an arrest; ethical issues related to resuscitation and organ donation; and the special emotional needs of the survivors of a cardiac arrest and their families.

At the end of each chapter, a section on nursing management emphasizes nursing diagnosis as the foundation for nursing care decisions and priorities. This section offers assessment guidelines and interventions for potential and actual complications, with recommendations for patient and family teaching and discharge planning. To provide continuity, each chapter ends with a summary of the case study and briefly discusses the patient outcome.

The final chapter covers care of patients who require mechanical ventilation. It discusses types of ventilatory assistance, therapeutic adjuncts to mechanical ventilation, and monitoring of potential complications. It concludes with guidelines for weaning the patient from the ventilator and thoroughly explores the relevant psychological issues and techniques for successful weaning.

Cardiopulmonary Emergencies offers a wealth of practical information that can help every nurse—from novice to expert—to provide superior care for patients with major cardiac or respiratory illness.

Sandra K. Goodnough, RN, PhD
Critical Care Consultant
Texas Woman's University
Houston

Linda S. Baas, RN, MSN, CCRN
Cardiac Clinical Nurse Specialist
Nursing Consultation Department
University of Cincinnati Hospitals

CHAPTER 1

Cardiac arrest

Cardiac arrest leads to biological death if resuscitation does not begin within minutes of shutdown of the body's breathing and circulation. Every year, sudden cardiac death takes an estimated toll of 300,000 lives in the United States.

Lifesaving response to cardiac arrest, which includes both basic life support and advanced cardiac life support, is typically handled by an efficiently organized resuscitation team. Successful team intervention can restore the patient's spontaneous respiration and circulation while preserving the function of vital organs.

During resuscitation, nursing concerns include continual assessment and monitoring, as well as participation in cardiopulmonary resuscitation (CPR). After successful resuscitation, nursing concerns include major legal, ethical, and psychosocial issues—for example, questions regarding life-support systems and subsequent quality of life for the patient. After resuscitation and throughout the patient's hospitalization, nursing management should include reassurance and emotional support for both the patient and family.

Case study: Part 1

Collapsed, unconscious, and with no signs of breathing—that's how the security officer described the man he discovered in the restroom of a downtown office building. The security officer notified the operator of the building's switchboard and immediately started CPR. The operator who took the call dispatched an emergency medical services (EMS) mobile intensive care unit (MICU) to the building. When the team arrived, they found the patient—a white man who looked about 35 years old—still unresponsive, with no spontaneous respirations or pulse. Traces of a white powder resembling cocaine were visible in his left nostril. The paramedics took over the CPR at once, established radio contact with the EMS base at the local hospital, and applied a cardiac monitor.

When they saw the chaotic rhythm of ventricular fibrillation on the ECG, they immediately defibrillated the patient at 200 joules; he didn't respond. After a second defibrillation, however, the monitor

Case study: Part 1 *(continued)*

showed a supraventricular tachycardia (SVT) rhythm with occasional premature ventricular contractions (PVCs).

    Although the patient's pupils were equal and reactive, he remained unresponsive. Still unable to detect respirations, the paramedics inserted an esophageal obturator airway attached to a bag-mask device. Then they performed manual ventilation at a rate of 12 ventilations/minute and administered a 100-mg bolus of lidocaine by a peripheral vein. As the van approached the emergency department (ED), the paramedics measured a pulse rate of 150 beats/minute and a mean blood pressure of 88 mm Hg. They also noted that the patient's skin was warm, dry, and pale.

Causes and characteristics

Cardiac arrest is the abrupt cessation of effective heart action resulting in failure to maintain adequate oxygenation of the brain and other vital organs. Sudden cardiac death (SCD) is defined as an abrupt loss of consciousness within 1 hour of the onset of acute cardiac symptoms in an individual with or without pre-existing heart disease, in whom the time and mode of death are unexpected. In adults, SCD includes cardiac arrest that is unexpected and independent of a preexisting heart condition. In infants and children, cardiopulmonary arrest is rarely a sudden, primary cardiac event; it is usually the end result of progressive deterioration of both respiration and circulation.

    Four factors must be present to satisfy the medical and legal requirements for SCD: prodromal signs and symptoms, onset of the terminal event, cardiac arrest, and biological death. However, progression through all four stages may not be identifiable, depending on the underlying cause. For instance, if the cause is a dysrhythmia, prodrome may not occur and onset of cardiac arrest may be instantaneous; if the cause is cardiac failure, all four stages may be identifiable. (See *Stages of progression: Sudden cardiac death.*)

    The underlying cause of most SCDs is coronary artery disease (CAD) and pathologic changes related to it. For example, intraventricular conduction disturbances are known to influence the incidence of SCD in patients with CAD. Anterior myocardial infarctions (MIs) and bundle branch block during the first 30 days after infarction are associated with a risk of ventricular

Stages of progression: Sudden cardiac death

Sudden cardiac death develops in the following sequential stages: prodromal signs and symptoms, onset of the terminal event, the cardiac arrest itself, and progression to biological death. These stages vary greatly. Some individuals, usually when the cause is dysrhythmia, have no prodromal signs and symptoms, with onset leading almost instantaneously to cardiac arrest; some, usually when the cause is cardiac failure, have an onset lasting up to 1 hour before cardiac arrest; and some survive for weeks after the cardiac arrest before progression to biological death if life-support systems are used. These modifying factors influence application of the 1-hour definition of the terminal event. The onset of the terminal event and the cardiac arrest itself are the major clinical factors; the time of biological death has major legal and social importance.

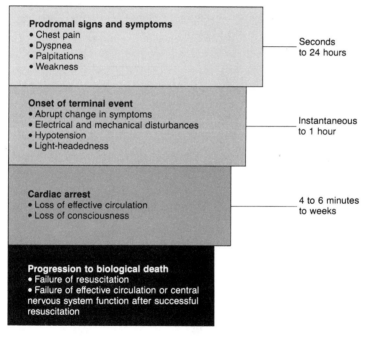

Prodromal signs and symptoms
• Chest pain
• Dyspnea
• Palpitations
• Weakness

Seconds to 24 hours

Onset of terminal event
• Abrupt change in symptoms
• Electrical and mechanical disturbances
• Hypotension
• Light-headedness

Instantaneous to 1 hour

Cardiac arrest
• Loss of effective circulation
• Loss of consciousness

4 to 6 minutes to weeks

Progression to biological death
• Failure of resuscitation
• Failure of effective circulation or central nervous system function after successful resuscitation

fibrillation. Hypertrophic cardiomyopathy is the most common cause of SCD in athletes under age 35; ischemic heart disease is the most common cause in athletes over age 35.

Other factors known to lead to cardiac arrest include drugs; surgery and invasive procedures; and physiologic factors, such

The deadly hours

Harvard Medical School researchers showed that of 2,203 persons who died within 1 hour of the onset of cardiac symptoms, 31% died in the morning, between 6 a.m. and noon. The peak hour, in which 6% of those struck died, was between 10 a.m. and 11 a.m. The "quiet" hour, in which only 3% died, was between 4 a.m. and 5 a.m.

These statistics match those reported for victims of nonfatal myocardial infarction and strokes. Coincidental? Probably not, say several researchers. Their explanations for the similarity in timing include increased blood pressure peaks and blood platelet adhesion (both of which are common in the morning), leading to loosening of fatty acid deposits inside blood vessels and subsequent thrombosis.

as metabolic abnormalities and reflex stimulation. (See *The deadly hours.*)

Whatever the cause, sudden cardiac arrest produces failure of cardiac muscle contraction. Consequently, electrical activity usually shuts down completely in about 20 to 30 minutes; brain cell death usually follows cardiac arrest in about 10 minutes.

Drugs

Toxic doses of sympathomimetic drugs may indirectly cause SCD by inducing ventricular fibrillation. Toxic levels of acetylcholine or other parasympathomimetic drugs are known to induce asystole, which can lead to SCD. Recent therapy with antiarrhythmic drugs (quinidine, disopyramide phosphate)—particularly those that prolong the QT interval (quinidine), decrease the fibrillation threshold, or increase myocardial irritability—has also been linked to SCD.

Abuse of cocaine is now known to sometimes cause SCD even in persons without a history of heart disease. Cocaine raises heart rate and blood pressure and increases the myocardial oxygen demand. Researchers believe cocaine could create a sudden increase in myocardial oxygen demand while simultaneously interfering with blood flow; this would explain, at least partially, the myocardial ischemia observed in cocaine users. (Cocaine has pronounced vasoconstrictor effects.) Further research may identify the mechanism by which cocaine induces cardiac arrest.

Surgery and invasive procedures

Cardiac arrest during surgery can result directly from the effects of general anesthetics and from hypovolemia, hypoxemia, hypercapnia, or respiratory acidosis, which may occur during surgery. It can also follow certain common surgical procedures that are associated with vagal stimulation, such as abdominal surgery involving traction on the gallbladder and eye surgery. With increased external ocular pressure, an afferent oculocardiac reflex that involves both the vagus and trigeminal nerves may cause dysrhythmias.

Certain invasive procedures or complications of diagnostic procedures, such as cardiac catheterization, can result in SCD. For example, insertion of a pacemaker or pulmonary artery catheter may irritate the ventricular myocardium, thereby causing ventricular fibrillation and triggering cardiac arrest. Endotracheal intubation, bronchoscopy, and colonoscopy also tend to precipitate lethal dysrhythmias through stimulation of vagal nerve fibers in the gastrointestinal (GI) and respiratory organs.

Physiologic factors

Central nervous system–related effects, notably those associated with the heart's electrical stability, have also been cited as contributory factors in SCD. Sympathetic nervous system imbalance is identified in some hereditary forms of prolonged QT-interval syndrome. Psychological stress, behavioral abnormalities, and emotional extremes have also been identified as risk factors in SCD. Curiously, auditory stimulation and auditory auras have also been linked to SCD.

Sudden death can also follow metabolic derangements, such as hypothermia and acid-base disorders, and fluid and electrolyte disturbances, such as hypovolemia, hypokalemia, hyperkalemia, hypocalcemia, and hypomagnesemia. In patients with diabetes, autonomic denervation increases the risk of "silent MI" and of SCD.

Previous CAD or certain other cardiac abnormalities may place a person at risk for SCD. For example, 75% of all patients who have died suddenly have a history of earlier MI. Other predisposing cardiac conditions include the following.

Ventricular ectopy or PVC. In persons over age 30, ventricular ectopy greater than 6/minute is a predisposing factor for CAD and for SCD. Survivors of MI who experience frequent or complex forms of PVCs are at an even greater risk. Complex forms of PVCs that carry an increased risk of SCD include multifocal PVCs, bigeminy, short coupling intervals (R-on-T phenomenon), and, especially, salvos of three or more ectopic beats.

Left ventricular dysfunction. This condition can be considered both a co-factor and an independent predictor for SCD. Left ventricular dysfunction with postmyocardial infarction PVCs greatly increases the risk of death, especially in the first 6 months after infarction. Complex postinfarction PVCs seem to carry a greater risk in patients with non-Q-wave infarctions than in those with transmural infarctions.

Reflex stimulation. Stimulation of vagal reflexes—for example, by straining (Valsalva's maneuver) — can precipitate cardiac dysrhythmia. Remember that increased vagal tone may not only propagate sinus bradycardia by slowing the heart rate, but may also depress atrioventricular (AV) conduction, causing atrial and ventricular slowing or asystole.

Individual characteristics

Certain individual characteristics may influence or increase the patient's risk of SCD. These include age, heredity, gender, psychosocial factors, or a history of cardiac disease (especially ventricular ectopy or left ventricular dysfunction).

Age. Two major high-risk age-groups are children between birth and age 6 months and adults between ages 45 and 75. In adults, the incidence of SCD related to CAD rises with advancing age; however, the incidence related to all other causes decreases with advancing age. In children older than those at risk for sudden infant death syndrome, SCD is associated with identifiable heart disease. SCD usually occurs in children who have undergone surgery for congenital cardiac disease (about 25%) or who have cardiac lesions, typically one of the following: congenital aortic stenosis, Eisenmenger's syndrome, tetralogy of Fallot, pulmonary stenosis or atresia, or hypertrophic obstructive cardiomyopathy.

Heredity. Although not a common cause of SCD, genetic predisposition is linked to such syndromes as hereditary and congenital QT-interval prolongation, hypertrophic obstructive cardiomyopathy, and familial SCD in children and adolescents. Progressive familial conduction system disease also carries a risk of SCD.

Gender. SCD is far more common in men than in women. Apparently, premenopausal women benefit from greater protection from coronary atherosclerosis.

Psychosocial factors. Certain life-styles place individuals at greater risk for SCD. Cigarette smokers between ages 30 and 59, for example, have a twofold to threefold increased risk of SCD. Because smoking lowers the threshold for ventricular fibrillation, it is the only CAD risk factor that is also an independent risk factor for ventricular fibrillation.

Obesity— often associated with high cholesterol levels, hypertension, physical inactivity, and heavy consumption of alcohol—is also thought to increase the risk of SCD, although controversy surrounds some of the supporting evidence for this view. Recent changes in health, work, home and family, and personal and social factors cause high levels of stress and increase the risk for SCD. Other significant psychosocial factors include social isolation, a history of psychiatric treatment, and a low educational level.

Cardiac history. A history of CAD, ventricular ectopy, or left ventricular dysfunction is associated with higher risk of SCD.

Pathophysiology

The underlying pathophysiologic cause of deadly tachydysrhythmia, severe bradydysrhythmia, or asystole typically includes complex interactions among coronary vascular events, myocardial injury, and variations in the autonomic, metabolic, and conductive state of the myocardium. Probably multiple pathophysiologic abnormalities combine to induce SCD. However, no single hypothesis explains the mechanisms of these interactions.

Lethal dysrhythmias usually arise as a consequence of acute myocardial ischemia—a condition marked by dramatic electrophysiologic changes, including those associated with transmembrane action potentials and refractory periods. Furthermore, reperfusion after transient ischemia may cause lethal dysrhythmias. Consequently, onset of acute ischemia is now known to cause immediate electrical, mechanical, and biochemical dysfunction of myocardial cells.

Several changes immediately follow ischemia at the cellular level: Myocardial cell membranes lose their selectivity, so potassium ions now flow out of the cell and calcium ions enter the cell, transmembrane resting potentials are reduced, acidosis results, and automaticity is enhanced in some tissues.

During reperfusion, a different series of changes occur: the continued influx of calcium ions, responses to alpha- or beta-adrenoceptor stimulation, and neurophysiologically induced afterdepolarization.

Myocardial tissue status at the time of ischemic injury is another important factor. Abnormal and chronically hypertrophied myocardial tissue, for example, seems more susceptible to the destabilizing electrical effects of acute ischemia. Hypokalemia is known to render the ventricular myocardium more susceptible to potentially lethal dysrhythmias. Such dysrhythmias

Common ECG rhythms in cardiac arrest

VENTRICULAR FIBRILLATION	**VENTRICULAR ASYSTOLE**	**ELECTROMECHANICAL DISSOCIATION**
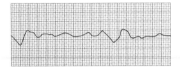	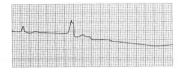	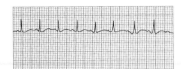

VENTRICULAR FIBRILLATION

Characteristics
- Ventricular rhythm rapid and chaotic, indicating varying degrees of depolarization and repolarization; QRS complexes not identifiable
- Patient unconscious at onset
- Absent pulses, heart sounds, and blood pressure
- Dilated pupils; rapid development of cyanosis

VENTRICULAR ASYSTOLE

Characteristics
- Totally absent ventricular electrical activity
- Possible P waves
- Possible severe metabolic deficit or extensive myocardial damage

ELECTROMECHANICAL DISSOCIATION

Characteristics
- Electrical activity but no pulse
- Organized electrical activity without any evidence of effective myocardial contraction
- Possible failure in the calcium transport system (can cause electromechanical dissociation)
- Possible association with profound hypovolemia, cardiac tamponade, myocardial rupture, massive myocardial infarction, or tension pneumothorax

then result from a triggering event imposed on a susceptible myocardium. For example, premature impulses in a chronically abnormal myocardium may trigger multiple uncoordinated reentrant pathways—that is, ventricular fibrillation. (See *Common ECG rhythms in cardiac arrest.*)

Ventricular fibrillation. This condition is often a direct result of ischemia. (Physiologically, ischemia is characterized by a sudden drop in the transmembrane resting potential, amplitude, and duration of the action potential in the affected area.) Before ischemic cells become completely unable to transmit electrical signals to neighboring cells, they show reduced excitability with slow conduction and electrophysiologically unstable membranes. In this situation, premature impulses generated between adjacent pockets of ischemic and normal heart tissue create a setting for reentry—slow conduction in a unidirectional block—which makes the myocardium vulnerable to reentrant dysrhythmias. Such a condition almost invariably leads to ventricular fibrillation.

Ventricular asystole. When the heart fails to maintain automatic pacing because of electrophysiologic disruptions at the sinus node or the AV junction, bradycardia and asystole may result. Bradydysrhythmias and asystolic arrests are more common in severely diseased hearts.

Electromechanical dissociation. With electromechanical dissociation (EMD), electrical rhythmicity continues in the absence of effective mechanical function. In the primary form, the muscular walls of the ventricles fail to sustain contractions although electrical activity continues. The secondary form results from sudden cessation of cardiac venous return, as in massive pulmonary embolism, acute malfunction of prosthetic valves, severe blood loss, or cardiac tamponade. EMD is the least common mechanism of SCD.

Case study: Part 2

As soon as the MICU arrived at the ED, the medical team connected the patient to another cardiac monitor. Again, the ECG showed SVT with occasional PVCs. They continued the lidocaine drip at an infusion rate of 2 mg/minute.

The patient's pulse rate and mean arterial blood pressure remained unchanged: 150 beats/minute and 88 mm Hg, respectively. His skin was still warm, dry, and pale; his pupils were equal and reactive; and he remained unresponsive without spontaneous respirations. The ED team intubated him and placed him on an MA2 mechanical ventilator. A nurse drew blood samples for analysis of serum electrolytes, cardiac enzymes, and arterial blood gases (ABGs). A chest X-ray and 12-lead ECG showed no abnormalities.

As the patient was being prepared for transfer to the intensive care unit (ICU), an ED nurse searched his belongings for identification and information concerning his medical history. Reaching into the pocket of his suit jacket, she felt a powdery substance, then discovered a small sterling silver pillbox with its top unhinged. Inside the box, she saw a small mound of white powder.

She also found a wallet and began looking for a Medic Alert card or other medical history information. She found none—but she did find a driver's license and business card. The patient, she learned, was Garon Gardner II, a 33-year-old corporate attorney for a downtown law firm. After finding Mr. Gardner's telephone number in the directory, she called his home. His wife Marilyn answered and said she'd be at the hospital as soon as possible.

In the meantime, the laboratory report arrived. ABG values were as follows: pH, 7.20; $Paco_2$, 50 mm Hg; Pao_2, 60 mm Hg; HCO_3^-, 15 mEq/liter; and Sao_2, 0.90 (90%).

Assessment and diagnosis

In the patient with SCD, emergency assessment and intervention must be performed simultaneously. This section will review confirmation of the four progressive stages of SCD: prodromal signs and symptoms, onset of the terminal event, cardiac arrest, and biological death.

Prodromal signs and symptoms

Common signs and symptoms of impending cardiac arrest or SCD include onset of chest pain, chest pain unrelieved by nitroglycerin, chest pain at rest, palpitations and dysrhythmias, shortness of breath at rest, dyspnea, increased orthopnea, diaphoresis, and sudden changes in blood pressure and level of consciousness. Other common but nonspecific symptoms are weakness or fatigue and restlessness. (See *Diagnostic profile: Laboratory tests.*)

Assessment of patients with prodromal signs and symptoms should be performed quickly and accurately. In emergency situations, assessment usually may have to proceed simultaneously with treatments, such as insertion of an intravenous (I.V.) line and administration of supplemental oxygen.

The patient's chief complaint will often guide you in obtaining a personal history. Phrase your questions so the patient can provide "yes," "no," or short responses—for example, "Do you have chest pain now?" or "Are you having difficulty breathing?" Take a few moments to look at your patient. Observe skin color. Is it cyanotic? Ruddy? Is his skin cool to the touch or clammy? Watch your patient's body language. Is he grimacing? Are his fists clenched? During such assessment, careful listening is vital. Commonly, the patient in prodromal stages subtly expresses a feeling of "impending doom." More often than not, this feeling reliably signals an impending emergency. Learn to listen for such clues and develop your own intuitive "sixth sense" that so often helps expert nurses give excellent care.

While obtaining the patient's history, remember that cardiac arrest or SCD may occur from noncardiac-related complaints. For this reason, check vital signs immediately and constantly monitor:
• cardiovascular system (heart rate, rhythm, and sounds; rate, rhythm, equality and presence of arterial pulses; neck veins for distention and pulsation; point of maximum impulse for thrills)

DIAGNOSTIC PROFILE

Laboratory tests

Tests that measure serum electrolytes and cardiac enzymes are commonly performed to help determine the cause of cardiac arrest or evaluate treatment. *Note:* Laboratory values may vary.

Serum electrolytes
Electrolyte profiles commonly measure potassium, sodium, chloride, calcium, phosphate, magnesium, blood urea nitrogen (BUN), carbon dioxide (CO_2) content, and glucose.
• Serum potassium
Physiologic values: 3.5 to 5 mEq/liter
Possible abnormalities: hyperkalemia, hypokalemia
• Serum sodium
Physiologic values: 135 to 145 mEq/liter
Possible abnormalities: hypernatremia, hyponatremia
• Serum chloride
Physiologic values: 95 to 105 mEq/liter
Possible abnormalities: hyperchloremia, hypochloremia (commonly associated with hypokalemia and metabolic alkalosis)
• Serum calcium
Total serum calcium values: 8.5 to 10.5 mg/dl or 4.0 to 5.5 mEq/liter
Serum ionized calcium values: usually 50% of total serum calcium

Possible abnormalities: acidosis, alkalosis
• Serum phosphate
Physiologic values: 2.5 to 4.8 mg/dl or 1.8 to 2.6 mEq/liter
Possible abnormalities: hyperphosphatemia, hypophosphatemia
• Serum magnesium
Physiologic values: 1.8 to 3.0 mg/dl or 1.5 to 2.5 mEq/liter
Possible abnormalities: hypermagnesemia, hypomagnesemia
• BUN
Physiologic values: 10 to 20 mg/dl
Possible abnormalities: hypovolemia, excessive protein intake, increased catabolism, overhydration, reduced protein intake
• CO_2 content
Physiologic values: 24 to 30 mEq/liter *Note:* CO_2 content reflects total serum bicarbonate and carbonic acid levels.
Possible abnormalities: metabolic alkalosis, metabolic acidosis
• Serum glucose
Physiologic values: 70 to 100 mg/dl
Possible abnormalities: osmotic diuresis, hypovolemia.

Cardiac enzymes
Enzymes and subtypes of enzymes (isoenzymes) can be detected in the circulation roughly 30 to 60 minutes after irreversible myocardial tissue injury. Clinicians typically examine the pattern of en-

zyme levels when they suspect myocardial infarction (MI). Elevated levels of creatine phosphokinase (CPK), lactic dehydrogenase (LDH), and serum aspartate aminotransferase (AST), formerly SGOT, indicate MI.
• CPK is considered the most accurate indicator of MI. The isoenzyme CPK-MB concentrates mainly in the heart; it rises markedly 4 to 8 hours after MI onset and may remain elevated for 72 hours.
Physiologic values: undetectable to 7 IU/liter
Possible abnormalities: myocarditis, cardiac trauma (possibly resulting from cardiopulmonary resuscitation)
• LDH levels peak 3 to 6 days following onset of chest pain.
Physiologic values: 48 to 115 IU/liter. The isoenzymes LDH_1 and LDH_2 concentrate primarily in the heart.
Possible abnormalities: anemia, leukemia, myocarditis
• AST concentrates in the heart, but it is not a reliable marker of cardiac dysfunction. Elevated AST readings can also result from liver disease, shock, and pulmonary embolism. Many hospitals no longer use AST levels as part of their cardiac enzyme analysis.

• respiratory system (breath sounds, respiratory rate and quality, and chest symmetry)
• renal system (urine output for amount, color, and odor)
• skin (color, temperature, turgor, nail bed capillary refill in the extremities)

• blood pressure (hypotension, hypertension, pulsus alternans, pulsus paradoxus)
• neurologic system (orientation to time, place, and person; restlessness).

Subtle changes, such as restlessness, drop in blood pressure, and clammy skin, can signal impending cardiac arrest.

The patient with prodromal signs and symptoms requires continuous assessment by cardiac monitor. Diagnostic studies may include a 12-lead ECG; serum laboratory studies, such as serum electrolyte levels and cardiac enzyme analysis; ABG analysis; and a chest X-ray. Additional tests may be appropriate, depending on the patient's history and physical examination.

Onset of the terminal event

The interval of 1 hour or less between acute changes in the prodromal signs and symptoms and actual cardiac arrest is the *onset of the terminal event.* During this interval, common changes in cardiac electrical activity may include fluctuating heart rate and advancing grades with ventricular ectopy—including R-on-T phenomenon, ventricular tachycardia, and ventricular fibrillation. These changes can produce slowing of electrical activity, resulting in bradycardia.

These changes, which produce corresponding deterioration of the patient's clinical status, usually result from decreased cardiac output. Watch for falling blood pressure and cooling of skin temperature, diminishing urine output, and change in level of consciousness. Expect to see the patient's skin color turn pale and possibly dusky. Restlessness will increase, and nail bed capillary refill will be prolonged. Other vital signs, such as heart rate and respiratory rate, will fluctuate with the patient's clinical condition, the cause of impending cardiac arrest, and the length of time between the onset of prodromal signs and symptoms and the actual cardiac arrest. If oxygen therapy, I.V. lines, and cardiac monitoring are not yet in place, they must be started immediately.

Cardiac arrest

Cardiac arrest is marked by an abrupt loss of responsiveness or consciousness caused by inadequate cerebral blood flow. The patient is pulseless and unresponsive and stops breathing. Cardiac arrest's other clinical features may include any of the following dysrhythmias: ventricular fibrillation (most common), brady-dysrhythmias, ventricular asystole, and electromechanical dissociation and ventricular tachycardia. Pupils may or may not dilate as a secondary response to inadequate cerebral blood flow.

If the patient is monitored and rhythm is ventricular fibrillation, defibrillation should be immediate, followed by assessment of the patient's airway, breathing, and circulation (ABCs). In assessing the airway, look and listen. Place your ear close to the patient's nose and mouth. If he is breathing, you should be able to hear his respirations and feel his breath on your cheek. If the airway is not patent, intervene immediately to open it.

Once the airway is patent, assess breathing. Evaluate its rate, depth, and quality. Observe the chest wall for symmetrical chest movements with respirations and use of accessory muscles. If breathing is inadequate, intervene immediately to provide adequate ventilation.

To assess circulation, check central pulses (femoral or carotid). If central pulses are strong and regular, check blood pressure. If no pulse is evident, begin CPR immediately and call a code according to your institution's policies. (See "Resuscitation techniques" on page 14 for more information on CPR.)

If the patient is in cardiac arrest, his history must be available to the code team members because it may help determine specific interventions. If the cardiac arrest occurs in a hospital setting, initiate CPR while another team member obtains the patient's history. Possible sources include medical records, the patient's personal identification, and family members. Relatives can also provide information about possible drug and food allergies, and use of prescribed and over-the-counter drugs.

If cardiac arrest occurs outside the hospital, a team member should interview the prehospital rescue team and members of the patient's family. Be sure to obtain a written record of the resuscitative effort. This record should include the duration of the cardiac arrest, the time interval between the onset of cardiac arrest and the beginning of resuscitation efforts, and life-support interventions and outcomes. In trauma victims, also record details about the cause of injury, which can help guide therapy.

BLS: An update

Basic life support (BLS) standards have changed. Periodic re-
fresher courses are recommended to keep your BLS
certification current. Both the
American Heart Association
(AHA) and the American Red
Cross offer BLS training and certification. Here are some recent
notes from the AHA:
• Cardiopulmonary resuscitation
(CPR) procedures differ very little for adults and children. Depending on the child's size, both
the nose and mouth are sealed
off during resuscitation. Also,
only use one hand for chest
compressions and go down 1" to
1½" (2.5 to 3.8 cm), rather than
the 1½" to 2" (3.8 to 5.1 cm)
used for adults.
• Disposable airway equipment
or resuscitation bags, along with
gloves and clear plastic face
masks with one-way valves, are
now suggested for use during
CPR because of the potential
risk of contracting such diseases
as hepatitis B and acquired immunodeficiency syndrome.

Don't forget the patient's family. They can be extremely anxious. For them, minutes seem like hours. While the code team is attempting resuscitation, another team member should establish a rapport with the family, making every effort to inform them at least every 15 minutes and offering appropriate reassurance without arousing false hope. The family needs to know that everything possible is being done. If possible, a private room with a phone should be made available to them. Some institutions now allow family members at the code scene, but this is controversial.

Progression to biological death

Uninterrupted ventricular fibrillation commonly leads to irreversible brain damage within 4 to 6 minutes and to biological death within 10 minutes. The time course of biological death varies with the patient's medical history, the nature of the arrest, and the elapsed time between the onset of symptoms and resuscitation efforts.

Case study: Part 3

Once in the ICU, Mr. Gardner's cardiac monitor showed an abrupt change to ventricular fibrillation. Immediate defibrillation with 200 joules elicited no response; a second attempt with 300 joules also failed. Fortunately, the third defibrillation with 300 joules produced conversion to sinus tachycardia with frequent PVCs. The patient's pulse was palpable at a rate of 126 beats/minute and his blood pressure measured 90/60 mm Hg.

The cardiologist ordered another 100-mg bolus of lidocaine and increased the infusion rate to 4 mg/minute. The patient remained unresponsive, but his pupils were equal and reactive. Because he still wasn't breathing spontaneously, the doctor continued mechanical ventilation. An indwelling catheter was inserted to measure urine output and monitor renal function.

Shortly after the patient's arrival in the ICU, the patient's family was escorted to the ICU waiting room. The patient's primary nurse and the ICU doctor discussed the patient's situation with them.

Resuscitation techniques

The interventions designed to resuscitate patients in cardiac arrest are classified as basic life support (BLS) and advanced cardiac life support (ACLS) techniques.

BLS techniques

BLS involves the administration of CPR to a patient who has an obstructed airway or is in respiratory or cardiac arrest. Its purpose is to maintain function of the patient's vital organs until definite interventions can begin. The ABCs of CPR mandate confirming unresponsiveness and absence of breathing and pulse before CPR can begin. CPR is warranted if pulse or spontaneous respirations are absent. (See *BLS: An update.*)

Once the cardiac arrest has been confirmed and CPR begun, the resuscitation or code team should be alerted. *Note:* Be sure to know and follow your institution's policy on cardiac arrest. The code team acts quickly and in unison, anticipating the patient's needs.

ACLS techniques

Once CPR has been initiated and other members of the resuscitation team begin to arrive, ACLS can begin. (See *Code team responsibilities,* at right, and *Code record,* page 16.) The goals of ACLS are to provide adequate ventilation; to begin, maintain, and support a hemodynamically effective cardiac rhythm; and to maintain and support restored circulation. The technical elements used to achieve these goals are BLS and the use of adjunctive equipment and special techniques, ECG monitoring to detect dysrhythmias, establishment and maintenance of I.V. access, and administration of pharmacologic and electrical therapies for emergency treatment of cardiac and respiratory arrests, for postarrest stabilization, and for treatment of overt or suspected acute MI. (For more information on ACLS and treatment of patients with suspected or overt acute MI, see Chapter 3, Myocardial infarction.)

Ventilation and oxygen. Critical to effective ventilation, supplemental oxygen must be delivered to a patient in cardiac arrest as soon as possible. Although normal room air contains 21% oxygen, mouth-to-mouth resuscitation provides only 16% to 17% oxygen. This amount is adequate to sustain life because it produces a partial pressure of alveolar oxygen of 80 mm Hg. However, this lower oxygen level, superimposed on the patient's low cardiac output, and the presence of intrapulmonary shunting and ventilation-perfusion abnormalities often cause a discrep-

Code team responsibilities

The code team usually must assume the following eight roles:
• Team leader has overall responsibility for running the code, overseeing resuscitation efforts, and directing any major lifesaving interventions.
• Basic rescuer 1 calls for another rescuer and starts one-person cardiopulmonary resuscitation (CPR).
• Basic rescuer 2 calls the code team and performs two-person CPR with basic rescuer 1.
• Nurse anesthetist, anesthesiologist, or respiratory therapist maintains a patent airway, intubates the patient as necessary, administers oxygen as directed, and monitors respiratory status.
• Medication nurse brings a code cart and prepares and administers all medications. *Note:* In some institutions, a pharmacist assists with medication preparation.
• Equipment nurse sets up adjunctive emergency equipment, takes vital signs, and helps with medications as needed.
• Go-between nurse stays flexible, helping out when needed.
• Recorder nurse documents resuscitation efforts and writes postarrest progress notes.

Code record

The code record describes the resuscitation effort and should include the following detailed information:
• patient biographical data
• time of arrest
• witnessed or unwitnessed arrest
• cardiac or respiratory arrest, or both
• time resuscitation was initiated
• drug therapy, including time, dose, route, and person administering
• cardiac rhythms generated
• countershocks delivered, including energy level and outcome
• presence of spontaneous pulses and respirations
• special procedures
• patient status and disposition at end of arrest
• time resuscitation ended
• names of all personnel participating in code.

ancy between partial pressures of alveolar and arterial oxygen. This discrepancy further complicates matters by producing hypoxemia, which then leads to anaerobic metabolism and metabolic acidosis. To prevent these conditions, which often interfere with drug and electrical therapy, delivery of 100% oxygen is recommended.

To deliver oxygen, a patient's airway must be patent at all times. Four adjunctive therapies are commonly used during a cardiac arrest to open the airway and keep it patent. These include an oropharyngeal airway, a nasopharyngeal airway, an esophageal obturator airway (EOA) or esophageal gastric tube airway (EGTA), and endotracheal intubation. Cricothyrotomy, transtracheal (or translaryngeal) catheter ventilation, and tracheotomy may be used occasionally. (See *Precautions for intubation.*)

Oropharyngeal airway. This semicircular piece of plastic, metal, or rubber tubing is placed between the tongue and the posterior wall of the pharynx to establish an open airway. It should be in place whenever a bag-valve-mask device or a manually cycled, oxygen-powered mechanical breathing device is used. An oropharyngeal airway should be used only in unconscious patients because it triggers gagging or vomiting in conscious or semiconscious patients.

Nasopharyngeal airway. An uncuffed plastic or rubber tube, a nasopharyngeal airway (also called a trumpet tube) is used in semiconscious patients or in those with conditions that prevent insertion of an oropharyngeal airway. The nasopharyngeal tube is inserted along the floor of the patient's nostril and past the tongue into the posterior pharynx.

EOA or EGTA. An EOA is a soft, cuffed plastic tube with several openings corresponding to the level of the pharynx. The tube, mounted onto a face mask, is placed into the esophagus, and the cuff is inflated with 30 cc of air (maximum) to seal off the esophageal opening and prevent air from entering the stomach. The pharyngeal openings allow air to pass through the holes and enter the trachea, thereby ventilating the lungs. The EGTA, a variation on the EOA, has an opening at the distal end of the tube that allows placement of a catheter for suctioning the stomach. It is used only in unconscious patients.

Endotracheal intubation. An endotracheal tube may be inserted (by specially trained personnel only) if the patient is

Precautions for intubation

Oropharyngeal airway
Correct placement of the tube within the patient's mouth is critical. Take care to keep the head in a chin-lift position and to ensure that the lips are not wedged between the airway and the teeth. Avoid airway obstruction: Do not trap the tongue in the back of the pharynx or press the epiglottis against the entrance of the larynx.

Nasopharyngeal airway
Avoid using a tube that's too long; if the tube enters the esophagus, gastric distention or hyperventilation might occur during ventilation. Use a water-soluble lubricant with a local anesthetic during insertion to protect mucous membranes, and keep the patient's head in a high head-lift position.

Esophageal or gastric tube
Be sure to verify correct placement of an esophageal obturator airway (EOA). If the esophagus has been correctly intubated, the rise and fall of the patient's chest wall will be evident. Verify correct placement of the EOA or esophageal gastric tube airway (EGTA) by mouth-to-tube or bag-valve-to-tube before ventilating the patient. If the tube has entered the trachea, chest wall extension and breath sounds will be absent and auscultation of the epigastrium will produce gurgling sounds. If this occurs, extract the airway immediately and initiate another ventilation method.

Esophageal airways should be used only in patients who are unconscious, older than age 16, and free of esophageal disease. Because removal of an esophageal airway is frequently followed immediately by regurgitation, the tube should be removed after insertion of an endotracheal tube in patients who remain semiconscious or unconscious. If the patient is conscious, alert, and breathing spontaneously, the esophageal airway should be removed. Before removal, the patient should be turned on his side with suctioning available and the balloon deflated.

Endotracheal intubation
During intubation, ventilation should not be interrupted for more than 15 seconds. If repeated attempts at intubation are necessary, adequate ventilation and oxygen must be provided between attempts. Aside from adequate ventilation, endotracheal intubation also allows administration of certain drugs and suctioning of the trachea. Once the endotracheal tube is in place, chest compressions should be spaced asynchronously at 12 to 15 per minute for an adult.

unconscious; it is the preferred method of ventilation in ACLS. The tube should be 7.5 to 8 mm in internal diameter for women and 8 to 8.5 mm for men. For children, use the diameter of the nail bed on the child's little finger to approximate the correct tube diameter. Tubes with cuffs are usually not used in children younger than age 8. Tube placement should be at least 3 cm above the carina and verified by X-ray. Breath sounds should be equal on both sides with no sounds proceeding from the stomach.

Other methods. If rapid entrance to the trachea is required in a patient with continued airway obstruction, a cricothyrotomy may be performed. Cricothyrotomy is a surgical procedure in which a #6 tracheostomy tube is inserted into an opening between the topmost prominence of the thyroid cartilage and the second prominence of the cricoid cartilage. Ventilation should be provided with positive-pressure ventilation at a high oxygen concentration.

An over-the-needle catheter can be inserted through the cricothyroid membrane (needle cricothyrotomy) to provide transtracheal catheter ventilation until a tracheotomy or endotracheal intubation can be performed for patients with an obstructed airway. Ventilation is provided by jet insufflation (a temporary means of periodic ventilation through a catheter). Subsequent ventilation is provided by an external high-pressure oxygen source connected by I.V. extension tubing to the catheter with a hand-operated release valve and a pressure-regulated adjustment valve. The hand-operated release valve sends oxygen flowing into the trachea. Releasing the valve after the lungs are inflated allows passive exhalation. The pressure-regulated valve should be adjusted to allow the minimum pressure that sustains lung inflation.

Tracheotomy provides an opening for insertion of a tracheal tube. Cricothyrotomy, transtracheal catheter ventilation, and tracheotomy must be performed only by specially trained personnel.

Administering oxygen

All patients with cardiac or respiratory arrest or hypoxemia should receive 100% oxygen as soon as possible. With respiratory support, oxygen will increase hemoglobin saturation and PaO_2. Oxygen may be administered by several methods: nasal cannulas or masks, bag-valve-mask devices, and oxygen-powered mechanical breathing devices. The choice of method depends on several factors, but mainly on whether or not the patient is breathing spontaneously.

Nasal cannulas or masks. A nasal cannula is a low-flow system that delivers humidified oxygen at 22% to 30% concentration. The simple face mask is another low-flow system; it delivers humidified oxygen at 40% to 60% concentration with a recommended flow rate of 8 to 10 liters/minute. A face mask with oxygen reservoir provides oxygen concentrations higher than 60% at a flow rate of 6 liters/minute. The oxygen reservoir bag lets the patient rebreathe exhaled air. This mask may be modified to allow partial or no rebreathing. To allow partial rebreathing, apply the mask snugly during exhalation, never letting the bag deflate totally during inhalation. A Venturi mask may be used for patients with chronic lung disease and moderate to severe hypoxemia. This high-flow system provides a fixed oxygen concentration of 24%, 28%, 35%, or 40% and an oxygen flow rate of 4, 4, 8, or 8 liters/minute respectively. *Note:* Nasal cannulas or masks should be used only in spontaneously breathing patients.

Bag-valve-mask devices. With a bag-valve-mask device, such as an Ambu bag, you can ventilate the patient with room air (21% oxygen). By providing 12 liters/minute from an additional oxygen source, you can raise the oxygen concentration to 40%. And if you add a plastic cap and a 3′ (0.9-m) reservoir of corrugated tubing with an open end, you can raise the oxygen concentration to about 90%.

To provide ventilation with a bag-valve-mask unit, use an oropharyngeal or nasopharyngeal airway with the unit to maintain a patent airway. To ventilate with oxygen (preferable when available), attach the bag to the mask and connect it to an oxygen source unit. (To ventilate with room air, just attach the bag to the mask.) Keep the patient's lower jaw elevated, and hyperextend his neck (unless contraindicated). Place the mask over his face. (If he has an endotracheal tube, EOA, or tracheostomy tube in place, remove the mask from the bag and attach the unit directly to the tube.) Use firm pressure to seal the mask tightly to his face, keeping his neck hyperextended. (Keep a child's neck in a neutral, or "sniffing," position.) Compress the bag with your free hand. Watch for the patient's chest to rise and fall with each compression.

Oxygen-powered mechanical breathing devices. Manually triggered oxygen-powered mechanical breathing devices can deliver 100% oxygen and may be used for a patient with cardiac or respiratory arrest. Like the bag-valve-mask devices, these devices require an oropharyngeal or nasopharyngeal airway. High-pressure (50-psi) oxygen sources power these devices. High instantaneous flow rates are controlled by a manual button. These devices can be used with a mask, an endotracheal tube, an esophageal airway, a tracheostomy tube, or as an inhalant for a spontaneously breathing patient who needs oxygen.

Consider the following precautions that apply to use of oxygen-powered mechanical breathing devices with masks:
• Know how to use them correctly to minimize mistakes.
• Use the special adaptor required for children.
• Watch for possible system failure caused by high airway resistance.
• Watch for gastric inflation or distention.

Suctioning

Rigid pharyngeal catheters clear secretions from the mouth and pharynx; tracheobronchial suction catheters clear secretions from the endotracheal tube or nasopharynx. Suctioning can cause complications that include sudden onset of hypoxemia resulting from decreased lung volume; this can worsen the patient's hemodynamic status or even lead to cardiac arrest. In some patients, suctioning can cause vagal stimulation, leading to bradycardia and hypotension. The suctioning catheter may trigger coughing by stretching the mucosa; such coughing can raise intracranial pressure and reduce cerebral blood flow.

Supplementary support of circulation

Methods to support circulation include the use of mechanical devices for chest compression, medical antishock trousers (MAST suit), and the intra-aortic balloon pump (IABP). Rarely, internal cardiac compression may also be used to support circulation.

Mechanical chest compressors. For use only in adults, mechanical chest compressors can free CPR personnel to deliver ACLS, ensure adequate compressions during transport, and ease rescuer fatigue during prolonged resuscitation. They can be manually operated or automatic. A manually operated compressor, called a cardiac press, is a simple hinged device. It should be equipped to depress the chest 1½" to 2" (4 to 5 cm). During use of the cardiac press, artificial ventilation can be administered during the upstroke of every fifth chest compression. An automatic mechanical chest compressor consists of a compressed gas–powered plunger fastened to a backboard. It can provide compression and ventilation during CPR. This device can provide acceptable ECGs and does not require removal for defibrillation.

Compressor ventilation should be provided only with endotracheal tubes, face masks, or EOAs, as appropriate.

MAST suit. Also called a pneumatic antishock garment, (PASG), a MAST suit is usually used to raise the mean arterial pressure by selectively increasing peripheral vascular resistance in the lower half of the body. While no evidence exists that a MAST suit increases the survival rate of cardiac arrest patients, it does produce a definite hemostatic effect; it is therefore potentially useful for hypovolemic shock caused by bleeding in the lower half of the body. If a MAST suit improves the patient's clinical status, it should be used until hypovolemia is corrected and then gradually deflated. Of course, if a MAST suit worsens the patient's condition, it should be deflated immediately.

IABP. Another adjunct to circulation, especially in patients with left ventricular power failure (low output syndrome), an IABP pump provides intra-aortic balloon counterpulsation. A balloon inserted into the aorta is inflated during ventricular diastole after closure of the aortic valve; this supplements blood flow and boosts perfusion pressure in the coronary artery. With ventricular systole, the balloon rapidly deflates, reducing afterload and, consequently, left ventricular work load. (See *Promising research: Experimental circulation support and monitoring.*)

Internal cardiac compression. Also known as direct cardiac massage, this technique for restoring circulation should be used only within a hospital setting and requires expertise in thoracotomy and respiratory support. Indications for open-chest cardiac compression include cardiac arrest associated with severe trauma, such as penetrating chest trauma and crushed-chest injury; open-heart surgery; thoracic deformity or lung disease that limits chest compressions; ruptured aortic aneurysm or cardiac tamponade; and severe hypothermia.

I.V. fluids. Because blood is shunted away from muscle and skin during cardiac arrest, emergency rescue should include direct administration of fluid and drugs into the circulatory system via an I.V. line placed in a peripheral vein to avoid interfering with CPR. If necessary, a central vein (internal jugular or subclavian) may be used and is preferred over intracardiac injection.

PROMISING RESEARCH

Experimental circulation support and monitoring

Four other circulatory techniques are currently being studied and may prove useful.

• The cardiopulmonary support system gains access to the circulatory system by cannulation of the femoral artery and thus provides emergency cardiopulmonary bypass without thoracotomy.

• Simultaneous compression-ventilation CPR (SCV-CPR) maintains high-pressure ventilation through endotracheal intubation with closed-chest compressions. Like standard CPR, this technique requires asynchronous breath support. It is promising because, in some patients, more blood flow results from increased intrathoracic pressure than from direct cardiac compression.

• Interposed abdominal compression CPR (IAC-CPR) involves alternating thoracic and abdominal compressions supported by standard asynchronous ventilation. IAC-CPR increases peripheral blood flow, but there is still no evidence that it enhances cerebral perfusion pressure.

• A conjunctival oxygen monitor may aid assessment of cerebral perfusion, which is a reliable indicator of the patient's circulatory status. This device uses a polarographic Clark electrode, which is mounted on a doughnut-shaped ocular conformer and fitted into the superior and inferior conjunctival fornices.

Electrocardiographic monitoring

Early detection and prompt treatment of dysrhythmias often prevent fatal outcomes. Therefore, continuous cardiac monitoring should be provided as soon as possible for the patient with prodromal signs and symptoms as well as for the patient in cardiac arrest. *Note:* Quick-look paddles on defibrillators may be used initially to avoid delay in initiating cardiac monitoring or interventions.

Dysrhythmias result from conduction disturbances leading to conduction delay or block and reentry or from an impulse formation disturbance. Impulse formation disturbances often result from altered automaticity: Enhanced automaticity may cause extrasystoles, premature beats, or tachycardia; depressed automaticity can lead to bradycardia or escape beats. Impulse formation disturbances can also occur when afterdepolarization and triggered activity cause repetitive ectopic firing from stimulation by a prior impulse. (See *Recognizing dysrhythmias,* pages 24 to 26.)

Competent participation in ACLS requires the ability to recognize ventricular tachycardia, ventricular fibrillation, asystole, symptomatic bradycardia, and electromechanical dissociation, which must commonly precede cardiac arrest. It also requires recognition of certain other dysrhythmias, including sinus tachycardia, premature atrial contraction, atrial tachycardias, atrial flutter, atrial fibrillation, junctional rhythm, premature junctional contraction, junctional tachycardias, AV block, ventricular dysrhythmias, and ventricular flutter.

Therapies for dysrhythmias

Defibrillation, synchronized cardioversion, precordial thump, and pacemakers are highly effective therapies for various dysrhythmias. They are useful during emergency treatment and postarrest stabilization. (See *Automatic external defibrillator,* page 27.)

Defibrillation. Passing an electrical current through a fibrillating heart to depolarize a critical mass of the myocardium can convert life-threatening dysrhythmias—specifically, ventricular fibrillation and ventricular tachycardia—into normal cardiac rhythm if the depolarized cells manage to repolarize uniformly. Uniform repolarization can restore organized, coordinated contractions if the sinoatrial node generates a normal electrical impulse. Defibrillation is the treatment of choice for ventricular fibrillation; it is used to treat ventricular tachycardia if the patient is unconscious or lacks sufficient circulation.

The effectiveness of defibrillation depends on the myocardial metabolic status. The longer fibrillation persists, the greater the resulting myocardial deterioration and the less likely that defibrillation will be successful. Because defibrillation may fail if the myocardium becomes too hypoxic, BLS may be necessary before defibrillation can be successful. Myocardial acidosis, hypothermia, electrolyte imbalances, and drug toxicity may also block a successful response to defibrillation.

Other factors can also prevent successful defibrillation: the number of and interval between previous shocks; the electrical current's energy level; the size, position, and pressure of the paddle electrodes; and electrical resistance. Remember, the longer the patient remains in ventricular fibrillation, the less likely the recovery. Repeated attempts at defibrillation lead to decreased transthoracic resistance. For adults, ACLS standards allow for the delivery of three electrical shocks of 200 joules (watt-seconds), 200 to 300 joules, and 360 joules, respectively. Such a series of electrical current should be powerful enough to restore rhythm without damaging the myocardium and without triggering another deadly dysrhythmia. For open-heart defibrillation, give only 5 joules for the initial shock and no more than 50 joules for any subsequent shock. (For children, ACLS standards recommend 2 joules/kg of body weight initially and 4 joules/kg for second attempts.) Defibrillation should begin as soon as possible with the three shocks delivered consecutively— even if it means interrupting BLS.

The paddle electrode size, position, and pressure are all significant factors. The paddle electrodes should be 1¾″ (4.5 cm) in diameter for infants and young children, 3″ (8 cm) for older children, and 4″ (10 cm) for adults. Each of the electrodes should be placed to maximize current flow through the heart. Standard procedure is to place one electrode anteriorly to the right clavicle, the other to the left of the nipple with the center of the electrode in the midaxillary line. Alternatively, one paddle may be placed anteriorly over the left precordium and the other posteriorly behind the heart. (See *Paddle placement for defibrillation,* page 28.)

(Text continues on page 26.)

Recognizing dysrhythmias

SINUS DYSRHYTHMIAS

Sinus tachycardia

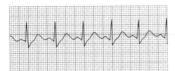

ECG characteristics. Regular rhythm; rate between 100 and 160 beats/minute.

Sinus bradycardia

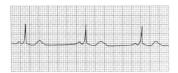

ECG characteristics. Regular rhythm; rate less than 60 beats/minute.

ATRIAL DYSRHYTHMIAS

Premature atrial contraction (PAC)

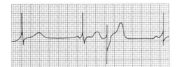

ECG characteristics. Premature and abnormal P waves, possibly lost in the previous T wave; PR intervals longer or shorter than normal; and normal QRS complexes, unless the patient has delayed or absent ventricular conduction. If the impulse arrives in the ventricles during their absolute refractory stage, no QRS complex follows the P wave (known as a nonconducted PAC).

Atrial tachycardias

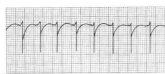

These dysrhythmias usually result from atrioventricular (AV) nodal reentry or enhanced automaticity of an ectopic focus. Enhanced automaticity probably causes atrial tachycardia with block and multifocal atrial tachycardia (MAT); an AV nodal reentry mechanism probably leads to paroxysmal atrial tachycardia (PAT, also known as paroxysmal supraventricular tachycardia, or PSVT).
ECG characteristics. Three or more successive atrial ectopic beats occurring at a rate between 160 and 220 beats/minute; upright P wave or a P wave that's lost in the previous T wave; and normal QRS complexes (in most cases). In MAT, ectopic P-wave configurations vary. Atrial rate varies from 100 to 150 beats/minute. PR and P-P intervals also vary.

Atrial flutter

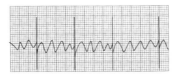

ECG characteristics. Saw-toothed flutter (F) waves ranging from 220 to 350 beats/minute; variable or constant ratio of atrial to ventricular contractions; and usually, normal QRS complexes.

Atrial fibrillation

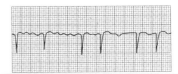

ECG characteristics. Absent P waves; irregular ventricular response (R-R interval); and chaotic fibrillatory (f) waves, indicating atrial tetanization from rapid atrial depolarizations (400 to 600 beats/minute). The rhythm is called coarse atrial fibrillation when waves appear pronounced, fine fibrillation when waves show less marked deflection. The atrial rate greatly exceeds the ventricular rate, because most impulses aren't conducted through the AV junction.

JUNCTIONAL DYSRHYTHMIAS

Junctional rhythm

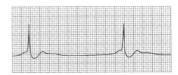

ECG characteristics. Slow, regular rhythm of 40 to 60 beats/minute; normal QRS complexes; and a P wave preceding the QRS complex, with a shortened PR interval, if the junctional impulse conducts antegradely to the ventricles. With retrograde conduction to the atria, the P wave follows the QRS complex or takes an inverted shape. If conduction occurs both antegradely and retrogradely, expect an absent or buried P wave. *Note:* A junctional escape beat appears late (after the next expected beat

Recognizing dysrhythmias *(continued)*

would normally occur), differentiating it from a premature or early beat.

Premature junctional contraction (PJC)

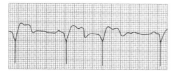

ECG characteristics. Inverted (or otherwise abnormally shaped) P waves before or after the QRS complex; or a P wave hidden in the QRS complex. If a normally shaped P wave appears, expect a shorter-than-normal PR interval. The QRS complex usually has a normal configuration and duration. PJCs appear before the next normally expected complex.

A noncompensatory pause reflecting retrograde conduction to the atria usually accompanies PJCs. (Because PJCs share some features with PACs, take care not to confuse the two dysrhythmias.)

Junctional tachycardias

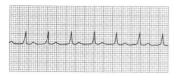

ECG characteristics. In accelerated junctional rhythm, a rate between 60 and 100 beats/minute (higher than the inherent rate of junctional tissue); in junctional tachycardia, a rate between 100 and 250 beats/minute. Expect a PQRS complex similar to that seen in junctional rhythm. Accelerated junctional rhythm usually has a gradual onset, whereas

junctional tachycardia usually begins and ends abruptly.

ATRIOVENTRICULAR HEART BLOCK (AV BLOCK)

Any delay or interruption in impulse conduction constitutes heart block. In AV block, the interruption occurs between the atria and ventricles, preventing the impulse from reaching the ventricles when it should.

AV block is classified by degree as follows.

First-degree AV block

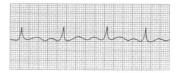

ECG characteristics. Prolonged but constant PR interval greater than 0.20 second.

Second-degree AV block
This condition blocks one or more—but not all—supraventricular impulses. Second-degree block occurs in two types: Type I (Wenckebach or Mobitz I) and Type II (Mobitz II).
• Type I second-degree AV block (Wenckebach or Mobitz I)

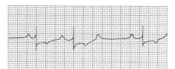

ECG characteristics. Constant P-P intervals; progressively lengthening PR intervals; progressively shortening R-R intervals, until a P wave appears

without a QRS complex (dropped beat). The next conducted beat has a short PR interval and the QRS complex usually appears normal.

Group beating ("the footprints of Wenckebach") usually distinguishes this dysrhythmia. In each group, the first PR interval is only slightly prolonged, with the largest increment falling between the first and second intervals. The R-R interval encompassing the dropped beat measures less than twice the shortest cycle.
• Type II second-degree AV block (Mobitz II)

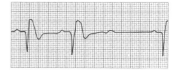

ECG characteristics. Constant P-P and PR intervals and sudden dropped beat. The interval containing the nonconducted P wave equals two normal P-P intervals. The QRS complex may be prolonged.

Third-degree AV block (complete heart block)

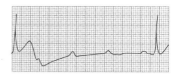

ECG characteristics. Constant P-P intervals, with no relationship between the P wave and QRS complexes. QRS configuration depends on where the ventricular beat originates. Ventricular rate is usually less than 45 beats/minute.

(continued)

Recognizing dysrhythmias *(continued)*

VENTRICULAR DYSRHYTHMIAS

Premature ventricular contraction (PVC)

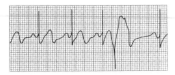

ECG characteristics. Wide (greater than 0.12 second), bizarre QRS complexes, because the impulse arises from the ventricle; absent P waves; slow rate; usually regular rhythm; and T waves in the opposite direction of the wide QRS complex. A long horizontal baseline, called a compensatory pause, usually follows the T wave. However, not all PVCs have compensatory pauses. (Those that don't are called interpolated PVCs). A compensatory pause exists if the P-P interval encompassing the PVC has twice the duration of a normal sinus beat's P-P interval.

Ventricular tachycardia

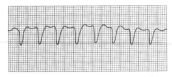

ECG characteristics. Wide, bizarre QRS complexes; regular rhythm; fast rate (100 to 180 beats/minute); absent P waves; and T waves pointing in the direction opposite to QRS complexes.

Ventricular flutter

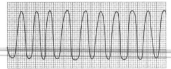

ECG characteristics. Wide, bizarre QRS complexes; regular rhythm; extremely rapid rate (200 to 400 beats/minute); and a regular up-and-down sweeping form with no discernible P or T waves.

Torsades de pointes

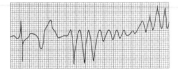

ECG characteristics. Wide, bizarre QRS complexes (the QRS polarity seems to spiral around the isoelectric line); rate ranging from 200 to 240 beats/minute; and no discernible P or T waves.

Because defibrillation can affect pacemaker function, patients with permanent pacemakers should be defibrillated with electrodes no closer than 5″ (13 cm) to the pacemaker generator.

Applying conductive, low-resistance gel serves several purposes: It establishes skin contact, reduces skin burns, and reduces skin resistance. Approximately 25 lb (11.3 kg) of twisting pressure should be applied to the electrodes to evenly distribute the conduction gel or paste, to develop transthoracic resistance, and to prevent paddle slippage. (See *Procedure for defibrillation,* page 28.)

Synchronized cardioversion. Another electrical therapy, synchronized cardioversion is used to treat patients with rapid ventricular and supraventricular dysrhythmias — conditions associated with low cardiac output and hypotension. It is not recommended for patients with dysrhythmias caused by digitalis toxicity. Synchronized cardioversion delivers an electrical current to the heart approximately 10 msec (milliseconds) after the peak of the R wave. The monitoring level must produce a tall, upright R wave before cardioversion can occur. Once an appropriate R wave is observed and the defibrillator is fired, the paddles should remain in position for several seconds to allow the synchronizer to discharge the energy. Patients who receive emergency synchronized cardioversion are usually responsive and should receive a sedative or analgesic. The energy level depends on the type of dysrhythmia. Ventricular and supraventricular tachycardia require less energy for conversion. Give no more than 50 joules initially for ventricular tachycardia (unless the patient is pulseless or unresponsive). Give 25 to 100 joules for atrial flutter and 75 to 100 joules for paroxysmal supraventricular tachycardia or atrial fibrillation. Energy levels for subsequent attempts, when necessary, are the same as those for defibrillation: 200 to 300 joules. The interval between shocks should be 3 minutes or longer.

Precordial thump. If a defibrillator is unavailable for a cardiac-monitored patient with ventricular fibrillation or in witnessed cardiac arrest, a single precordial thump may convert the cardiac rhythm. The thump is delivered with a sharp, quick blow over the midsternum with a fist. If it is not effective, defibrillation and BLS should begin immediately. *Note:* Precordial thump is not part of BLS. It is an ACLS technique that is used only for cardiac-monitored patients.

Pacemaker therapy. For patients with severe bradycardia or idioventricular rhythm during cardiac arrest, a pacemaker can be another effective form of electrical therapy. The pacemaker delivers an impulse to stimulate myocardial cells to depolarize and contract. The device consists of a pulse generator, containing a power source and electronic circuitry, and one or two pacing leads, each with an electrode on its tip. Artificial pacing generates an impulse and creates an electrical circuit between two electrodes within the heart.

Automatic external defibrillator

Patients with ventricular fibrillation or ventricular tachycardia have a 70% chance of surviving if defibrillation occurs within 3 minutes of onset. This survival percentage drops dramatically if defibrillation is delayed for 20 minutes—only 3% survive. Because of this timing, patients identified at high risk for cardiac arrest can take advantage of a device called an automatic external defibrillator (AED). AEDs can be used in the home as well as in the prehospital setting. Family members can easily be trained in the use of an AED.

The AED consists of a computer dysrhythmia recognition unit with a cardiac defibrillation unit. External, adhesive conduction pads are used to sense the cardiac rhythm as well as to deliver the countershocks. An AED can be used only for an adult patient who is unconscious, pulseless, not breathing, and stationary, in areas free of flammable gases. As with all defibrillator equipment, there should be no contact with the patient during the procedure.

Paddle placement for defibrillation

ANTERIOR-LATERAL PLACEMENT

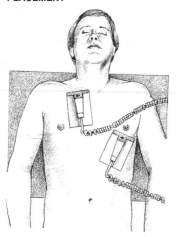

ANTERIOR-POSTERIOR PLACEMENT

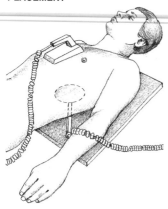

Procedure for defibrillation

Step One
Apply conductive, low-resistance gel or paste to the electrode paddles (or saline-soaked pads to the patient).

Step Two
Turn on the defibrillator, checking to make certain that the machine is not in the synchronous mode.

Step Three
Select the appropriate energy level and activate the capacitor. Then charge the defibrillator (which may take a few seconds).

Step Four
Once the capacitor has reached the appropriate energy level, make sure the patient's cardiac rhythm is unchanged (still ventricular fibrillation or ventricular tachycardia). Quickly assess the patient's level of consciousness.

Step Five
Order the area cleared. To avoid electrical shock, check to make sure that no one—including yourself—is in contact with the bed, the equipment, or the patient.

Step Six
Position the paddles and apply firm pressure (25 lb).

Step Seven
Reassess the patient's cardiac rhythm: Make sure the patient is in ventricular fibrillation or ventricular tachycardia.

Step Eight
Discharge (fire) the defibrillator. On most machines, this involves depressing both buttons on both paddles. If the shock is delivered, you should be able to see chest muscle contraction. If not, recheck the machine's power supply to ensure the synchronizer circuit is off, the machine is plugged in, and, if a battery is used, that it is sufficiently charged.

Step Nine
Assess the patient's pulse and ECG immediately after defibrillation. If ventricular fibrillation or ventricular tachycardia persists, a second attempt should be made as quickly as the machine will allow.

Step Ten
Document the procedure, including the energy level used and the response obtained. Include an ECG strip on the documentation record.

Most temporary pacemakers (in which the pulse generator lies outside the body) have bipolar leads. Both pacing electrodes sense spontaneous cardiac activity; one electrode also stimulates the heart. Temporary pacing is commonly used in SCD or cardiac arrest. The primary indications for temporary cardiac pacing are AV block, certain AV conduction defects, and symptomatic bradydysrhythmias or tachydysrhythmias.

Temporary cardiac pacing is occasionally indicated to overdrive, or suppress, atrial or ventricular tachydysrhythmias. Overdrive pacing is used to stimulate the myocardium at a rate above the patient's own intrinsic cardiac rhythm, thereby suppressing impulse formation. Four methods of temporary cardiac pacing are available.

Transthoracic pacing is an emergency procedure designed to gain access to the right ventricle. A large-bore needle is placed between the fourth and fifth intercostal spaces and the left sternal border. A pacing wire is inserted through the needle until it is embedded in the ventricle wall. The needle is removed and the wire connected to a temporary pacemaker. This procedure commonly produces complications that include cardiac tamponade, coronary artery laceration, and pneumothorax.

Epicardial pacing, in which one lead is secured to the epicardium and the other to the subcutaneous tissue, is often performed prophylactically during open-heart surgery. If dysrhythmias occur postoperatively, the leads will be in position and available for connection to a temporary pacemaker. These temporary leads can be removed through the skin when no longer needed.

Transvenous endocardial pacing is the most widely used cardiac pacing method. Pacing and catheter wires are threaded through the brachial, femoral, subclavian, or jugular vein into the heart. The catheter wire is then advanced into the right atrium and through to the tricuspid valve until it is secured in the right ventricle wall. *Note:* Some pulmonary artery catheters have pacemaker leads for endocardial pacing.

Noninvasive temporary pacing transmits an electrical stimulus to the myocardium through large electrodes that are placed on the patient's anterior and posterior chest. Although some muscle twitching occurs when the impulse is delivered, most patients will find the sensation tolerable. Unlike transvenous pacemakers, noninvasive pacemakers do not require special skills; operating personnel need only be familiar with the equipment.

Permanent pacemakers (in which the pulse generator usually lies inside the body) are usually inserted under a local anesthetic in an operating room or a special procedures de-

Recognizing pacemaker spikes

The sharp vertical line on each ECG strip represents the pacemaker spike—that is, the electrical impulse sent to the heart. A QRS complex following a spike demonstrates that capture has occurred.

ATRIAL PACING

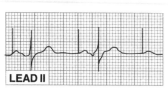

LEAD II

Atrial pacing is typified by a spike before every P wave.

VENTRICULAR PACING

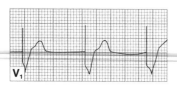

V₁

In ventricular pacing, a spike will appear in front of every QRS complex.

ATRIAL AND VENTRICULAR PACING

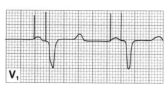

V₁

If both atria and ventricles are being paced, spikes will appear before both QRS complexes and P waves. *Note:* Epicardial, transcutaneous, and transvenous unipolar pacing are usually evident in the ECG as large spikes. Transvenous bipolar pacing will usually show small spikes.

partment. In a procedure similar to placement of a temporary transvenous endocardial pacemaker, the pacemaker lead is advanced transvenously into the heart chamber and anchored into the endocardial trabeculae. Methods of embedding include flange-tine or fin-tipped devices, spring-release barbs, screws, or clamps at the lead's tip. The pulse generator is implanted subcutaneously under the clavicle or sometimes under the abdominal wall. Permanent pacemakers are programmed after the pacing lead is implanted; reprogramming may be necessary if the patient's pacing needs change after insertion.

Pacemaker settings. These include the rate, stimulation threshold (or capture level), and sensitivity control. The *rate* depends on the patient's myocardial profile—that is, the need for pacing. The most desirable setting is the lowest setting that will control the dysrhythmia and, at the same time, produce maximum cardiac output at rest.

The *stimulation threshold*—the energy required to stimulate the heart—can be determined by slowly raising the energy output control until a QRS complex occurs after every pacer spike. (See *Recognizing pacemaker spikes.*) This one-to-one capture level (one QRS complex for every spike) indicates whether the electrode is positioned correctly. If less than 1 ma (milliampere) is needed for the capture event, the position is indeed correct. Because eating, sleeping, certain drugs (anesthetics and mineralocorticoids), and the development of fibrosis around the catheter tip commonly increase the energy demands for stimulation, the threshold level is usually set two to three times above the stimulation threshold. Conversely, exercise, low blood glucose levels, and treatment with glucocorticoids or sympathomimetics lower the stimulation threshold.

The *sensitivity control,* which ranges from 1 to 20 mV (millivolts), represents the amplitude (millivolt size) of an R or P wave that is sensed by the pacemaker. If the sensitivity control reads asynchronous, the pacer will function at a fixed rate without sensing.

Malfunction of a temporary or permanent pacemaker can contribute to SCD or cardiac arrest. To identify and correct malfunction quickly, take a simple, systematic approach. First, assess the patient's vital signs and level of consciousness. Second, confirm that the temporary pacemaker is turned on for those patients with temporary pacemakers. Assess the battery light indicator, rate of pacing, mode of pacing, energy output, and sensitivity control levels. Finally, check the insertion site for wire placement and the connection between the pacemaker terminals and electrodes.

Drug therapies in ACLS

The primary goal of drug therapy during ACLS is to achieve myocardial electrical stability; the secondary goal, to maintain normal hemodynamic status. Such drugs are primarily administered I.V.—by bolus, infusion, or both. Peripheral veins will deliver these drugs to the central circulation within 2 minutes. A faster response can be achieved by elevating the patient's extremities and administering large volumes of flush solution.

If venous access is unavailable, the endotracheal tube offers an alternate route for several drugs that are commonly used in cardiac emergencies: epinephrine hydrochloride, atropine sulfate, and lidocaine hydrochloride. The extensive surface area of the lungs allows for quick, efficient absorption into the circulatory system. This administration route also tends to prolong the duration of action because of the depot effect—that is, sustained absorption by the alveoli.

In addition to oxygen, which is of utmost priority, the following drugs, or classes of drugs, are commonly used in emergency cardiac situations. (See also *ACLS drug update,* pages 32 and 33.)

Morphine. Commonly used for pain associated with acute MI, morphine also reduces anxiety and helps treat pulmonary edema by increasing venous capacitance, decreasing venous return, and inducing mild arterial vasodilation. To reduce the risk of respiratory depression or hypotension, morphine is best administered in small I.V. doses (2 to 5 mg) repeated frequently (once every 5 minutes) until the desired effect is achieved.

Sodium bicarbonate. Once administered routinely in cardiac emergencies, sodium bicarbonate has not been found to improve survival except in patients with preexisting acidosis. In fact, it often inhibits the release of oxygen and interferes with simultaneously administered catecholamines (epinephrine, for example). Because of these effects, sodium bicarbonate should

(Text continues on page 34.)

ACLS drug update

Most of the drugs in this chart act either to control heart rhythm and rate or to improve cardiac output and blood pressure through peripheral vasoconstriction and inotropic or chronotropic cardiac effects.

Drug and indication	Dosage and administration	Special considerations
amrinone lactate Congestive heart failure	Give one 0.75 mg/kg dose I.V. over 2 to 3 minutes, followed by 5 to 10 mcg/kg/min by I.V. infusion.	• Amrinone may exacerbate myocardial ischemia in dosages greater than 20 mcg/kg/min.
atropine sulfate Sinus bradycardia with hemodynamic compromise; sinus bradycardia with frequent ventricular ectopic beats; ventricular asystole	*For bradycardia:* 0.5 mg I.V. every 5 minutes to a total of 2 mg. *For asystole:* 1 mg I.V.; repeat after 5 minutes if asystole persists.	• Atropine may be given endotracheally. • Doses below 0.5 mg have parasympathomimetic effects and therefore may slow heart rate. • Use cautiously in acute myocardial ischemia or infarction; excessive rate increases may widen areas of ischemia or infarction.
bretylium tosylate Resistant ventricular tachycardia or fibrillation	*For resistant ventricular tachycardia:* 5 to 10 mg/kg diluted to 50 ml with dextrose 5% in water (D₅W) and injected I.V. over 8 to 10 minutes. Follow loading dose with a continuous I.V. infusion at 1 to 2 mg/min. *For resistant ventricular fibrillation:* 5 mg/kg I.V. bolus followed by defibrillation. If indicated, increase dose to 10 mg/kg and give at 15- to 30-minute intervals to a maximum of 30 mg/kg.	• Don't use as a first-line drug. Use only if lidocaine and defibrillation fail to convert ventricular fibrillation, if lidocaine fails to prevent ventricular fibrillation from recurring, or if lidocaine and procainamide fail to control ventricular tachycardia associated with pulse. • Bretylium may take 2 minutes to reach central circulation.
dobutamine hydrochloride Heart failure	Give 2.5 to 10 mcg/kg/min I.V.	• Dobutamine may induce reflex peripheral vasodilation. • As ordered, give with sodium nitroprusside for synergistic effect. • Monitor heart rate closely. An increase of 10% or more may exacerbate myocardial ischemia (a common problem at dosages above 20 mcg/kg/min). Hemodynamic monitoring is required.
dopamine hydrochloride Shock	Give 2 to 5 mcg/kg/min I.V. initially and titrate according to response.	• At low dosages (1 to 2 mcg/kg/min), dopamine dilates renal and mesenteric vessels without increasing heart rate or blood pressure. At higher dosages (2 to 10 mcg/kg/min), it primarily stimulates beta receptors, increasing cardiac output without peripheral vasoconstriction. At dosages above 10 mcg/kg/min, it stimulates alpha receptors, causing peripheral vasoconstriction. • Don't give dopamine in same I.V. line as sodium bicarbonate. The alkaline solution may inactivate dopamine. • Hemodynamic monitoring is required.
epinephrine hydrochloride Cardiac arrest	Give 0.5 to 1 mg (5 to 10 ml of a 1:10,000 solution) I.V. or 1 mg (10 ml of a 1:10,000 solution) endotracheally. Repeat every 5 minutes during resuscitation efforts.	• Intracardiac injection is contraindicated unless I.V. and endotracheal routes are unavailable. Intracardiac injection interrupts resuscitation efforts and risks such complications as coronary artery laceration, cardiac tamponade, and pneumothorax. • Don't give in same I.V. line as sodium bicarbonate or any other alkaline solution.

ACLS drug update (continued)

Drug and indication	Dosage and administration	Special considerations
isoproterenol hydrochloride Hemodynamically significant bradycardia unresponsive to atropine, in a patient with a pulse	Add 1 mg isoproterenol to 500 ml of D_5W. Give 2 to 10 mcg/min by I.V. infusion. Titrate according to heart rate and rhythm response.	• Isoproterenol is not indicated in cardiac arrest. • Isoproterenol's potent inotropic and chronotropic effects increase cardiac output and work load, exacerbating ischemia and dysrhythmias in patients with ischemic heart disease. • Use this drug only as a temporary measure until pacemaker therapy begins.
lidocaine Ventricular tachycardia or fibrillation; premature ventricular contractions (PVCs) that are frequent, close-coupled, multifocal or arranged in short bursts of two or more in succession; myocardial infarction (to prevent ventricular fibrillation)	Give 1 mg/kg by I.V. bolus, followed by 0.5-mg/kg boluses every 8 to 10 minutes, as necessary, to a total of 3 mg/kg.	• Lidocaine may be used prophylactically when myocardial infarction is suspected but not confirmed. • In ventricular fibrillation, lidocaine improves response to defibrillation. • Give only bolus doses during resuscitation efforts. After resuscitation, give a continuous infusion at 2 to 4 mg/min. (Reduce dosage and monitor drug blood levels after 24 hours, as ordered.) • Monitor for signs of central nervous system toxicity.
nitroglycerin Congestive heart failure; unstable angina	Give 10 mcg/min I.V. Increase in increments of 5 to 10 mcg/min, as needed.	• Most patients respond to 200 mcg/min or less. Mean dosage range is 50 to 500 mcg/min. • Monitor for hypotension, an adverse reaction that exacerbates myocardial ischemia. Hemodynamic monitoring is required.
norepinephrine Severe hypotension with low total peripheral resistance	Add 4 or 8 mg norepinephrine injection to 500 ml of D_5W or dextrose 5% in normal saline solution. Administer the resulting concentration (8 and 16 mcg/ml, respectively) I.V., titrating according to patient response.	• Norepinephrine is contraindicated in hypovolemia. • Cardiac output may increase or decrease after norepinephrine administration, depending on vascular resistance, left ventricular function, and reflex responses. • Don't give in same I.V. line as alkaline solutions. • Monitor blood pressure with an intra-arterial line, because standard measurements may be falsely low.
procainamide hydrochloride Ventricular dysrhythmias, such as PVCs or tachycardia, when lidocaine is contraindicated or ineffective	In an emergency, give 20 mg/min up to a total dose of 1 g. Usual dosage is 50 mg I.V. every 5 minutes until desired response is achieved, up to a total of 1 g. Maintenance infusion rate is 1 to 4 mg/min.	• Reduce dosage in patients with renal failure. • Guard against too-rapid infusion, which causes acute hypotension. Use particular caution in patients with acute myocardial infarction. • Monitor for widening QRS complex. If QRS complex widens more than 50%, notify doctor and discontinue infusion, as ordered.
sodium nitroprusside Heart failure; hypertensive crises	Add 50 mg to 1,000 ml of D_5W. Initially, give 10 to 20 mcg/min.	• Wrap drug container in opaque material; light causes drug deterioration. (You needn't wrap I.V. tubing, however.) • Hemodynamic monitoring is required.
verapamil hydrochloride Atrial dysrhythmias, especially paroxysmal supraventricular tachycardia with AV node conduction	Give 5 mg I.V. initially, followed by 10 mg in 15 to 30 minutes if dysrhythmia persists and patient hasn't responded adversely to initial dose.	• Monitor patient for hypotension, severe bradycardia, congestive heart failure, and facilitated accessory conduction in patients with Wolff-Parkinson-White syndrome.

Evaluating ABG levels after cardiac arrest

Arterial blood gas (ABG) measurements establish acid-base status and evaluate pulmonary gas exchange efficiency, blood oxygenation, and respiratory function. ABGs include the following measurements:

• **pH.** This reflects the blood's acidity index, based on the negative logarithm of hydrogen ion (H) concentration.

• **$PaCO_2$.** The partial pressure, or tension, of carbon dioxide in arterial blood reveals respiratory acid-base status.

• **HCO_3^-.** The arterial blood bicarbonate concentration is used to evaluate acid-base balance.

• **Base excess.** Several bases, including bicarbonate, plasma proteins, and hemoglobin, are all reflected in this measurement. Base excess contributes in the evaluation of metabolic acid-base component.

• **PaO_2.** The partial pressure, or tension, of oxygen in arterial blood corresponds to the lungs' oxygenating potential; it helps guide oxygen administration.

• **SaO_2.** Oxygen saturation in arterial blood tells the actual percentage of hemoglobin that has complexed with oxygen; it is a sensitive gauge for respiratory function.

Other blood gas tests

Transcutaneous blood gas monitoring and pulse oximetry are noninvasive procedures. Transcutaneous blood gas monitoring calculates the oxygen and carbon dioxide transcutaneous partial pressures ($TcPO_2$ and $TcPCO_2$) when the skin is warmed with electrodes. In normovolemic and normotensive patients, $TcPCO_2$ and $TcPO_2$ levels correspond with $PaCO_2$ and PaO_2 levels. Pulse oximetry measures SaO_2 with light-emitting diodes in a sensor attached to the patient's body. Pulse rate and amplitude are also measured. A photodetector records the relative absorption of red and infrared light by arterial blood with each heartbeat.

---

not be administered during an early code sequence. It should be used only to correct abnormal ABG levels or when all other ACLS interventions have been tried—and only at the discretion of the code team leader. (See *Diagnostic profile: Evaluating ABG levels after cardiac arrest.*)

Diuretics. Furosemide is the diuretic most commonly administered during ACLS. Furosemide inhibits reabsorption of sodium chloride in the proximal and distal renal tubules and the loop of Henle and produces desirable vascular effects: It produces vasodilation in patients with acute pulmonary edema within 5 minutes of injection. Furosemide is also used to treat cerebral edema after cardiac arrest.

Digitalis. Various forms of digitalis are sometimes used to decrease the ventricular rate of patients with rapid atrial rates (atrial flutter, atrial fibrillation, or paroxysmal supraventricular tachycardia).

Beta-adrenergic receptor blocking agents. These agents, which compete directly with beta-adrenergic receptor stimulators for beta-receptor sites, are indicated for recurring supraventricular tachycardia and occasionally for malignant ventricular dysrhythmias. Because they may exert cardiac-depressive effects, these agents should be used with special caution in cardiac arrest or asthma.

Calcium. The routine use of calcium during ACLS is not recommended. In some cases of hyperkalemia, hypocalcemia, or calcium channel blocker toxicity, calcium chloride may be given in doses of 2 ml of a 10% solution (2 to 4 mg/kg), repeated as necessary. Calcium gluceptate may be given in a dose of 5 to 7 ml; calcium gluconate, in a dose of 5 to 8 ml.

Failure of resuscitation

If attempts to resuscitate are unsuccessful, management will focus on the decision to terminate ACLS measures. The order to terminate is a medical decision that depends on the doctor's assessment of the patient's cardiovascular condition. *Note:* In some states, the Nurse Practice Act allows nurses to pronounce death. Be sure to know your state's practice. Clinical criteria that establish the adequacy of cerebral function include reactivity of the pupils, level of consciousness, and the presence of spontaneous breathing. Most nurses know the ominous prognostic signs — such as deep unconsciousness, absence of spontaneous breathing and brain-stem reflexes, and pupils that remain fixed and dilated for 15 to 30 minutes — but these signs cannot be used to establish clinical death. (See *DNR orders.*)

According to current guidelines, CPR may be terminated when BLS and ACLS have failed to restore cardiovascular function. However, the doctor must also consider the state's legal definition of death because the legal and clinical definitions of death may differ. Because the heart can tolerate hypoxemia longer than the brain, cardiovascular function can be reestablished in a person who has lost brain function. (See *Ethical dilemmas: Defining death,* page 36.)

Also complicating the definition of death and the decision to terminate ACLS is the issue of organ donation. Hospitals are now required to ask the patient's family about organ donation. The decision to donate organs will influence the timing of ending life support and pronouncing death.

DNR orders

Ideally, life-support issues, such as do-not-resuscitate (DNR) orders, should be discussed with the patient and family before the need. DNR orders should be documented and communicated to the appropriate staff. Living wills—whether legally binding in your state or not—can at least suggest what the patient would have decided for himself. The judgment concerning DNR orders should be based on the individual patient. Input from nurses and doctors as well as the family or the patient's legal guardian should be gathered. Consider these guidelines:
• When discussing DNR orders, the primary focus should be on the patient. A collaborative discussion will draw out sustained disagreement, which may be in the patient's best interest.
• The Joint Commission on Accreditation of Healthcare Organizations (JCAHO) recently approved new standards on withholding resuscitation. Most significantly, the doctor must document in the patient record the decision to withhold treatment; written DNR orders are mandatory. After such an order, performing CPR can violate the patient's right to die with dignity.
• Unless a DNR order is written on the patient's chart, CPR is mandatory. Only a doctor has the legal right to decide to withhold CPR. The nurse could be challenged on a verbal DNR order; in court the doctor could disclaim verbal DNR orders.
• After a DNR order is written, the patient's condition must be evaluated at least daily and continuation of the DNR order written.
• To avoid litigation, meticulously follow your hospital's policies and procedures concerning DNR orders.

▼ ETHICAL DILEMMAS

Defining death

Clinical death has been legally defined as the cessation of circulation and vital functions, including respiration and pulsation. However, new methods for sustaining life have created problems that require a revised definition of death.

• Cellular death follows some time after clinical death. Brain cells, for example, begin to die 4 to 6 minutes after the onset of anoxia. Biological death, then, has been defined as death of brain cells. A legal definition of death, however, cannot simply cite brain death because it is possible to maintain cardiopulmonary function in patients who have lost brain activity.

• In 1968, the Ad Hoc Committee to Examine the Definition of Brain Death (Harvard University) proposed a revised definition for death based on irreversible coma. The major criteria were outlined as follows:

—Total unresponsiveness to externally applied stimuli

—No spontaneous respiration

—No spontaneous muscular movement in response to pain, touch, sound, or light as observed by the doctor for 1 hour

—No elicitable reflexes: pupils fixed and dilated; no ocular movement; no blinking; no postural activity; no swallowing, yawning, or vocalization; no corneal or pharyngeal reflexes

—A flat EEG for a full 10 minutes and again when repeated in 24 hours. Note two exceptions: hypothermia (body temperature below 90° F [32.2° C]) and central nervous system depression (such as that induced by barbiturates).

• All criteria must be met before pronouncing a patient dead in states where brain death is recognized by statutory law. Criteria similar to those drawn up by the Ad Hoc Harvard Committee should be incorporated into written guidelines where statutory law does not recognize brain death. The current recommendation for patients who meet the criteria for brain death is that life-support measures be withdrawn. The decision to withdraw supportive therapy when all criteria for brain death have been met is considered mandatory—just as if cardiopulmonary function has ceased.

• A dilemma still persists with the definition of total brain death: The criteria for brain death do not address the issue of irreversible brain damage that involves cortical death. The cerebral cortex, which controls such higher brain functions as thought and consciousness, dies sooner than the lower brain stem (medulla and midbrain), which controls respiration, circulation, and parts of the nervous system. If the brain stem continues to function, a patient can suffer cortical death and still not fulfill the criteria for total brain death. For example, the patient may have a persistently flat EEG but may resume spontaneous respiration and is therefore not dead by definition. Another patient who has a flat EEG and whose cardiac function depends solely on mechanical ventilation, however, can be pronounced dead. An alternate definition of death may resolve this problem.

After the doctor has pronounced death, management focuses on postmortem care and emotional support for the patient's family. Remember that cardiac arrest is most often sudden and unexpected; it does not allow the patient's family to prepare for death or for the ensuing ethical and legal issues that it may be forced to confront. Usually the family needs to know that someone cares, understands, and is willing to help. Taking the time to be that someone is an important aspect of nursing care.

Case study: Part 4

In the ICU, a complete assessment of Mr. Gardner's body systems was done to provide a clinical baseline. The cardiac monitor showed sinus tachycardia with only occasional PVCs. His pulse rate was 116 beats/minute, and his blood pressure was 108/64 mm Hg.

Over the next 24 hours, Mr. Gardner showed signs of improvement—some muscle movement and attempts at spontaneous ventilation. The cardiologist ordered the lidocaine drip reduced to 2 mg/minute. The patient was monitored for the return of ventricular ectopy on the ECG, which didn't occur. Mr. Gardner's pupils were equal and reactive. He'd begun to respond to verbal stimuli and had a Glasgow Coma Scale rating of 15.

When the new ABG report showed adequate ventilation, Mr. Gardner was removed from the ventilator. The patient continued to breathe spontaneously, so the doctor ordered extubation and oxygen administration via mask.

Nursing management

Nursing management after resuscitation varies according to the initial outcome of the resuscitation effort. It can vary, depending on the patient's status, from simple monitoring and observation to the complex management of multiple organ system failure. This section will address postresuscitation status, assessment, and long-term management.

Postresuscitation status

Nursing care after cardiac arrest requires continuous monitoring and observation for 48 to 72 hours and thorough evaluation of postresuscitation status, including a baseline postarrest assessment of each organ system. Physical examination should emphasize detection of neurologic deficits. Clinical laboratory investigations should include a 12-lead ECG, a chest X-ray, and determinations of urine output, serum chemistry, and ABG and electrolyte levels. A pulmonary artery catheter may be indicated to monitor hemodynamic status (pulmonary capillary wedge pressure [PCWP] and cardiac output). At this time, the precipitating cause of the cardiac arrest should also be investigated. (See *Resuscitation after hypothermia.*)

If an I.V. infusion was not started during the resuscitation, it should be started at this time with dextrose 5% in water. Any

Resuscitation after hypothermia

Victims of hypothermia (body temperature below 86° F [30° C]) may appear clinically dead because of marked depression of brain function. Bradycardia and vasoconstriction make palpation of peripheral pulses difficult. Hypothermia is associated with decreased cerebral blood flow, decreased oxygen requirements, decreased cardiac output, and decreased arterial pressure.

To assess the patient, check his airway, breathing, and circulation, and check pulse for up to 1 minute to determine pulselessness. To prevent further heat loss, wrap the patient and apply external heat with warm packs or warm, moist oxygen. Transport the patient to a facility with ACLS as quickly as possible. Keep the patient still; excessive movement can trigger ventricular fibrillation. Perform only essential procedures.

Treatment is aimed at rewarming. Rewarm the patient's core by heated, humidified ventilation; peritoneal dialysis; thoracotomy; and extracorporeal blood warming with partial bypass. Because hypothermia reduces the body's metabolism, monitor emergency drug dosages closely for toxicity. *Note:* a hypothermia victim may be unresponsive to life-support interventions until body temperature reaches normal.

Resuscitation after near-drowning

Consider the following points during rescue of a victim of submersion:
• Hypoxemia is the main consequence of prolonged submersion without ventilation. Initial ventilation consists of the mouth-to-mouth or mouth-to-nose technique and should begin before the victim is even out of the water.
• There is no need to clear the lower airway of aspirated water unless foreign matter is obstructing the airway. Most victims aspirate only a modest amount of water; some do not aspirate at all because of laryngospasm or holding their breath. Suction is the best method to remove aspirated water because other means could cause gastric aspiration.
• If a neck injury is suspected, float the victim in a supine position while supporting the neck. He should be moved onto a firm surface before being removed from the water.
• Next, assessment of circulation. Central pulses may be difficult to palpate due to vasoconstriction and low cardiac output. Chest compressions should begin if no pulse is felt.
• All submersion victims should be taken to a medical facility for follow-up care. Life-support measures should be continued en route and aggressively continued at the hospital. Full neurologic recovery has occurred in near-drowning victims who survived prolonged submersion in cold water.

I.V. lines that were started without sterile technique during resuscitation should also be replaced. Depending on the rhythm during arrest, administer appropriate drug therapy. For example, for ventricular fibrillation or ventricular tachycardia, administer a lidocaine bolus followed by a lidocaine infusion; for bradycardia, administer atropine sulfate or assist with insertion of a pacemaker. Administer morphine for pain. Assess and monitor hemodynamic status, vital signs, and urine output for a full 48 to 72 hours.

Organ system failure may begin immediately after the cardiac arrest or may develop later. Patients who are in good post-resuscitation condition are awake, are responsive, and breathe spontaneously. Typically, patients who have multisystem failure may or may not breathe spontaneously; their hemodynamic status, cardiac rhythm and rate, systemic blood pressure, and organ perfusion may be unstable; and they may be comatose or may show declining responsiveness.

In prolonged resuscitation efforts, hypotension is common. (See *Resuscitation after near-drowning*.) If blood pressure does not rise promptly after circulation is restored, pharmacologic intervention (with dopamine, for example) is indicated. To provide adequate cerebral perfusion, arterial systolic pressure should be maintained at no lower than 90 mm Hg— or a mean arterial pressure between 50 and 60 mm Hg—without exacerbating ischemia or inducing cardiac dysrhythmias.

Body system assessment

Because cardiac arrest can interrupt blood flow to any organ system, it can cripple organ function temporarily or permanently. To detect such injury, assess each organ system in detail.

Respiratory system. Auscultate breath sounds to determine if they are bilateral and equal. If the patient is intubated, unilateral breath sounds on the right could mean the endotracheal tube is in the right primary bronchus and needs to be adjusted. However, unilateral breath sounds may also signal pneumothorax or air, blood, or fluid in the pleural space. Also listen for characteristic types of breath sounds. Crackles suggest aspiration or pulmonary edema.

Chest X-rays are necessary for thorough respiratory assessment. They can confirm location of the endotracheal tube, confirm placement of I.V. or hemodynamic monitoring catheters and pacemaker wires, and identify fractured ribs, pneumothorax, and pulmonary edema. If the patient's condition suggests accumulation of pleural fluid, bilateral decubitus films may be ordered. If possible, X-ray films should be compared to the patient's previous chest X-rays.

If the patient's respirations are inadequate or absent, begin mechanical ventilation. Adjust ventilation according to the PaO_2, $PaCO_2$, and pH values. ($PaCO_2$ and pH are examined to assess ventilation as well as acid-base balance.) Check ABG levels 20 minutes after any changes in mechanical ventilation to assess the adequacy of the ventilator settings (because reaching a steady state in ventilation and $PaCO_2$ takes 20 minutes). *Note:* An intra-arterial catheter may be inserted to facilitate repeated arterial blood sampling. Systemic blood pressure can also be monitored from this arterial line.

If the patient has an endotracheal tube in place, suction the tube, trachea, and bronchi every 1 to 2 hours. Measure and record the volume and pressure in the endotracheal tube cuff every 4 hours. Keep in mind that elevated cuff pressure can damage the trachea.

Cardiovascular system. Carefully monitor blood pressure for signs of hypotension or hypertension and pulse for heart rate and rhythm. Auscultate for abnormal heart sounds, such as S_3 (often heard with congestive heart failure) or S_4 (often heard with a noncompliant left ventricle). ECG monitoring or 12-lead ECG may show any dysrhythmias or myocardial damage, such as myocardial ischemia or infarction. Watch for reperfusion dysrhythmias, which may signal myocardial postischemic reperfusion injury. Also assess neck veins for distention. Hemodynamic monitoring via a pulmonary artery catheter may be indicated if the patient is unstable. Cardiac output and pulmonary artery pressure measurements, such as PCWP, should be obtained and used as a guide for therapy.

If PCWP and cardiac output are low, continue infusion of fluids. Administer morphine, diuretics, and vasodilators, as ordered, if PCWP is elevated above the optimum range (15 to 18 mm Hg) and the patient is symptomatic or shows signs of pulmonary edema.

Assess peripheral vascular resistance based on cardiac output and mean arterial blood pressure. Subsequent interventions vary according to a combination of factors. Infusion of fluids is indicated if the patient has increased systemic vascular resistance with hypotension and oliguria. But vasodilators are indicated if the patient has increased systemic vascular resistance without hypotension but with decreased cardiac output and pulmonary congestion. Inotropic drugs are indicated if PCWP is elevated with decreased cardiac and urine output. Relevant diagnostic tests, such as electrolyte levels and cardiac enzyme analysis, help assess cardiovascular status; however, elevated cardiac enzyme values may result from resuscitative efforts.

Renal system. After resuscitation, urine output may be reduced or absent, requiring catheterization. Urine output is a vital part of renal assessment; therefore, record hourly intake and output. Tests for serum and urine electrolyte levels, osmolality, and albumin, creatinine, and BUN levels are required but should be scheduled for 12 to 24 hours after diuretic therapy begins.

Monitor carefully for signs of acute renal failure (ARF), which may occur postarrest. ARF, the rapid deterioration of renal function, causes nitrogen waste products to accumulate in the blood and usually results in hypovolemia and decreased cardiac output caused by cardiac arrest. Early dialysis is the treatment of choice for patients with ARF.

GI system. Assess GI function by auscultating for bowel sounds. If bowel sounds are absent, a nasogastric tube should be inserted. Because a high incidence of stress ulceration and GI bleeding occurs after cardiac arrest, prophylactic antacids and a histamine blocker should be administered to control gastric acidity. Watch for signs of mesenteric ischemia, which may result from hypovolemia after cardiac arrest.

Nervous system. Assessment of the central nervous system usually begins with checking the patient's pupils. Persistently dilated pupils may indicate cerebral death, even if spontaneous respirations and heart beat are present. (See *Keeping the brain alive.*) Keep in mind, however, that various drugs can affect pupil size; atropine, for example, causes pupils to dilate.

Regularly assess the patient's level of consciousness. To increase venous drainage, elevate the head of the bed to 30

Keeping the brain alive

To prevent brain damage, rescuers must restore cerebral perfusion as quickly as possible with basic and advanced life support. Some BLS and ACLS interventions that restore cardiac function, however, can affect brain function adversely. Intracranial pressure (ICP) is increased, for example, when fluids are administered to raise arterial pressure.

Cerebral ischemia during the immediate postarrest period causes brain damage that can persist even if perfusion returns. Secondary problems may arise during reperfusion, including vasospasm, increased blood viscosity, hypermetabolism, and increased cellular calcium. To protect brain function during cerebral resuscitation:
• Monitor level of consciousness.
• Elevate the head of the bed 30 degrees to prevent increased ICP, but be sure to avoid head turning or neck constriction. Minimizing suctioning and administering corticosteroids and diuretics will also help control increased ICP.
• Maintain optimum oxygenation and circulation during early resuscitation.
• With a mechanical ventilator, maintain moderate hyperventilation (PaCO$_2$ at 25 to 30 mm Hg), moderate hyperoxygenation (PaO$_2$ >100 mm Hg), and normal pH (7.3 to 7.6).
• Using I.V. colloids and crystalloids, blood products, and vasopressors or antihypertensives, maintain mean arterial pressure at 90 to 100 mm Hg, systolic blood pressure at >100 mm Hg), and normal blood volume.
• Reduce metabolic demands by administering sedatives and by maintaining normothermia or even slight hypothermia.
• Monitor hematocrit, osmolality, and serum glucose, electrolyte, and albumin levels.

degrees for comatose patients. Such patients should receive ophthalmic methylcellulose drops every 1 to 2 hours; cover their eyes with pads and adhesive to prevent corneal abrasions. Coma may be induced by hyperosmolality, which in turn may result from overuse of sodium bicarbonate during resuscitative efforts. Serum osmolality should be kept at 280 to 295 mOsm/kg H$_2$O.

Watch for signs of cerebral edema, which can result from cerebral hypoxia during cardiac arrest. Treatment to reverse cerebral edema may include mannitol, furosemide, or methylprednisolone administration, or it may involve hyperventilating the patient to produce a PaCO$_2$ level between 28 and 30 mm Hg.

To maintain a cerebral perfusion pressure of 80 to 100 mm Hg, the mean arterial pressure should be elevated if blood pressure is low; and intracranial pressure (ICP) reduced for patients with high mean arterial pressure. Factors that can raise ICP, such as endotracheal suctioning, require careful monitoring.

Psychological assessment

Evaluation of a resuscitated patient should include psychological assessment. Many resuscitated patients experience a phenomenon known as a near-death experience. Near-death experiences

Near-death experiences

Many resuscitated patients have so-called near-death experiences (NDEs)—perceptions or recollections of events during the moment of clinical death.

Each person describes an intensely personal experience but most involve at least some of these characteristics:
• Feeling separated from the body (the most common characteristic) and a total absence of pain. Patients might also report hearing and watching everything that was said and done and describe it all in detail.
• Moving through a dark tunnel or space and hearing loud noises and music unlike anything ever heard before.
• Meeting deceased family or friends who welcome them.
• Meeting a superior being, often a religious figure.
• Seeing their lives pass before them.
• Reaching a boundary and knowing, if they could cross it, they would not have to go back to their bodies, but understanding the need to return.
• Having a sudden sense of understanding universal truths and losing their fear of dying.
• Changing their understanding of life and their values. Many be-

come more altruistic or more loving and have a heightened sense of spiritual purpose.

A few patients may have a negative experience, of having felt isolated in a void.

An NDE can also cause conflicts when it changes philosophy and life-style. Patients who never feel comfortable enough to tell anyone about their experiences may need help in integrating the NDE into their everyday lives. This is where you can help.

Ways you can help
• Be alert to signs of an NDE. Listen for verbal clues, like "I had the funniest dream" (although the patient doesn't look on it as a dream or as funny at all). Many don't even say that. But look for certain clues in patients who've pulled through a life-threatening crisis: They might seem angry on awakening and become withdrawn or suddenly calm or silent.
• Explore your own attitude toward NDEs. Whether you believe in the phenomenon or not, it's your responsibility to support the patient— emotionally and spiritually. Listen without trying to "talk him out of it."
• Allow the patient to express his emotions. Don't show surprise at anything he says. And don't

pump him for details about the experience; let him proceed at his own pace. To create rapport, try "active listening."
• Avoid labeling the NDE or the patient. Don't be tempted to explain it as an effect of medication, a reaction to stress, or the patient's way of handling his fear of death. This reinforces the patient's fear that he'll be considered crazy.
• Don't give the impression of abandoning the patient. The patient may feel rejected at having been "returned" to life and may be afraid of being rejected by the staff, too.
• Provide human contact during and after unconsciousness. While any patient is unconscious, continue to orient him to his name, time, and place. Also, let him know what's going on with his body—for instance, if he's intubated or in traction. Touch him frequently.
• Give the patient information about NDEs. Above all, reassure the patient that he's not the only person ever to have had this experience.
• Refer him to an appropriate professional who understands this phenomenon for follow-up counseling, if necessary.

are defined as perceptions or recollections of feelings and experiences during clinical death. (See *Near-death experiences.*)

Especially common is the patient's anxiety about a recurrent arrest. Such anxiety can itself increase catecholamine release, lower the fibrillation threshold, and cause fibrillation. To cope, the patient may use denial, projection, and displacement. To help the patient cope more effectively, encourage verbalization of feelings and provide information about risk factors.

Automatic implantable cardioverter-defibrillator

The automatic implantable cardioverter-defibrillator (AICD), used to treat patients with recurrent life-threatening dysrhythmias, consists of a small pulse generator implanted in the patient's abdomen. One of the unit's leads senses heart rate at the right ventricle; the second lead, which senses morphology, and thus rhythm, defibrillates at the right atrium; the third lead defibrillates at the apical pericardium. The AICD can be programmed to suit each patient's needs, and it uses far less energy (25 joules on the first attempt) than does an external defibrillator (360 joules).

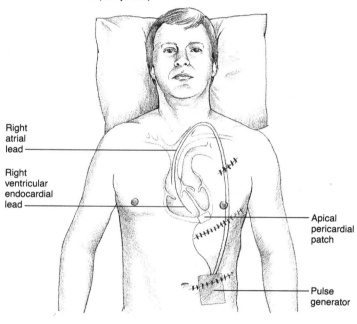

Right atrial lead

Right ventricular endocardial lead

Apical pericardial patch

Pulse generator

Long-term management
Management of the survivor of cardiac arrest depends on the cause and pathophysiologic factors that provoked the arrest, on the success of the resuscitative efforts, and on any complications.

Medical goals. The long-term goal of medical management is prevention of lethal dysrhythmias by the following methods:
• implantable devices, such as an automatic implantable cardioverter-defibrillator to control recurrent ventricular tachycardia or ventricular fibrillation; or a permanent pacemaker (see *Automatic implantable cardioverter-defibrillator*)

Cough CPR

Cough cardiopulmonary resuscitation (CPR), as the name implies, involves a series of regularly spaced deep breaths, followed by deep forceful coughs every 1 to 3 seconds. Potentially lethal ventricular tachycardia or fibrillation can thus be converted into a normal sinus rhythm. Deep breathing decreases intrathoracic pressure and promotes venous return to the heart, whereas coughing raises intrathoracic pressure and propels blood forward. Increased aortic pressure and reflex coronary vasodilation help to improve myocardial perfusion and maintain consciousness. Cough CPR is a useful form of CPR that can be taught to patients who frequently experience life-threatening ventricular dysrhythmias.

• antiarrhythmic drug therapy (dosage determined by monitoring serum plasma levels, evaluating exercise testing, or evaluating electrophysiologic stimulation studies)
• surgical techniques (map-guided endocardial resection and encircling endocardial ventriculotomy to control recurrent sustained ventricular tachycardia, especially in patients unresponsive to drug therapy).

Nursing goals. Long-term nursing management aims to prevent cardiac arrest through patient teaching, discharge planning, and home care. It should involve the patient and his family. (See *Cough CPR.*)

Before discharge, the patient should be able to demonstrate knowledge of risk factors associated with his cardiac arrest. He should know the underlying causes and the steps he must take to diminish this risk. He should have a detailed review of all medications, as well as instruction in other treatments—such as pacemaker care and correct use of the automatic external defibrillator at home. Patient teaching should also emphasize appropriate medical follow-up.

Be sure patient and family know signs and symptoms of impending cardiac arrest, what procedures they should take if arrest occurs, and how to activate the local EMS system in their area. Encourage family members to learn BLS techniques. It may also be appropriate to discuss with the patient ethical and legal issues, such as do-not-resuscitate orders and death with dignity.

Case study: Part 5

Five days after Mr. Gardner was admitted to the hospital, he was discharged with a diagnosis of cardiac arrest secondary to cocaine overdose. Before discharge, he was told how cocaine use could lead to cardiac arrest: By increasing the heart rate and reducing the fibrillation threshold, cocaine increases myocardial oxygen demand. His doctor also discussed the schedule of follow-up care by a cardiologist and a psychologist. Mr. Gardner was encouraged to enter a drug rehabilitation program.

CHAPTER 2
Angina

Chest pain caused by angina pectoris is one of the most common warning signs of cardiac disease. Angina causes paroxysmal pain in the chest and adjoining areas, usually stemming from coronary artery obstruction and atherosclerosis.

Although angina doesn't always progress to acute myocardial infarction (MI), it requires prompt and aggressive treatment to prevent myocardial damage and progression of coronary artery disease (CAD). Because angina can be fatal (unstable and variant angina) or chronic (stable angina), early diagnosis and correct treatment can be lifesaving and can reduce the psychological and economic burdens associated with this frightening disease.

An array of cardioactive drugs, new diagnostic tests, and surgical treatments is available to help detect and treat angina. Using these successfully also involves good nursing management: thorough patient and family teaching, continuous and precise monitoring, evaluating response to treatment, assessing for complications, and teaching changes in life-style that can prevent future anginal attacks.

Case study: Part 1

Carl Neimann, a 40-year-old single musician, knew he was out of shape. So when he first began having chest pains while lifting his portable keyboards, he chalked it up to lack of exercise and the approach of middle age. Six months before, when his doctor told him he had moderate hypertension, he hadn't taken the matter too seriously. The low-sodium, low-cholesterol diet the doctor put him on was inconvenient—especially when his band went on the road. But he figured he could live with it as long as he cheated every so often.

The chest pain, though, was getting hard to tolerate. It had started 3 weeks earlier, then recurred a week later, also when he lifted his keyboards. Both times, the pressing feeling in his chest subsided when he put the keyboards down.

Case study: Part 1 *(continued)*

Today, however, the discomfort radiated to his neck, left shoulder, and left jaw and he became nauseated, anxious, and diaphoretic. When lying down brought only partial relief, he had a friend drive him to the hospital.

Causes and characteristics

Angina pectoris—commonly known as angina—is a clinical syndrome of ischemic heart disease characterized by spasmodic, recurring pain in the chest and adjoining areas. The pain occurs because an imbalance between myocardial oxygen needs and myocardial oxygen delivery causes myocardial ischemia.

The primary cause of angina is atherosclerotic heart disease. Patients with atherosclerosis-induced angina usually have advanced occlusion or stenosis of at least 75% of one or more of the three main coronary arteries. This drastic constriction of the arteries diminishes blood flow to the myocardium, decreasing its ability to offset demands for extra oxygen during exercise and stress.

Another common cause of angina is physiologic stress, which narrows blood vessels by a sympathetic nerve response and increases heart rate and myocardial oxygen requirements. Strenuous exercise can also trigger angina by increasing the heart's oxygen demand, especially in patients suffering from compromised blood flow. Other precipitating factors include exposure to cold weather; drinking cold beverages, which causes vasoconstriction; eating a heavy meal, which redirects blood to the mesentery from the heart and other large organs; systemic hypertension; cardiac dysrhythmias (especially tachydysrhythmias); anemia; fever; hyperthyroidism (thyrotoxicosis); hypotension; and polycythemia.

Angina may sometimes result from severe aortic stenosis or regurgitation, idiopathic hypertrophic subaortic stenosis, syphilitic stenosis of the coronary ostia, syphilitic aortitis, coronary arteritis, congenital anomalies of the coronary arteries, cardiomyopathy, mitral valve disease, systemic lupus erythematosus, or polyarteritis nodosa. In addition, in 5% to 10% of patients, angina results from coronary artery spasm. This syndrome, called variant or Prinzmetal's angina, occurs in both normal and severely stenosed coronary arteries.

Pathophysiology

The coronary arteries deliver oxygen-rich blood to the myocardium so that it may pump blood efficiently to body organs and tissues. When the body is at rest, the heart uses about 75% of the oxygen supply from the circulation; the remaining 25% is used by other organs. Because the heart has few oxygen reserves, it depends on increased coronary blood flow to meet its increased oxygen needs during stressful times.

Coronary blood flow is controlled by the amount of pressure in the aorta and the amount of vascular resistance in the coronary arteries. Atherosclerotic lesions in the coronary vascular system cause diminished blood flow. Although increased aortic pressure may augment myocardial perfusion by overcoming the vascular resistance caused by the obstruction, the increase may not be enough to meet myocardial oxygen demands. The heart adapts to these increased oxygen demands by dilating the collateral vessels, but just how this works isn't clear.

What controls myocardial oxygen demand? The heart rate, ventricular wall tension, and the heart's contractile state. When angina occurs, heart rate, systemic blood pressure, and left ventricular end-diastolic pressure all rise. Coronary atherosclerotic lesions cause segmental myocardial dysfunction during an angina attack despite enhanced collateral circulation. But once myocardial demands decrease and coronary blood flow increases, the heart returns to normal. (See *How angina develops*.)

Myocardial ischemia commonly results in angina, which occurs in three forms: stable, unstable, and variant. However, in some patients, significant myocardial ischemia does not produce chest pain and is said to be silent.

Stable angina. Also called chronic, classic, or exertional angina, stable angina is usually caused by coronary artery atherosclerosis. It is triggered by strenuous activity, emotional stress, or cold weather and typically lasts only 1 to 5 minutes, building gradually and reaching maximum intensity quickly. Pain is usually relieved by rest or nitroglycerin. Patients often describe the pain of stable angina as a strangling, crushing, viselike, tight, heavy, or squeezing sensation in the chest. However, a few pa-

How angina develops

Angina develops when stress stimulates the sympathetic nervous system, narrowing blood vessels and increasing heart rate, contractility, and blood pressure.

The myocardial cells secrete potassium, histamine, and serotonin, activating pain nerve endings; as their metabolism converts from aerobic to anaerobic, the lactic acid produced activates pain nerve endings even more.

Pain travels from the heart to other parts of the body by sparking nerve reflexes that stimulate the autonomic nervous system.

Angina can provoke excessive release of norepinephrine, causing platelet aggregation and thromboxane A_2 release.

When metabolism becomes anaerobic, decreasing production of adenosine triphosphate permits sodium to collect inside cells and potassium to collect outside. This chain reaction blocks the depolarization-repolarization sequence of the heart, which is essential for normal contraction.

The role of platelet aggregation in ischemia

Platelet aggregates probably help trigger ischemic attacks. Sudden reductions in coronary blood flow distal to areas of coronary artery stenosis may be caused by platelet groups obstructing a partly closed coronary artery.

Platelets interact with the coronary vascular endothelium by generating the proaggregatory and vasoconstrictive agent thromboxane A_2, while the endothelium creates antiaggregatory prostacyclin. Other factors that may aid platelet aggregation include changes in sympathetic vascular tone and activation of alpha$_2$-adrenergic and serotoninergic platelet receptors.

Patients with unstable angina who've had pain within the preceding 24 hours show elevated levels of thromboxane A_2 metabolites in their plasma and urine. So local thromboxane release may be linked to unstable angina. Platelet inhibitors, such as aspirin, sulfinpyrazone, prostacyclin, ibuprofen, and indomethacin, apparently prevent reductions in coronary blood flow, but heparin, nitroglycerin, and papaverine don't. Again, this implies that such reductions of blood flow are controlled by platelet aggregation, not vasospasm or fibrin deposition.

Aspirin, which inhibits platelet aggregation, can prevent death and nonfatal acute myocardial infarction in patients with unstable angina.

tients feel only mild pressure. Other symptoms include shortness of breath, diaphoresis, faintness, anxiety, and nausea. Most patients feel the pain in the substernal area, with radiation to the left arm, jaw, neck, and occasionally the right arm and back.

Unstable angina. Also called preinfarction angina, crescendo angina, acute coronary insufficiency, intermediate coronary syndrome, or impending MI, unstable angina is more severe than stable angina. It usually results from progression of atherosclerosis; it commonly precedes an acute MI and follows an unpredictable course. An attack may last up to 30 minutes and may be triggered by a condition of unusual myocardial oxygen demand (such as anemia, infection, thyrotoxicosis, or cardiac dysrhythmias), coronary artery spasm, stress-related catecholamine release, or platelet aggregation, or it may occur for no apparent reason. (See *The role of platelet aggregation in ischemia.*)

Patients complain of dyspnea, nausea, vomiting, and diaphoresis and say that the pain radiates into previously uninvolved areas. Nitroglycerin may not give enough relief, so some patients need narcotics to relieve the pain.

Typically, unstable angina shows one or more of the following features:
• angina of new onset, caused by minimal exertion
• increasingly severe, prolonged, or frequent angina in a patient with relatively stable, exertion-related angina
• angina both at rest and with minimal exertion.

Most patients with unstable angina have severe obstructive CAD. Unstable angina is a complicated syndrome with complicated treatments. It may also be a warning of impending MI. The risk of MI is greatest in the first year after onset of new angina or after progression from stable to unstable angina.

Variant angina. Also called Prinzmetal's angina, atypical angina, or vasospastic angina, variant angina usually occurs when patients are at rest, not during physical exertion or emotional stress. It may occur at the same time every day in a particular patient—often between midnight and 8 a.m. (probably because levels of endogenous circulating catecholamines increase in the early morning hours). Patients with this type of angina show ST-segment elevations on an ECG but often show no CAD risk factors. Many have dysrhythmias and conduction abnormalities.

Diagnosing the three angina types

Stable (chronic) angina

The resting ECG usually isn't definitive in diagnosing stable angina; however, an exercise stress test provokes the characteristic ST-segment depression of ischemic heart disease.

Ischemia is also assessed by Holter monitoring, which reveals ST-segment depression during certain activities. Exercise thallium scans differentiate between ischemic and infarcted heart tissue. Exercise radionuclide angiography, coronary catheterization, and coronary angiography also show evidence of coronary artery disease (CAD).

Unstable angina

Transient ST-segment depression or elevation or T-wave inversions on the ECG are common in unstable angina. Usually, these resolve when pain is relieved. But if ECG changes persist for more than 6 hours, a non-Q-wave infarction may have occurred.

Coronary catheterization and coronary angiography reveal CAD. Thallium scanning and technetium-99m pyrophosphate scanning may show myocardial perfusion defects. If cardiac enzyme tests show abnormal elevations, the diagnosis would be acute myocardial infarction, not unstable angina.

Variant angina

An ECG is the definitive test in diagnosing variant angina. During anginal pain, an ECG shows characteristic elevations in ST segments that are usually normal at rest. In variant angina, ST-segment changes commonly occur in inferior leads because of right coronary artery involvement. Because variant angina usually occurs at rest, exercise testing is of limited value. The ergonovine test and coronary angiography are rarely used because of the associated risk.

Signs and symptoms of variant angina include syncope, dyspnea, and palpitations. A few patients have both variant and stable angina. Nitroglycerin usually relieves the pain quickly.

Variant angina is caused by coronary artery spasm, which results in a sudden, brief narrowing of an epicardial or large septal coronary artery. Unless myocardial oxygen supply increases, this narrowing causes myocardial ischemia, evidenced by elevated heart rate or blood pressure. Both normal and diseased coronary arteries may become constricted, occasionally in more than one site. If the spasm occurs in a diseased artery, it's often near atherosclerotic plaques. (See *Diagnosing the three angina types.*)

Other causes include endothelial injury (which turns the dilator response to various stimuli into a vasoconstrictor response) and hypercontractility of vascular smooth muscle, caused by higher concentrations of blood-borne vasoconstrictors in areas of neovascularized atherosclerotic plaques.

Silent myocardial ischemia. Although the classic symptom of ischemic heart disease is the typical chest pain of angina, some patients have "silent" myocardial ischemia—with no chest pain at all. Although they're diagnosed as having ischemia by ECGs, exercise tests, or radionuclide tests, even those with documented CAD may show no symptoms. Perhaps these patients have exceptionally high pain thresholds. Or the syndrome may be related to decreased myocardial oxygen supply secondary to vasospasm rather than increased oxygen demand as in classic angina.

Silent myocardial ischemia occurs in three types of patients:
• those with no symptoms of angina who have ST-segment shifts during exercise testing or ambulatory ECG monitoring
• those who are asymptomatic postinfarction and who have ST-segment changes during exercise testing or ambulatory ECG monitoring
• those who have multiple episodes of silent ischemia during 24-hour Holter monitoring.

Silent ischemia is especially hazardous because neither the patient nor the doctor may be aware of its presence until a fatal event occurs or until an old MI is detected on a routine ECG. (See *Origins of anginal pain.*)

Case study: Part 2

Except for hypertension, Carl Neimann had no previous medical problems. However, he did have a family history of heart disease and hypertension and had smoked about 10 cigarettes a day for the last 15 years.

On physical examination, the emergency department (ED) nurse found the patient to be well nourished and in moderate distress. Mr. Neimann described the pain, located just below the sternum and radiating to the left shoulder and jaw, as a crushing feeling, as if "someone is sitting on my chest." The nurse measured a blood pressure of 150/100 mm Hg, a pulse rate of 85 beats/minute, and a temperature of 98.6° F (37° C). A cardiac examination revealed a point of maximum impulse at the fifth intercostal space and midclavicular line.

All heart sounds were normal and the lungs were clear on auscultation. On inspection, the nurse noted several xanthomas around the patient's eyes.

An ECG taken during a pain episode revealed a normal sinus rhythm and normal QRS, PR, and QT intervals. Leads II, III, and aV$_F$, however, showed ST-segment and T-wave abnormalities. A chest X-ray revealed a normal cardiac silhouette and no lung field infiltrates. The patient was diagnosed as having unstable angina.

Because unstable angina is unpredictable and presents a great risk of MI, Mr. Neimann was admitted for further observation and treatment. He was very upset about being admitted because it meant a substantial loss of income.

Assessment and diagnosis

Cardiac-related chest pain may mimic the pain of other disorders, including indigestion. You must quickly and correctly determine its origin so that you can intervene appropriately. This section will review the collection of critical data that verify underlying cardiac disease: patient history, physical examination, and diagnostic tests and results.

Patient history

With angina patients, a careful history usually reveals more than the physical examination. Although the questions you ask during your history can uncover critical information, the most important point to remember is: If your patient complains of chest pain, assume that he has had an MI. However, remember that chest pain may be caused by something other than angina. (See *Recognizing causes of chest pain,* page 52.) Also remember that patients with possible angina may need emergency intervention during assessment—so be prepared to provide it.

Your history should include questions in these categories: quality, location, and duration of the discomfort; what provokes the discomfort; what relieves it; and what are the associated symptoms.

Quality of chest discomfort. Most patients with angina complain of chest pain or discomfort, but some use other terms. Be sure to ask your patient to describe the feeling in his own words. Although he may not call it pain, his description may be

Origins of anginal pain

What, exactly, stimulates the sympathetic afferents and starts the chain reaction that ends in chest pain?

Some researchers think this reaction is caused by such agents as adenosine, bradykinin, histamine, or serotonin released from cells after a transient ischemic attack. Acidosis or high potassium levels in the involved tissues may elicit release of these substances, which act on the intracardiac sympathetic nerves. The nerves' sensory endplates are receptors of a network of unmyelinated nerves that are located between cardiac muscle fibers and around coronary vessels, and that go to the cardiac plexus and up to the sympathetic ganglia at level C7 to T4. Impulses are then transmitted to corresponding spinal ganglia, through the spinal cord to the thalamus, and finally to the cerebral cortex.

Patients feel the pain of myocardial ischemia in different parts of the chest, because it's referred to the corresponding peripheral dermatomes that supply afferent nerves to the same part of the spinal cord as the heart. One explanation is that a common pool of secondary neurons is activated by somatic and visceral afferent impulses. Overwhelming visceral stimuli may excite adjoining intermediate neurons that receive somatic impulses. So, for example, pain impulses can be referred to the medial aspects of the arm through connections to the brachial plexus and can be referred to the neck through connections with the cervical roots.

Recognizing causes of chest pain

Cause and characteristics	Location	Aggravating factors	Alleviating factors
Cardiovascular origin			
Angina pectoris: aching, squeezing, pressure, heaviness, burning; usually subsides within 10 minutes	Substernal; may radiate to jaw, neck, arms, and back	Eating, exertion, smoking, cold, stress, anger, hunger, lying down	Rest, nitroglycerin *Note:* Unstable angina appears even at rest.
Acute myocardial infarction: pressure, burning, aching, tightness; diaphoresis, weakness, anxiety, nausea; sudden onset; lasts ½ to 2 hours	Across chest; may radiate to jaw, neck, arms, and back	Exertion, anxiety	Analgesics, particularly morphine sulfate
Pericarditis: sharp; may be accompanied by friction rub; sudden onset; continuous pain	Substernal; radiating to neck and left arm	Deep breathing, supine position	Sitting up, leaning forward, anti-inflammatory agents
Dissecting aortic aneurysm: excruciating, tearing; possible blood pressure difference between right and left arms; sudden onset	Retrosternal, upper abdominal, or epigastric; radiating to back, neck, and shoulders	None	Analgesics, but emergency surgery is usually indicated
Pulmonary origin			
Pulmonary embolus: sudden, knifelike; cyanosis, dyspnea, or cough with hemoptysis	Over lung area	Inspiration	Analgesics
Pneumothorax: sudden; severe; dyspnea, increased pulse rate, decreased breath sounds, or deviated trachea	Lateral thorax	Normal respiration	Analgesics, chest tube
Gastrointestinal origin			
Esophageal spasm: dull, pressurelike, squeezing	Substernal, epigastric	Food, cold liquids, exercise	Nitroglycerin, calcium channel blockers
Hiatal hernia: sharp, severe	Lower chest, upper abdomen	Heavy meal, bending, lying down	Antacids, walking, semi-Fowler's position
Peptic ulcer: burning after eating; hematemesis or tarry stools; sudden onset; usually subsides in 15 to 20 minutes	Epigastric	Lack of food or highly acidic foods	Food, antacids
Cholecystitis: gripping, sharp; with possible nausea and vomiting	Right epigastric or abdominal; radiating to shoulders	Fatty foods, lying down	Rest, analgesics, surgery
Musculoskeletal origin			
Chest wall syndrome: sharp; tender to the touch; gradual or sudden onset; continuous or intermittent	Anywhere in chest	Movement, palpation	Time, analgesics, heat
Other origin			
Acute anxiety: dull, stabbing; hyperventilation or dyspnea; sudden onset; transient or may last for several days	Anywhere in chest	Increased respiratory rate, stress or anxiety	Slowing of respiratory rate, stress relief

characteristic of angina. He may describe the feeling as pressure, tightness, heaviness, aching, crushing, squeezing, burning, vise-like, constricting, or suffocating. If he describes the pain as shooting, knifelike, sharp, stabbing, fleeting, or tingling, it's probably not angina. Also ask him to rate the pain on a scale of 0 to 10, with 0 being no pain and 10 being the worst pain imaginable.

Location of discomfort. Anginal pain is usually substernal, but it may be retrosternal. It may radiate to the neck, jaw, teeth, back, shoulders, arms, elbows, and wrists, usually on the left side. When pain travels down the arm, it usually affects the fourth and fifth fingers. Patients also occasionally describe pain in the posterior thorax or intrascapular areas. Ask the patient to point to the area of discomfort. Does it move? Is the pain reproducible by applying direct pressure to the area? Localized pain usually isn't related to the heart; if the patient can point to the painful area with one finger, it's probably not angina.

Also ask the patient to outline the discomfort area with his finger. This area is usually about fist-sized, and many patients clench a fist to their midsternal area when describing the discomfort (Levine's sign). (See *Sites of referred ischemic pain,* page 54.)

Duration of discomfort. Ask your patient if he has ever had this kind of pain before and, if so, how long it lasted. Anginal pain is usually steady, gradually changing in severity, and transient. Angina from physical effort usually lasts 1 to 5 minutes if the precipitating factor is relieved. Angina from emotional stress may last up to 15 minutes because emotions are harder to control than physical activity. The longer the pain lasts, the greater the chance of irreversible ischemia.

Precipitating factors. Ask the patient to recall what he was doing when or just before the pain started. *Physical exertion* can cause angina by increasing myocardial work load and oxygen demand. Angina usually occurs during the exertion, not afterward, but in some patients, the symptoms disappear during exertion ("second-wind" angina pectoris). Exercising, walking up stairs, or having sexual intercourse can provoke an attack. Holding the arms above shoulder level for long periods or simply getting out of bed in the morning ("early morning syndrome") can cause an attack in some patients who have no discomfort during more strenuous effort.

Sites of referred ischemic pain

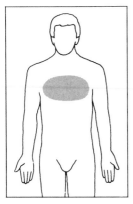

UPPER CHEST

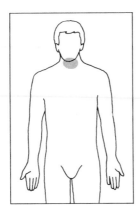

NECK AND JAW

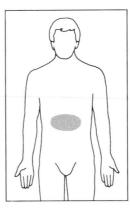

EPIGASTRIC

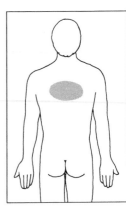

INTRASCAPULAR

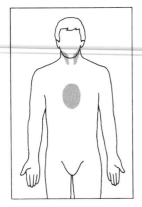

BENEATH STERNUM, RADIATING TO NECK AND JAW

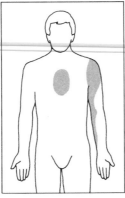

BENEATH STERNUM, RADIATING DOWN LEFT ARM

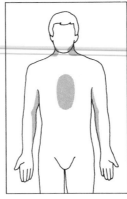

EPIGASTRIC, RADIATING TO NECK, JAW, AND ARMS

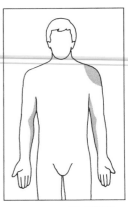

LEFT SHOULDER, INNER ASPECT OF BOTH ARMS

Emotional tension can also trigger angina. Anger, fear, enthusiasm, worry, stress, disturbing thoughts, and nightmares can increase catecholamine levels in the blood, which in turn increase heart rate, contractility, and myocardial oxygen demand.

Exposure to cold—cold weather, cold wind on the face, cold bed sheets, or cold drinks—can trigger angina by increasing myocardial work load. Shoveling snow, which combines physical exercise and cold, often causes angina. Exposure to hot weather may also cause angina.

Smoking, which stimulates adrenaline release and causes coronary artery spasm, also triggers angina. So does *heavy eating;* by increasing gastrointestinal oxygen demand, it increases cardiac output to the gut, putting more demand on the heart. Angina may also occur during rapid-eye-movement sleep when the sympathetic nervous system is stimulated and heart rate, blood pressure, and contractility rise, increasing myocardial oxygen demand. Lastly, angina can occur at rest, for no apparent reason. When this happens, the ischemia is probably caused by insufficient myocardial oxygen supply.

What relieves the discomfort. Ask the patient what he does for relief during an attack. Does the discomfort disappear when he stops physical effort and rests? Nitroglycerin usually stops anginal pain in 1 or 2 minutes. Performing Valsalva's maneuver may also relieve angina by slowing the heart rate, so many patients learn this technique. Many patients are so accustomed to angina that they simply slow down or stop an activity, without anyone else realizing what's happening. If angina occurs when a patient's lying down, just sitting up might relieve it. Patients with extended periods of myocardial ischemia often pace the floor for relief.

Associated symptoms. Ask your patient to describe any symptoms besides chest pain that he has noticed during angina attacks. The most common include nausea; vomiting; diaphoresis; dyspnea; exhaustion; pale or dusky complexion; cool, clammy skin; and palpitations (reflecting increased heart rate and possible dysrhythmias). Cardiac dysrhythmias may also occur when ischemia affects certain areas of the heart.

However, some patients with ischemic heart disease have no symptoms at all. Why this happens isn't known, but one group—patients with diabetes—seems to have silent ischemia more often, perhaps because of autonomic denervation.

Physical examination

Upon examination, the patient may be asymptomatic or show various risk factors for coronary atherosclerosis. Assess the following for signs of atherosclerosis.

Skin and eyes. Look for xanthomas—skin plaques caused by lipid deposits. Then check for xanthelasma, intracellular lipid deposits on the eyelids, which is probably caused by high triglyceride levels and low high-density lipoprotein levels. Also examine the eyes for corneal arcus—a gray opaque line surrounding the margin of the cornea—more common in middle-aged men than women. Finally, check the patient's light reflex. Abnormal reflexes can signal retinal arteriolar changes, which suggest CAD.

Ears. Check the earlobes for diagonal creases, which are common in patients with CAD, except in native Americans, Orientals, and children with Beckwith-Weidemann syndrome. Young patients with CAD usually develop a unilateral crease, which later becomes bilateral.

Cardiovascular status. The patient's blood pressure may be chronically elevated and prompt an angina attack, or it may rise suddenly along with heart rate during an angina attack. Other important signs to look for include arterial pulse and venous system abnormalities, such as bruits. Findings for the heart are usually normal unless the patient has a valvular dysfunction, such as aortic or mitral stenosis. Auscultation may reveal a systolic murmur of mitral regurgitation caused by papillary muscle dysfunction. Auscultation may also reveal a fourth heart sound, paradoxical splitting of the second heart sound, and pulsus alternans; however, they are not specific to ischemic heart disease. A third heart sound is rarely heard during an anginal episode, except in patients with major left ventricular dysfunction caused by myocardial ischemia.

Diagnostic tests and results

Various diagnostic tests may help determine the extent of myocardial ischemia or damage, the type of angina, and the kind of treatment needed and its effectiveness. Although different patients need different tests, those most often performed include electrocardiography (ECG), exercise ECG, radionuclide imaging, cardiac catheterization, and coronary angiography. (See *Imaging tests.*)

Electrocardiography. An ECG records the heart's electrical activity or potential, but not its contractions (mechanical activity). This activity is recorded through electrodes attached to the patient's chest; the ECG machine converts the activity into waveforms and prints them on graph paper. The standard, or 12-lead, ECG usually records electrical activity from 12 different angles, or leads.

This test is mandatory for patients with chest pain or other anginal symptoms, and it should be performed during or after the attack. Performed during the attack, the test can disclose evidence of myocardial ischemia: ST-segment depression and T-wave inversion often appear in ECGs taken during anginal attacks but may disappear when angina subsides. Some patients have transient ST-segment depression of 1 mm or more during angina attacks or episodes of silent ischemia. All of these problems are common signs of myocardial ischemia. However, a resting ECG is of limited use in diagnosing angina associated with atherosclerotic heart disease, except in the case of an old MI.

The ECG is especially valuable in diagnosing variant angina. During a typical attack, transient ST-segment elevations appear in the leads corresponding to the ischemic areas. Some patients also have ST-segment depression. Variant anginal pain can occur at any time and isn't always caused by exercise or other factors that raise myocardial oxygen needs. But after the symptoms diminish, ST segments usually return to normal. (See *Ambulatory electrocardiogram monitoring,* page 58.)

Exercise ECG. An exercise ECG, also called a graded exercise test or stress test, reliably identifies and assesses CAD and the patient's functional ability to work or exercise. The test compares 12-lead ECGs during and after exercise to resting ECGs; it works by increasing the patient's myocardial oxygen needs and then evaluating the ability of his coronary arteries to meet them. The test also assesses intramyocardial oxygen tension, the heart's ability to increase its rate appropriately, and its ability to increase the strength of contraction and stroke volume of the left ventricle appropriately.

This test can be performed in a doctor's office, a clinic, or the central heart station of a hospital. The patient is monitored while performing a multiple-stage test (such as the Bruce test)

Imaging tests

Chest X-rays, magnetic resonance imaging, and positron emission tomography yield valuable information about the location and size of the heart and its chambers and the location of devices, such as pacemakers or pulmonary artery monitoring catheters. X-rays also reveal the size of the great vessels, detect calcium in the heart or the vessels that supply it, and detect changes that may accompany heart disease, such as pulmonary congestion from heart failure.

Chest X-rays can uncover several anomalies that may be connected with atherosclerotic coronary heart disease and its complications. For example, the test may reveal coronary artery calcification, which almost always indicates coronary atherosclerosis.

Magnetic resonance imaging (MRI)
This noninvasive test, also called nuclear magnetic resonance, produces high-resolution, three-dimensional tomographic images. MRI allows visualization of valve leaflets and structures, pericardial abnormalities and processes, ventricular hypertrophy, cardiac neoplasm, infarcted tissue, anatomic malformations, and structural deformities.

Positron emission tomography (PET)
This noninvasive scanning test shows physiologic activity. Although it's used mainly for diagnosing central nervous system disorders, the test also provides information about myocardial perfusion, myocardial metabolism of fatty acids and sugars, amino acid uptake, and infarction size.

Ambulatory electrocardiogram monitoring

An ambulatory electrocardiogram monitor (AEM), commonly called a Holter monitor, records the electrical activity of the heart constantly, usually for 24 hours. AEM is useful in pinpointing anginal attacks or episodes of myocardial ischemia because it gauges the effects of physical and psychological stress on the heart during normal activity. It's also useful in assessing patients with suspected atherosclerotic heart disease, silent ischemia, or coronary spasm.

During the test, the patient wears a tape recorder around his waist to record the ECG continuously. Chest electrodes are attached to measure heart current. The patient is instructed to record his activities during episodes of angina so that when the monitoring is over, a computer can analyze the tape and compare any irregularities with the corresponding activity in the patient's diary. Advise the patient to keep his diary up to date and log any symptoms he has while wearing the monitor. Tell him to perform his usual daily activities, but warn him not to get the monitor wet.

or, occasionally, a single-stage test (such as the Master two-step test). Most commonly, the multiple-stage test is performed; exercise becomes increasingly more strenuous, gradually increasing cardiovascular work load.

During the multiple-stage stress test, the patient walks slowly on a treadmill or pedals on a bicycle ergometer with no resistance. Blood pressure is recorded after a few minutes of warm-up, then the bicycle pedal resistance or the treadmill speed or incline is increased gradually to increase the work load. The patient continues exercising until he reaches a predetermined heart rate or until one of the following conditions occurs:
• ST-segment depression within the first 3 minutes of exercise
• continual ST-segment depression 8 minutes after exercise
• downward-sloping or 2-mm ST-segment depression for at least 0.8 second
• hypotension.

The patient then cools down by walking or pedaling slowly for a few minutes. The doctor examines him and takes another 12-lead ECG. The patient is released when his pulse rate returns to within 20 beats/minute of his starting pulse rate or when it is less than 100 beats/minute after 10 minutes.

Exercise ECG is used mainly for patients with stable angina; it usually isn't recommended for patients with unstable angina. The test has limited diagnostic value for patients with coronary vasospasm because spasm rarely occurs during exercise. In addition, the test can help diagnose silent ischemia in asymptomatic patients.

Exercise ECGs don't require a great deal of preparation on the patient's part, but you will need to explain the following points.

Fasting. Because a full stomach can decrease the available blood supply to the heart and cause nausea and vomiting, tell the patient to fast for 2 hours before the test, after eating a light meal. He shouldn't fast all night because he won't have enough energy to take the test.

Smoking. Tell him to avoid smoking for at least 2 hours before the test, because nicotine constricts the blood vessels and raises heart rate and blood pressure. Also, the carbon monoxide in cigarette smoke diminishes the blood's oxygen-carrying ability, which is vital to cardiac function.

Drugs. If the patient's taking a drug that influences the cardiovascular system and might interfere with his diagnosis of CAD, the doctor will probably discontinue the drug temporarily a few days before the test. However, if the patient's having a stress test to check functional capacity after an acute MI or coronary artery bypass graft (CABG) surgery, or if he's a candidate for a cardiac rehabilitation exercise program, he'll continue the medication so that the doctor can accurately determine his exercise tolerance.

What to wear. Advise the patient to dress comfortably for the test in shorts, a sweatsuit, or other loose-fitting clothing and to wear sneakers or other walking shoes to prevent slipping on the treadmill or bicycle pedals. Women should wear a bra for comfort.

What to do during the test. Tell the patient not to worry if he perspires during the test—it's normal. Inform him that he can stop the test whenever he needs to regain his sense of control. Also tell him to report any chest or leg discomfort or breathlessness immediately; many patients believe that any cardiac symptoms they have during the test will be recorded on the ECG, so they don't bother to report any discomfort.

After the test. When the test is over, caution the patient not to take a hot shower for 1 to 2 hours. Explain that a hot shower, which opens peripheral blood vessels, causes pooling of blood in his arms and legs, which can cause syncope.

Used with an exercise ECG, cardiokymography helps identify cardiac problems electromagnetically. This noninvasive test measures heart-wall contraction patterns before and after an exercise ECG. Although cardiokymography is still experimental, it's thought to be as accurate as a thallium scan. (See *Rapid atrial pacing.*)

Radionuclide imaging. Noninvasive radionuclide imaging tests check coronary artery blood flow and ventricular contraction with special cameras, computers, and radiopharmaceuticals injected intravenously. As these drugs decompose, they emit gamma rays, which are recorded by a scintillation camera and analyzed by a computer to create an image of the drugs' concentration in certain areas of the body. These images help differentiate healthy tissue from damaged or diseased tissue and point out heart regions that don't contract normally. In patients

Rapid atrial pacing

Rapid atrial pacing is sometimes used instead of exercise ECG to diagnose angina because it checks left ventricular function without causing changes in cardiac output, afterload, and circulating catecholamine levels. Because this test produces tachycardia without increasing blood pressure or cardiac output, the doctor can monitor possible ischemic attacks while the patient's at rest. So it's especially useful in patients with intermittent claudication, resting angina, or severe pulmonary disease; in patients who've just had cardiac surgery; and in those who have complications when they exercise to their maximum heart rate.

To perform this test, the doctor threads one end of a pacing wire into the patient's right atrium and attaches the opposite end of the wire to a pulse generator. He usually begins pacing at 100 beats/minute, increasing by 20 beats every 2 minutes until he reaches 160 beats/minute. He performs an ECG after each 2-minute increase to detect ST-segment depression or other signs of ischemia. If the patient has chest pain or ST-segment depression, the test is stopped. Test results are positive when an ST-segment depression of 1 mm occurs 0.08 second after the J point (where the QRS complex ends and the ST segment begins).

Thallium scanning

This test, also called cold-spot imaging and perfusion imaging, assesses myocardial blood flow and myocardial cell status. It can detect regions of ischemic myocardium and infarcted tissue and evaluate coronary artery and ventricular function and pericardial effusion. It can also disclose a myocardial infarction (MI) in its first few hours.

Here's how the test works: Thallium-201, a radioactive isotope that emits gamma rays and closely resembles potassium, is injected I.V. It penetrates healthy myocardial tissue quickly, but it's slow to enter damaged cells and areas with poor blood flow and doesn't enter scarred or infarcted areas lacking blood flow. A scintillation camera counts the gamma rays and displays an image showing areas with heavy isotope uptake (hot spots) as light and those with poor uptake (cold spots) as dark.

The doctor may order an exercise thallium scan, followed by a resting thallium scan, to isolate normal from infarcted tissue. On the camera, the ischemic myocardium is shown as a reversible defect (the cold spot disappears), and the infarcted myocardium appears as a nonreversible defect (the cold spot remains).

In an exercise thallium scan, the patient undergoes a stress test, and the doctor injects thallium-201 at the peak of exercise. Images are taken immediately after exercise and after 3 hours of rest. Dipyridamole may be added.

Dipyridamole thallium testing
Dipyridamole may be given I.V. during exercise thallium scanning. While the patient lies supine, the doctor infuses dipyridamole at a rate of 0.15 mg/kg/minute over 4 minutes. He records vital signs and takes an ECG every minute. After the infusion, the patient walks in place for 2 to 3 minutes, and the doctor injects thallium-201 I.V. while the patient continues walking for 2 minutes more. Then imaging is done, with the patient again in a supine position.

Oral dipyridamole can be substituted for the I.V. form if necessary.
Nursing considerations:
Before this test, the patient must fast overnight and avoid coffee and tea, which contain theophylline, a dipyridamole antagonist. If the patient has an adverse reaction, theophylline (aminophylline) can reverse it, so be sure this drug is on hand during the test.

Multiple-gated acquisition (MUGA) scanning
MUGA scanning, also called radionuclide ventriculography, blood pool imaging, gated heart study, or wall motion study, can be used to diagnose congestive heart failure and to evaluate:
• left ventricular function
• the extent of muscle damage after an MI
• the general level of cardiac function
• a patient's response to therapy
• the degree of cardiac muscle damage.

In this test, the patient is given an injection of a radiopharmaceutical that adheres to red blood cells and enters the circulatory system. A scintillation camera scans heart wall motion and the movement of these tagged blood cells; the resulting images depict blood flow through the heart. First-pass scans record radioactivity in the heart during one cardiac cycle.

MUGA scanning records several hundred cardiac cycles until a repetitive image pattern shows the patient's heart wall motion. These studies also compare end-diastolic and end-systolic counts of tagged red blood cells, allowing an estimated ejection fraction, which indicates overall ventricular strength. This test is safe for patients with congestive heart failure or recent MIs and those too unstable for coronary angiography; however, frequent extrasystoles or irregular rhythms may distort or invalidate test results.

---

with angina, these tests help detect or assess CAD and assess responses to treatment.

Radionuclide imaging tests commonly performed for angina patients include thallium scanning, multiple-gated acquisition (MUGA) scanning, and technetium-99m pyrophosphate scanning. (See *Thallium scanning*.) The latter test is sometimes used to detect MI in patients with unstable angina, but it's used more often in patients with acute MI. (See Chapter 3, Myocardial infarction.)

Cardiac catheterization. Cardiac catheterization is an indispensable diagnostic test that can be used to identify, measure, and verify almost every kind of intracardiac problem. In angina patients, this test is used to measure cardiac output, assess left ventricular and aortic pressures, evaluate coronary atherosclerosis, assess valvular function, and determine whether the patient is a good candidate for CABG surgery or percutaneous transluminal coronary angioplasty (PTCA). Unfortunately, the test involves a risk of serious complications: ventricular fibrillation, bradycardia, hypotension, MI, dissection of the coronary arteries, cerebrovascular accident, and local disorders of the cannulated artery. (See *Cardiac catheterization complications*, page 62.)

Before catheterization, record the patient's baseline vital signs. Also note anxiety and activity levels, the presence of chest pain and its pattern, and the location and intensity of peripheral pulses. In addition, check the patient's chart for any allergies (especially to iodine or shellfish, which can indicate sensitivity to the contrast material) and notify the doctor.

Make sure the patient has signed the consent form, and ask if he understands why the test is being performed. Explain that he'll be receiving a local anesthetic but that he'll probably also be given a mild sedative. Warn that he might feel lightheaded, warm, or nauseated for a few minutes after the contrast material is injected. Also inform him that the insertion site may be sore afterward but that the doctor will order pain medication, if necessary. Warn him to tell you immediately if he has any chest pain after the procedure.

If the patient's test is scheduled for early morning, withhold food and fluids after midnight. However, don't withhold any medications without checking with the doctor.

After catheterization, check the patient's dressing often for bleeding—the most serious risk. If it occurs, remove the pressure dressing and apply firm pressure with your hands. If the catheter was inserted through the femoral artery, tell the patient to keep his leg straight for at least 6 hours, and immobilize it with a

Cardiac catheterization complications

Cardiac catheterization imposes more patient risk than most other diagnostic tests. Such complications occur infrequently, but they are potentially life-threatening.

Complication and possible cause	Signs and symptoms
Left- or right-side catheterization	
Hematoma or blood loss at insertion site Bleeding at insertion site from vein or artery damage	Bloody dressing, limb swelling or increased girth, decreased blood pressure, tachycardia
Dysrhythmias Cardiac tissue irritated by catheter	Irregular heartbeat, palpitations, ventricular tachycardia, ventricular fibrillation
Myocardial infarction Emotional stress induced by procedure Dislodged plaque traveling to a coronary artery (left-side catheterization only) Occlusion of diseased artery by dye or catheter	Chest pain, possibly radiating to left arm, back, or jaw; cardiac dysrhythmias; diaphoresis, restlessness, or anxiety; thready pulse; nausea and vomiting
Reaction to contrast medium Allergy to iodine	Fever; agitation; hives, itching; difficulty breathing
Hypovolemia Diuresis from angiography contrast medium	Hypotension, tachycardia, pallor, diaphoresis
Infection (systemic) from insertion site Poor aseptic technique Catheter contamination	Fever, tachycardia, chills and tremors, unstable blood pressure; swelling, warmth, redness, soreness, or purulent discharge at insertion site
Cardiac tamponade Perforation of heart wall by catheter	Dysrhythmias, tachycardia, decreased blood pressure, chest pain, diaphoresis, cyanosis, distant heart sounds
Pulmonary edema Excessive fluid administration	Early stage: tachycardia, tachypnea, dependent crackles, diastolic (S_3) gallop. Acute stage: dyspnea; rapid, noisy respirations; cough with frothy, blood-tinged sputum; cyanosis with cold, clammy skin; tachycardia; hypertension
Left-side catheterization	
Arterial embolus or thrombus in limb Injury to artery during catheter insertion Plaque dislodged from artery wall by catheter	Slow or faint pulse distal to insertion site; loss of warmth, sensation, and color in arm or leg distal to insertion site; sudden pain in extremity
Cerebrovascular accident or transient ischemic attack Dislodged blood clot or plaque traveling to brain	Hemiplegia, paresis; aphasia; lethargy; confusion or decreased level of consciousness
Right-side catheterization	
Thrombophlebitis Vein damaged during catheter insertion	Hard, sore, cordlike, and warm vein (may look like a red line above catheter insertion site); swelling at site
Pulmonary embolism Dislodged blood clot	Dyspnea, tachypnea, tachycardia, chest pain, pink sputum
Vagal response Vagal irritation in sinoatrial node, atrial muscle tissue, or atrioventricular junction	Hypotension, bradycardia, nausea

sandbag. Elevate the head of the bed no more than 30 degrees. If the patient was catheterized through the brachial artery, tell him to keep his arm straight for at least 3 hours, and immobilize it with a sandbag.

Monitor the patient's vital signs every 15 minutes for at least the first hour after catheterization. Also check the patient's skin color, temperature, and pulses distal to the catheter insertion site. Check the peripheral pulses for changes, and notify the doctor if any occur. After cardiac catheterization, advise your patient to drink plenty of fluids to flush out the hypertonic contrast material. Check urine output carefully, especially in patients with impaired renal function. Also ask the doctor about restarting any medications withheld before the test.

Coronary angiography. This valuable diagnostic test is used to locate and evaluate coronary artery obstruction. It may be combined with cardiac catheterization. The procedure is called cineangiography when movie film is used to record the process of the contrast material filling the blood vessel.

During the test, the doctor inserts a cannula into a peripheral artery, then threads a catheter to the aortic root, the starting point of the coronary arteries. The catheter is curved at the end to ease insertion into the right or left coronary artery. The doctor injects contrast material through the catheter, and while the blood vessels fill, the process is recorded on X-rays or moving films. Next, the doctor may do a ventriculogram. (See *Cardiac function tests,* page 64.) Afterward, he removes the catheter and applies direct pressure for at least 15 minutes to help prevent hematomas and hemorrhage.

Because the contrast material completely fills the coronary arteries for a few minutes, oxygen problems may occur in the part of the myocardium supplied by the artery being tested. Therefore, the doctor may give the patient sublingual nitroglycerin before injecting the contrast material. This dilates the coronary arteries and the peripheral vascular beds, decreasing left ventricular work load.

Patient teaching for coronary angiography patients is similar to that for cardiac catheterization patients. The patient will need to hold his breath so that his diaphragm is away from the

Cardiac function tests

Ventriculography

Ventriculography used with cardiac catheterization or coronary angiography can help locate ventricular aneurysms or other sites of poor contractility and check mitral valve competence. This test measures stroke volume and ejection fraction. The ejection fraction is the amount of blood ejected from the left ventricle per beat; it is indicated as a percentage of the total ventricular volume. The fraction is usually about 65%, plus or minus 8%. A fraction below 50% usually signals severe ventricular dysfunction; one below 35% signals profound dysfunction.

Digital subtraction angiography (DSA)

DSA assesses coronary arterial flow, myocardial perfusion, and left ventricular function and wall movement. It combines coronary angiography with computer processing to create high-resolution images of the cardiovascular system. DSA has several advantages over other tests, including:
• fewer complications linked to

arterial puncture (contrast material is injected into a vein)
• a sharp picture of arterial structures
• fewer complications overall because the dilute, low-dose contrast material doesn't depress cardiac and kidney function
• outpatient use.

Coronary flow and perfusion evaluation

This test uses the same principles as DSA, but it can also evaluate coronary artery blood flow, check myocardial perfusion and anatomy, and judge the extent of coronary lesions.

After contrast material is injected through the coronary artery into the cardiac tissue, a multicolored image is displayed on a computer screen, with each color denoting blood flow during later cardiac cycles. The finished picture, called a contrast-medium-appearance picture, shows how long the contrast material takes to reach cardiac tissue.

area being photographed. He may be required to cough during the procedure to help eject the contrast dye from the coronary arteries by increasing positive pressure in the chest.

Complications are also similar to those for cardiac catheterization. But besides these risks, the patient undergoing coronary angiography can also have an acute MI during or immediately after the test. The stress of the test may also cause more angina symptoms.

One last caution: Don't take blood pressures or draw blood from the arm used in the procedure, and hang a sign in the patient's room to warn others of this precaution.

Ergonovine test. This highly sensitive test is used to diagnose coronary artery spasm in patients with variant angina. To perform the test, the doctor administers I.V. ergonovine, an ergot alkaloid, in gradually increasing doses (0.05 to 0.40 mg). The drug causes direct vascular smooth muscle constriction, inducing coronary artery spasm. The vessels that tend to have spontaneous spasms are most sensitive to the drug. Chest pain and ST-segment depression on an ECG indicate a positive test. Because this test involves substantial risk, it's used only on patients with normal or nearly normal coronary arteries.

Ergonovine tests are usually administered in the cardiac catheterization laboratory, where angiographic equipment, resuscitation equipment, and trained staff are available to diagnose the spasm and administer intracoronary nitroglycerin, if necessary. Two other tests useful in diagnosing angina include angioscopy and angiodynography. (See *Promising research: New tests.*)

Echocardiography. Echocardiography detects the causes and complications of ischemic heart disease. This test records ultrasonic waves reflected from the patient's heart and allows visualization of heart size and shape, myocardial wall thickness and motion, and cardiac valve structure and function. It assesses overall left ventricular function and can identify some MI complications as well as mitral valve prolapse; mitral, tricuspid, or pulmonic valve insufficiency; cardiac tamponade; pericardial diseases; cardiac tumors; prosthetic valve function; subvalvular stenosis; ventricular aneurysms; cardiomyopathies; and congenital abnormalities.

During the test, conductive jelly is spread on the patient's chest at the third or fourth intercostal space just left of the sternum, making an "acoustic window." A transducer is placed on the chest to transmit ultrasound waves to the heart. The waves reflect back to the transducer, where they're reabsorbed and sent to an oscilloscope, which displays these ultrasonic echoes on a screen.

Two types of echocardiography are used most often: M-mode and two-dimensional. In *M-mode echocardiography,* a single ultrasonic beam goes to the heart, creating a columnar

---

PROMISING RESEARCH

New tests

Angioscopy
Fiber-optic angioscopy allows the doctor to visualize the coronary arteries and detect any atherosclerotic plaque formation and thrombi. The test provides a topographic, cross-sectional view of the arterial obstruction and helps the doctor select the most appropriate therapy, such as percutaneous transluminal coronary angioplasty or coronary artery bypass graft surgery.

Angiodynography
This is a new diagnostic approach that determines the rate of blood flow in the arteries to assess the extent of arterial blockage. This test uses ultrasound (high-frequency sound waves bounced off internal structures) and a computer to create color-enhanced moving images; flow rate is represented by the intensity of color on the screen. This technique can help lower-risk patients avoid angiography, an invasive test.

In the future, angiodynography may be used to check the status of a transplanted organ (success is determined by the amount of blood it receives) and to evaluate if cancer therapy is successful when the amount of blood supplying the tumor decreases.

view of cardiac structures. In *two-dimensional echocardiography,* the beam traces an arc, producing a fan-shaped, cross-sectional image of cardiac structures and showing how they relate spatially. The scanning area in this test is an arc of 30 degrees and appears as a real-time television display. A Doppler study may be performed concurrently to detect murmurs and other sounds that indicate conditions that may cause or complicate angina.

Two other types of echocardiography, transesophageal and epicardial, may also be performed.

Transesophageal echocardiography. In this test, a small, phase-arrayed ultrasonic device mounted on the end of a gastroscope is inserted into the patient's esophagus and advanced until it rests directly behind the heart. This provides real-time images of the heart beating.

Epicardial echocardiography. During cardiac surgery, epicardial echocardiography may be used with coronary angiography to visualize the coronary artery wall and lumen. In this test, the doctor holds a small probe over the exposed epicardial coronary artery, slowly scans along the vessel, and stops to record images of its interior.

Blood studies

Other tests commonly performed to evaluate angina include serum cholesterol and serum lipid measurements, and cardiac enzyme analysis.

Case study: Part 3

I.V. morphine relieved Mr. Neimann's chest pain. He was then admitted to the cardiac care unit (CCU), where he was placed on a cardiac monitor. When the patient continued to have frequent episodes of chest pain, he received additional I.V. morphine. An ECG performed during these episodes showed ST-segment depression and T-wave inversion in leads II, III, and aV_F, diagnostic of myocardial ischemia. Once the pain subsided, these changes reverted to a nondiagnostic state.

The cardiologist ordered 10 mg of isosorbide dinitrate every 4 hours. Gradually, Mr. Neimann's condition improved. During the next 2 days, cardiac enzyme evaluation and radionuclide imaging failed to reveal any myocardial necrosis.

Despite his improved clinical status, Mr. Neimann was often restless and worried. He told the CCU nurse that he was concerned about missing so many performances because loss of work along with increasing hospital bills would be a great economic burden on him. The staff was concerned that his increasing stress over his financial situation could exacerbate his angina.

Treatment options

Because angina results from an imbalance between myocardial oxygen supply and demand, treatments aim to increase the oxygen supply, decrease its demands, or both. Although different types of angina require different treatments, one or more of the following therapies are usually used: modification of CAD risk factors through life-style changes, drug therapy, and myocardial revascularization. (See *Comparing angina treatments.*)

Modification of CAD risk factors

Controlling CAD risk factors is critical in the treatment of angina and can reduce the disparity between myocardial oxygen demand and supply. The five biggest risk factors are cigarette smoking, hypertension, high serum cholesterol level, obesity, and stress. Sedentary life-style is also a risk factor, but physical activity must be closely monitored to keep from provoking angina.

Certain life-style changes can help reduce the risk of angina attacks. Patients learn by trial and error exactly what precipitates an angina attack. They should then avoid or modify activities or situations that regularly cause angina.

Avoiding exertion and fatigue. Adequate rest reduces the risk of angina attacks. If angina is frequent or severe, the doctor may greatly restrict exercise or even prescribe bed rest until symptoms subside. With most patients, though, simply decreasing work hours and increasing rest periods reduces symptoms. Patients can climb stairs more slowly or rest along the way. They can modify recreational activities to be less demanding. For example, those who play golf can use a cart instead of walking on the golf course. Patients with chronic stable angina should take daily naps every day to avoid fatigue.

Many angina attacks follow increases in the heart's mechanical activity, caused by increases in myocardial oxygen consumption; therefore, patients should avoid sudden bursts of

Comparing angina treatments

Treatment for all types of angina involves modifications in risk factors and the patient's life-style. But medical or surgical treatments and goals vary with the type of angina.

Stable angina
Interventions
• Drug therapy with nitrates, beta-adrenergic blocking agents, or calcium channel blocking agents

Unstable angina
Interventions
• Admission to cardiac care unit, bed rest, and administration of oxygen
• Drug therapy with I.V. nitroglycerin or other nitrates; narcotics, such as morphine; beta-adrenergic blocking agents; calcium channel blocking agents; or possibly long-term aspirin therapy
• Myocardial revascularization by percutaneous transluminal coronary angioplasty (PTCA) or coronary artery bypass graft surgery
• Possibly intra-aortic balloon counterpulsation to help reverse myocardial ischemia or injury

Variant angina
Interventions
• Drug therapy with nitrates or calcium channel antagonists
Note: Beta-adrenergic blockers constrict coronary vessels, so they're not used.
• Possibly drug therapy with prazosin, a selective alpha-adrenoceptor blocker
• Possibly myocardial revascularization by PTCA if patient has coronary artery spasm and an obstructive lesion

activity, especially on arising in the morning. Because the anginal threshold is lower at this time, patients should shower, shave, dress, and perform other morning activities slowly and use nitroglycerin prophylactically, if necessary.

Modifying sexual intercourse. This activity raises the heart rate to about 120 beats/minute, approximately equal to climbing one flight of stairs at a normal pace. Most patients with chronic stable angina can continue having an active sex life if they take a few precautions. For example, they should delay intercourse until at least 2 hours after a meal and take an extra dose of a short-acting beta blocker an hour before having intercourse and nitroglycerin 15 minutes before.

Controlling environmental factors. Other beneficial changes include wearing a face mask or scarf over the mouth and nose in cold weather and having air conditioning installed. (Hot, humid weather can prompt an angina attack.) Patients should also avoid eating large meals and should never exercise right after a meal because blood flow then is diverted to the digestive organs.

Avoiding stress. Patients with angina should avoid extremely stressful situations or emotional outbursts, which increase myocardial oxygen needs and cause coronary vasoconstriction.

Increasing beneficial exercise. Most doctors recommend walking. Patients who want to try more vigorous activities should join a supervised exercise program and gradually increase their exercise capacity. Patients with stable angina can participate in physical activities that don't cause angina, but as a precaution, they should take nitroglycerin beforehand. Isotonic exercise (involving the large muscle groups) is more beneficial than isometric exercise, which may actually increase myocardial oxygen demand.

Drug therapy

Medications used to treat angina increase blood flow and decrease myocardial oxygen demand. The aims of drug therapy include:
• decreasing the length and intensity of pain during an attack
• prophylactically decreasing the number of attacks and improving the patient's work capacity
• averting or delaying the onset of MI.

The following drugs may be used alone or in combination: nitrates, beta-adrenergic blocking agents, and calcium channel blocking agents. (For information on thrombolytic therapy, see Chapter 3, Myocardial infarction.)

Nitrates. The main drugs prescribed for both angina and coronary spasm, nitrates dilate the vascular smooth muscles, causing veins and also some arteries to distend. Venous dilation reduces venous return to the right side of the heart (preload); this, in turn, decreases wall tension, which decreases oxygen demand. The slight arterial dilation causes a small dip in blood pressure. Nitrates may also increase coronary blood flow in some patients with coronary obstruction and increase collateral blood flow to the ischemic myocardium. These drugs have the opposite effect in patients with normal coronary arteries—they decrease coronary blood flow. *Note:* If nitroglycerin doesn't relieve angina, the doctor may order morphine sulfate. Morphine reduces the pain threshold and anxiety, causes drowsiness and venous pooling, and decreases the heart's oxygen demand. (See *Administering nitrates,* pages 70 and 71.)

Beta-adrenergic blocking agents. Beta blockers are used alone or with nitrates to treat stable and unstable angina. According to recent studies, combined therapy may be more effective in treating stable angina than either drug alone.

The drugs work by obstructing catecholamine binding at receptor sites, thereby blocking the effects of catecholamines. They constrain both inotropic and chronotropic actions created by beta-adrenergic stimulation. Beta blockers' clinical effect, then, is a decrease in myocardial contractility, resting and exercise heart rate, and myocardial oxygen use. In patients with CAD, most of these drugs increase exercise endurance and diastolic filling time, thus increasing coronary perfusion time.

Beta blockers have also been used to treat coronary spasm, but this use is controversial. The drugs may control variant angina symptoms by impeding the adrenergic effect that may cause coronary spasm. On the other hand, they may diminish coronary blood flow and increase coronary vascular resistance, rendering them ineffective in treating spasm because they don't have vasodilatory effects on coronary blood flow. (See *Administering beta-adrenergic blocking agents,* pages 72 and 73.)

(Text continues on page 73.)

Administering nitrates

When administering any of the nitrates, keep the following points in mind:
• Oral dosage forms are absorbed best if taken on an empty stomach (1 hour before or 2 hours after meals) and with a full glass of water. Advise the patient to swallow tablets whole and to chew chewable tablets thoroughly before swallowing.

• With buccal dosage forms, the tablet should be placed between the upper lip or cheek and gum. The dissolution rate varies but will usually range from 3 to 5 hours. Hot liquids increase the dissolution rate and should be avoided.
• Don't use the buccal form at bedtime to avoid risking aspiration.

NITROGLYCERIN (GLYCERYL TRINITRATE)

Trade names
Klavikordal, Niong, Nitro-Bid, Nitro-Bid IV, Nitrocap, Nitrocap T.D., Nitrodisc, Nitro-Dur, Nitrogard, Nitroglyn, Nitrol, Nitrolin, Nitrolingual, Nitronet, Nitrong, Nitrospan, Nitrostat, Nitrostat IV, Nitrostat SR, NTS, Transderm-Nitro, Tridil

Nursing considerations
• Use only sublingual form to relieve acute angina attack. Although a burning sensation was formerly an indication of drug's potency, many current preparations don't produce this sensation.
• To apply ointment, spread in uniform thin layer to any hairless part of the skin except distal parts of arms and legs because absorption will not be maximal at these sites. Don't rub in. Cover with plastic film to aid absorption and to protect clothing. If using Tape-Surrounded Appli-Ruler (TSAR) system, keep TSAR on skin to protect patient's clothing and ensure that ointment remains in place.
• When administering drug as I.V. infusion, use special nonabsorbent tubing supplied by manufacturer because regular

plastic tubing may absorb up to 80% of drug. Also prepare infusion in glass bottle or container.
• If drug causes headache (especially likely with initial doses), administer aspirin or acetaminophen, as ordered.
• Sublingual dose may be administered before anticipated stress or at bedtime if angina is nocturnal.
• Drug may cause orthostatic hypotension. To minimize this, have patient change to upright position slowly, go up and down stairs carefully, and lie down at the first sign of dizziness.
• Instruct patient to avoid alcohol because severe hypotension and cardiovascular collapse may occur.
• Tell patient to notify doctor if blurred vision, dry mouth, or persistent headache occurs.
• Warn patient not to stop taking drug abruptly because this may cause withdrawal symptoms.
• Remove transdermal patch before defibrillation. Because of the patch's aluminum backing, electric current may cause patch to explode.
• When terminating transdermal nitroglycerin treatment for angina, gradually reduce dosage and frequency of application over 4 to 6 weeks.

• To prevent withdrawal symptoms, reduce dosage gradually after long-term use of oral or topical preparations.
• Store drug in cool, dark place in tightly closed container. To ensure freshness, replace supply of sublingual tablets every 3 months. Remove cotton from container because it absorbs drug.
• Instruct the patient to take sublingual tablet at first sign of angina attack. Tell him to wet tablet with saliva, place it under the tongue until completely absorbed, and sit down and rest. If no relief occurs, he should call doctor or go to hospital emergency department. If he complains of tingling sensation with drug placed sublingually, he may try holding tablet in buccal pouch.
• If patient is receiving nitroglycerin lingual aerosol (Nitrolingual), show him how to use this device correctly. Remind him not to inhale spray but to release it onto or under tongue, then to wait about 10 seconds before swallowing.
• Warn patient to move to an upright position slowly because drug may cause dizziness or flushing.

Administering nitrates (continued)

ISOSORBIDE DINITRATE

Trade names
Dilatrate-SR, Iso-Bid, Isonate TR, Isordil, Isotrate, Onset-5, Sorbide TD, Sorbitrate, Sorbitrate SA

Nursing considerations
• Additional dose may be given before anticipated stress or at bedtime if angina is nocturnal.
• Drug may cause orthostatic hypotension. To minimize this, have patient change to upright position slowly, walk up and down stairs carefully, and lie down at first sign of dizziness.
• Instruct patient to avoid alcohol because severe hypotension and cardiovascular collapse may occur.
• Tell patient to notify doctor if blurred vision, dry mouth, or persistent headache occurs.
• Do not discontinue drug abruptly because this may cause withdrawal symptoms or coronary vasospasm.
• Advise patient to sit when self-administering sublingual tablets.

He should lubricate tablet with saliva or place a few milliliters of fluid under tongue with tablet. If patient experiences tingling sensation with drug placed sublingually, he may try to hold tablet in buccal pouch. Advise patient that burning sensations may indicate potency. Dose may be repeated every 10 to 15 minutes to a maximum of three doses. If no relief occurs, patient should call doctor or go to hospital emergency department.

PENTAERYTHRITOL TETRANITRATE

Trade names
Duotrate, Naptrate, Pentol, Pentritol, Pentylan, Peritrate, Peritrate SA

Nursing considerations
• Medication may cause headache, especially at first. Administer aspirin or acetaminophen.
• If necessary, administer additional doses before anticipated stress or at bedtime for nocturnal angina.
• Do not administer drug for relief of acute angina attacks.
• Do not discontinue drug abruptly after long-term therapy because this may cause withdrawal symptoms or coronary vasospasm.
• Warn patient that drug may cause dizziness or flushing. Instruct patient to change positions gradually to avoid excessive dizziness.

ERYTHRITYL TETRANITRATE

Trade name
Cardilate

Nursing considerations
• Additional dose may be administered before anticipated stress or at bedtime if angina is nocturnal.
• Do not discontinue drug abruptly because coronary vasospasm may occur.
• Instruct patient to wet sublingual tablet with saliva, place it under tongue until completely absorbed, and sit down and rest.

AMYL NITRITE

Nursing considerations
• Keep patient sitting or lying down during and immediately after inhalation. Crush ampule (has a woven gauze covering) between fingers, and hold to nose for inhalation.
• Monitor for orthostatic hypotension; do not allow patient to make rapid postural changes while inhaling drug.
• Amyl nitrite is highly flammable; keep away from open flame and extinguish all cigarettes before use.
• Amyl nitrite therapy alters the Zlatkis-Zak color reaction, causing a false decrease in serum cholesterol levels.
• Explain that ampule must be crushed to release drug.
• Warn patient to use drug only when seated or lying down.

Administering beta-adrenergic blocking agents

When administering beta-adrenergic blocking agents, keep the following points in mind:
• Check apical pulse rate daily; hold medication and notify doctor if extremes occur (for example, a pulse rate below 60 beats/minute).
• Monitor blood pressure, ECG, and heart rate and rhythm frequently; be alert for progression of atrioventricular block or severe bradycardia.
• Weigh patients with congestive heart failure regularly; report gains of more than 5 lb (2.25 kg) per week.
• Signs of hypoglycemic shock are masked; watch diabetic patients for sweating, fatigue, and hunger.

• Glucagon may be prescribed to reverse signs and symptoms of beta blocker overdose.
• Warn patient not to discontinue drug suddenly; abrupt discontinuation can exacerbate angina or precipitate myocardial infarction.
• Explain potential adverse effects and importance of notifying doctor of any unusual effects.
• Teach patient to minimize dizziness from orthostatic hypotension by taking dose at bedtime and by rising slowly and avoiding sudden position changes.
• Advise patient to check with doctor or pharmacist before taking nonprescription cold preparations.

ATENOLOL

Trade name
Tenormin

Nursing considerations
• Give single daily dose at same time each day.
• Dosage may need to be reduced in patients with renal insufficiency.

• Stress importance of not missing doses, but tell patient not to double the dose if one is missed, especially if taking once a day.
• Advise patient to check with doctor before taking nonprescription cold preparations.
• Atenolol may increase or decrease serum glucose levels in

diabetic patients.
• Atenolol also may cause changes in exercise tolerance and ECG; it has reportedly elevated platelet count, blood urea nitrogen (BUN) levels, and serum levels of potassium, uric acid, AST (SGOT), ALT (SGPT), alkaline phosphatase, lactic dehydrogenase, and creatinine.

METOPROLOL TARTRATE

Trade name
Lopressor

Nursing considerations
• Metoprolol may be administered daily as a single dose or in divided doses. If a dose is missed, patient should take only the next scheduled dose.
• Give drug with meals to en-

hance absorption.
• Dosage may need to be reduced in patients with impaired hepatic function.
• When used in low dosages (for example, daily dosages of less than 100 mg), most patients with asthma or bronchitis can safely use this drug without fear of worsening their condition.

• Avoid late-evening doses to minimize insomnia.
• Observe patient for signs of mental depression.
• Metoprolol may elevate serum transaminase, alkaline phosphatase, lactic dehydrogenase, and uric acid levels.

NADOLOL

Trade name
Corgard

Nursing considerations
• Dosage adjustments may be necessary in patients with renal impairment.

• Discontinue drug if patient develops heart failure.

Administering beta-adrenergic blocking agents (continued)

PROPRANOLOL HYDROCHLORIDE

Trade name
Inderal, Inderal LA

Nursing considerations
• Propranolol may elevate serum transaminase, alkaline phosphatase, and lactic dehydrogenase levels, and it may elevate BUN levels in patients with severe heart disease.
• Discontinue if signs of heart failure or bronchospasm develop.
• Give drug with meals to enhance absorption.

• Restoration of normal sinus rhythm after atrial fibrillation may cause thromboemboli; anticoagulant therapy is recommended before initiation of propranolol therapy.

Calcium channel blocking agents. Calcium channel blockers are widely prescribed for unstable angina and coronary spasm because of their vasodilator effect. Although their onset of action is slower than nitrates, their duration of action is much longer. Calcium channel blockers work by obstructing calcium ion movement across myocardial and vascular smooth muscle, causing coronary artery and collateral vessel vasodilatation; decreased myocardial contractility, which reduces myocardial oxygen demand; peripheral artery vasodilatation, which reduces systemic blood pressure; and decreased cardiac conduction. (See *Administering calcium channel blockers,* page 74.)

Myocardial revascularization
Myocardial revascularization is performed by two methods: PTCA and CABG surgery. Patients must understand that this treatment won't cure their angina, only ease the symptoms, and that they must also alleviate risk factors by changing their life-styles.
Percutaneous transluminal coronary angioplasty. PTCA, commonly called angioplasty, is used to dilate occluded coronary arteries. In this procedure, the doctor inserts a balloon-tipped catheter through the coronary artery lesion and inflates it briefly. The balloon compresses the atheromatous material on the vessel wall, enhancing myocardial perfusion and performance without the need for CABG surgery. (See *PTCA procedure,* page 76.)

Administering calcium channel blockers

When administering calcium channel blockers, keep the following points in mind:
• Monitor cardiac rate and rhythm and blood pressure carefully when initiating therapy or increasing dosage.
• Tell patient to check with doctor before discontinuing drug; gradual withdrawal may be necessary.
• Instruct patient to notify doctor if he experiences any of the following: irregular heartbeat, shortness of breath, swelling of hands and feet, pronounced dizziness, constipation, nausea, or hypotension.
• Advise patient to take a missed dose as soon as possible, but not if it's almost time for next dose. Warn patient not to double the dose.
• Sublingual nitroglycerin may be administered concomitantly, as needed, if patient has acute angina symptoms.
• Patients may experience annoying hypotensive effects during titration of dose. Urge compliance.
• Monitor these patients closely.

DILTIAZEM HYDROCHLORIDE

Trade name
Cardizem

Nursing consideration
• If diltiazem is added to therapy of a patient receiving digoxin, monitor serum digoxin levels and observe patient closely for signs of toxicity (especially elderly patients, those with unstable renal function, and those with serum digoxin levels in the upper therapeutic range).

NICARDIPINE

Trade name
Cardene

Nursing considerations
• Initial doses or dosage increase may exacerbate angina briefly. Reassure patient that this symptom is temporary.
• Monitor blood pressure regularly, especially if patient is also taking beta blockers or antihypertensives.

NIFEDIPINE

Trade name
Procardia

Nursing considerations
• Initial doses or dosage increase may exacerbate angina briefly. Reassure patient that this symptom is temporary.
• Nifedipine is not available in sublingual form. However, liquid in oral capsule may be withdrawn by puncturing capsule with needle, and the drug may be instilled into the buccal pouch. Or, a punctured capsule may be chewed.
• Monitor blood pressure regularly, especially if patient is also taking beta blockers or antihypertensives.
• Although rebound effect has not been observed when drug is stopped, dosage should be reduced slowly under doctor's supervision.
• Instruct patient to swallow capsules whole without breaking, crushing, or chewing them.
• Mild to moderate increase in serum concentrations of alkaline phosphatase, lactic dehydrogenase, AST (SGOT), and ALT (SGPT) have been noted.

VERAPAMIL HYDROCHLORIDE

Trade names
Calan, Isoptin

Nursing considerations
• If verapamil is added to therapy of patient receiving digoxin, digoxin dose should be reduced by half with subsequent monitoring of serum drug levels.
• During long-term therapy combining verapamil and digoxin, monitor ECG periodically for atrioventricular (AV) block and bradycardia because of possible additive effects on the AV node.
• Obtain periodic liver function test results.
• Patients with severely compromised cardiac function and those receiving beta blockers should receive lower verapamil doses.

How does PTCA improve vascular patency? This isn't fully understood. What actually occurs is a "controlled injury" to the vessel, which results in such tissue changes as compression, splitting, plaque redistribution, and stretching of the wall. The vessel's fibrous cap is broken, and the exposed matter lying beneath the cap is removed by phagocytosis. As the vessel heals, endothelialization takes place simultaneously with plaque activation, causing the diameter of the occluded segment to enlarge and blood flow to improve through the formerly constricted area. Before the procedure, various medications are used prophylactically, including antibiotics, aspirin, nifedipine, heparin, dipyridamole, low-molecular-weight dextran, nitroglycerin, and investigational drugs.

Before undergoing PTCA, patients must meet the criteria for CABG surgery, in case PTCA fails or complications occur that necessitate immediate surgery. The patient should know this before signing the surgical consent form, and the open-heart surgical team should be on call.

PTCA is performed on lesions in the three coronary vessels except for the left main coronary artery, but the typical surgical candidate usually has one or two proximal or midvessel stenoses. Ideally, the lesions should be noncalcified smooth plaque with sharp margins or irregular borders, located in arteries with a 50% to 95% reduction in blood flow. However, patients with distal and calcified lesions and multivessel disease may also benefit from PTCA. Most patients chosen for the procedure have stable angina that has caused life-style changes or unstable angina of less than 6 months' duration that hasn't responded to medical intervention. Emergency PTCA may be performed during acute unstable angina attacks or in the first 4 to 6 hours after the onset of chest pain in MI. During an MI, the doctor may also inject a thrombolytic drug into the heart to encourage thrombolysis and recanalization.

Because of advanced skill and technology, patients with multivessel disease may also be candidates for PTCA. To make sure the procedure will be successful, the most serious lesion is usually dilated first. If dilation of this lesion isn't successful, the patient will need CABG surgery instead.

PTCA procedure

Percutaneous transluminal coronary angioplasty (PTCA) offers some patients a nonsurgical alternative to coronary artery bypass graft (CABG) surgery. In this procedure, a tiny balloon catheter is used to dilate a coronary artery that's been narrowed by atherosclerotic plaque. The procedure for PTCA resembles that for cardiac catheterization. The doctor threads a guiding catheter through a femoral or brachial artery, then backward into the ascending aorta and into the ostium of the right or left coronary artery.

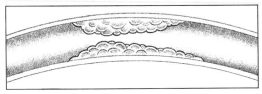

1. Cross-section of a coronary artery narrowed by plaque formation.

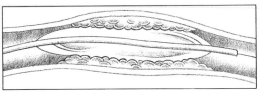

4. Once in position, the balloon is inflated with a mixture of contrast material and saline solution. The inflated balloon opens up the narrowed artery by splitting and compressing the plaque material and slightly stretching the artery wall.

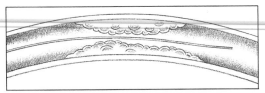

2. A guide wire is advanced from the balloon dilatation catheter through the coronary artery until its tip is beyond the narrowing.

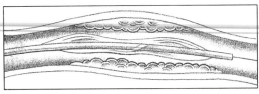

5. After the balloon reaches 3 to 6.5 atmospheres of pressure, it's deflated. The balloon is repeatedly inflated until the distal perfusion pressure falls about 20%. The catheter is then removed from the artery.

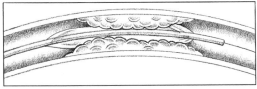

3. The balloon catheter is advanced over the guide wire until the balloon is wedged into the narrowing.

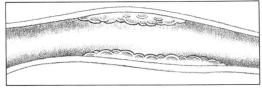

6. PTCA has widened the narrow part of the artery, and blood flow to the heart is improved.

Some doctors prescribe I.V. nitroglycerin before PTCA and keep patients on the drug during the procedure. Sublingual nifedipine and I.V. or intracoronary nitroglycerin may also be administered if coronary spasm occurs or is suspected. In addition, patients usually receive heparin during the procedure to ward off thrombus formation. Some patients also require calcium channel antagonists after PTCA, and some receive antiplatelet drugs or warfarin.

When PTCA is successful, coronary stenosis decreases 20% or more, and the pressure gradient across the lesion also diminishes.

Although most PTCAs are uneventful, complications occasionally occur. These include acute vessel occlusion during the procedure, which can cause an acute MI or arterial dissection. In addition, about 25% to 30% of patients have recurrent stenosis, usually within 6 months. Endovascular stents are now being used to help prevent restenosis or to stabilize arterial dissection while the patient is transported to surgery. (See *Reducing restenosis.*)

Coronary artery bypass graft surgery. CABG surgery is also called bypass surgery, direct myocardial revascularization, aortocoronary bypass surgery, and saphenous vein bypass. Unlike medical treatments that reduce myocardial oxygen needs, this surgical procedure increases myocardial oxygenation by bypassing the blockage in the coronary artery and restoring blood flow to the myocardium. A grafted saphenous vein or internal mammary artery is used to bypass the occluded artery, which may be the left main coronary artery, the left anterior descending artery, the distal right coronary artery, the posterior descending artery, or the marginal branch of the circumflex artery.

CABG surgery doesn't cure atherosclerosis, but it does alleviate symptoms and improve and lengthen the patient's life. It's usually recommended for patients with:
• chronic disabling angina that doesn't respond to medical treatment
• unstable angina that doesn't respond to medical treatment
• significant stenosis of the left main coronary artery (Significant stenosis is defined as a 50% or greater narrowing of the artery's diameter, coinciding with a 75% or greater decrease in the cross-

Reducing restenosis

Although the initial success rate for percutaneous transluminal coronary angioplasty (PTCA) is about 81%, 25% to 40% of patients have restenosis after 6 months. To reduce this rate, researchers are trying several approaches:
• supplementing diet with fatty acids (fish oil). Recent studies suggest that fish oil limits smooth muscle proliferation and collagen synthesis in blood vessels.
• inserting a stent—a flexible, elastic, stainless-steel mesh tube—after PTCA. The stent expands to fit the interior of the previously occluded vessel.
• administering drugs, including ciprostene (a prostacyclin analog), recombinant hirudin (an anticlotting protein originally derived from leeches), and monoclonal antibodies that block clotting receptors on platelets.

Lowering the risk of PTCA

Researchers are trying to lower the risks of percutaneous transluminal coronary angioplasty (PTCA) and extend its use. Methods under investigation include the following.

Fluosol-DA
This fluorocarbon oxygen transport fluid protects the heart from temporary ischemic damage during PTCA. Many times, balloons must be inflated for 45 seconds or more, causing ischemia and other complications. Injecting Fluosol-DA into the coronary artery beyond the occlusion can prevent ischemia.

Retroperfusion
This new technique for retrograde rather than antegrade reperfusion reduces ischemia by pumping oxygenated blood through a coronary sinus catheter. The pump draws blood from the femoral artery and pumps it through a jugular catheter into the great cardiac vein. Pumping is coordinated with the PTCA catheter in the left anterior descending coronary artery; arterial blood is pushed into the myocardium and held there during alternate balloon inflations. This procedure reduces chest pain and improves myocardial perfusion.

Another retroperfusion technique, the Bard cardiopulmonary support (CPS) system, allows for cardiopulmonary bypass during surgery with thoracotomy. This technique uses catheterization of the femoral artery and vein to access the patient's circulation. When connected to the CPS system, it can control circulation and cardiac output in high-risk angioplasty patients.

sectional area of the vessel. A 90% or greater decrease in area is considered critical stenosis.)
• CAD in three vessels
• angina that continues after an MI.

Some doctors have tried CABG surgery on patients with developing MI to try to restrict infarct size and save left ventricular function. This strategy is most successful within 6 hours after symptoms begin and in patients with subendocardial, rather than transmural, infarcts. In addition, recent research indicates the need for emergency surgery in post-MI patients with significant congestive heart failure from acute rupture of the ventricular septum or papillary muscle and for patients with congestive heart failure, angina, or systemic emboli from a left ventricular aneurysm.

Before recommending CABG surgery, the doctor considers the patient's signs and symptoms, test results, operative risks, quality of life before surgery, and the surgery's cost. He also considers the patient's sex and physical size: Twice as many women die from CABG surgery as men. Their smaller size and the smaller diameter of grafted coronary arteries may contribute to this higher mortality. In both men and women, mortality decreases when physical size increases. (For information about experimental angioplasty techniques, see *Promising research: Lowering the risk of PTCA, New therapy: Atherectomy,* and *Laser angioplasty.*)

Case study: Part 4

Three days after admission, Carl Neimann was transferred to the intermediate CCU. The move didn't please him—he'd been anticipating discharge, not a transfer. In the new unit, he told his primary nurse that he was sick of being in the hospital. He even hinted that he might sign out against medical advice. A staff conference consisting of his primary nurse, doctor, social service worker, and a crisis intervention nurse was called to find effective ways of dealing with his stress level and financial concerns.

After using some of the agreed upon interventions, the patient agreed to begin an exercise program and cardiac rehabilitation. Gradually, he increased his activity and tolerated it well. Still, he always seemed eager to get the exercise sessions over with.

Then, during an exercise ECG 2 days later, trouble arose. After exercising at 150 km/minute for just 2½ minutes, Mr. Neimann's heart

New therapy: Atherectomy

An experimental, nonsurgical technique, percutaneous transluminal atherectomy removes atherosclerotic plaque from arterial walls with a special catheter. A tiny rotating blade encased in the catheter either slices away the plaque or pulverizes it.

Atherectomy may have several advantages over balloon angioplasty: It doesn't cause as much trauma to the vessel wall, and it decreases the rate of restenosis.

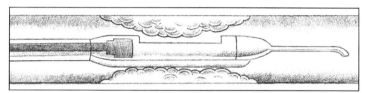

Window of atherectomy catheter's metal housing is placed next to plaque.

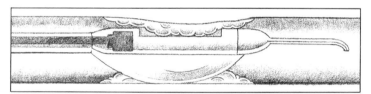

Balloon on opposite side is inflated, forcing window against lesion.

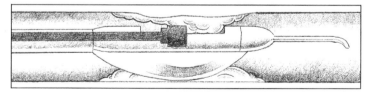

Rotating blade shears off plaque.

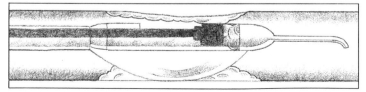

Plaque is then pushed into catheter tip.

Laser angioplasty

An experimental technique, laser angioplasty vaporizes plaques and thrombi that block atherosclerotic arteries. An argon laser is inserted through a fiber-optic catheter into a diseased artery, and when the laser nears the problem area, the doctor switches it on and off in rapid bursts for a predetermined time. Between bursts, he rotates the catheter, advancing it until he has opened the vessel completely.

So far, the best results have been in thrombi-obstructed arteries.

Researchers have found that limiting exposure time helps minimize intimal surface damage and that pulsed lasers and excimer laser systems (which operate in the near-ultraviolet range) may reduce thermal injury in nearby tissues. Combined with better visual control, this could make the technique safer.

Another experimental technique uses an excimer laser to clear completely blocked coronary arteries during open-heart surgery. This procedure was first done in Canada in 1987 and is now being tested on animals in the United States.

Another investigational procedure, laser-balloon angioplasty, combines laser energy with a conventional balloon catheter. During balloon inflation, the arterial wall absorbs heat from the laser, producing a smooth lumen that researchers hope will be less vulnerable to restenosis.

Preoperative nursing care

Is your angina patient scheduled for coronary artery bypass graft surgery? Then do the following preoperatively.
• Complete the nursing history.
• Assess for clinical signs and symptoms of compromised organ function.
—*Neurologic:* decreased level of consciousness, neurologic deficits, weakness, impaired verbal response.
—*Cardiovascular:* abnormal heart rate and rhythm, abnormal heart sounds, unequal blood pressure in both arms, decreased or absent peripheral pulses, edema, neck vein distention, bruits.
—*Respiratory:* abnormal breath sounds, tachypnea.
—*Renal:* decreased urine output.
—*Gastrointestinal:* abdominal distention, absent bowel sounds.
—*Immunologic:* increased temperature, any localized infections.
• Be sure all diagnostic tests are completed and all problems are reported to the doctor.
• Monitor the patient's response to medical treatment aimed at minimizing postoperative complications. Treatment includes pulmonary hygiene, administering electrolytes, and other pharmacologic interventions.
• Teach deep-breathing and coughing exercises to prevent pneumonia and leg exercises to prevent venous stasis.
• Tell the patient and his family what to expect postoperatively, and discuss their concerns and anxieties over the surgery.

Case study: Part 4 *(continued)*

rate reached 100 beats/minute and he developed severe substernal chest pain and 2 mm of ST-segment depression on the ECG. When the test was stopped and sublingual nitroglycerin administered, the pain subsided after 10 minutes.

The cardiologist recommended cardiac catheterization and coronary angiography to determine the cause of the poor exercise tolerance. An angry and frustrated Mr. Neimann reluctantly agreed.

Despite this setback, Mr. Neimann was beginning to acknowledge his illness. The episode of severe chest pain frightened him, finally convincing him that his condition was serious. Mr. Neimann resigned himself to an extended hospital stay. When several band members visited and offered to lend him some money, he became less anxious and more cooperative.

Cardiac catheterization and coronary angiography, performed 2 days after the exercise ECG, revealed a 75% narrowing of the first diagonal branch of the left anterior descending coronary artery. The next day Mr. Neimann consented to a PTCA.

Nursing management

Continuing nursing assessment and interventions are based on the patient's signs and symptoms, his medical treatment and drug therapy, and whether he has had PTCA or CABG surgery. (See *Preoperative nursing care* and *Patient-teaching checklist: CABG surgery.*)

Signs and symptoms

If the patient continues to complain of chest pain, he will need to be evaluated to determine whether his condition is deteriorating or whether he needs a different treatment approach. The doctor will probably review the patient's history and do another ECG. Then he'll compare the two test results, looking for changes that might indicate the myocardial ischemia is progressing to MI. For example, does the second ECG show T-wave inversion (indicating myocardial ischemia)? Has ST-segment elevation increased (indicating myocardial injury)? Are pathologic Q waves present (indicating MI)? (For more information on ECG changes, see Chapter 3, Myocardial infarction.)

When evaluating the patient's complaint of chest pain, ask him to rate his pain on the 1-to-10 scale mentioned earlier.

PATIENT-TEACHING CHECKLIST

CABG surgery

If your patient's having coronary artery bypass graft (CABG) surgery, be sure to cover the following points in your patient and family teaching:

☐ Anatomy and physiology of the heart
☐ Pathophysiology of patient's coronary artery disease
☐ Risk-factor modification and life-style changes
☐ Preoperative routine— diagnostic tests; preoperative procedure (for example, shower with antibacterial soap, nothing by mouth after midnight, daily weights, anesthesiology assessment, medications, including sedatives, analgesics, and antibiotics); medication tapering or discontinuation
☐ Surgical procedure
☐ Postoperative routine— endotracheal tube and mechanical ventilation; ECG monitoring, including pacing wires; hemodynamic monitoring, including arterial lines; I.V. lines; diagnostic tests, including arterial blood gas measurements and chest X-ray; daily weights; pain medication; relaxation techniques; communication techniques while intubated; coughing, deep breathing, and chest physiotherapy; incisional care; chest tubes, including stripping and milking procedure; urinary catheter placement; fluid or weight gain; leg exercises; progression of care (for example, extubation, diet, out-of-bed routine)
☐ Transfer to intermediate care unit
☐ Location of waiting room.

If possible, arrange for the patient and family to visit the cardiac care unit, or familiarize them with the unit using audiovisual materials.

Compare this latest rating to his previous rating. Also ask the patient to describe any new physical limitations since this recent onset of chest pain. Do activities that were tolerated well before now cause chest pain, or do activities that caused chest pain before now cause it more readily?

Drug therapy

When assessing and planning interventions for the patient receiving drug therapy, focus on whether his present therapy is meeting his needs. To do this, evaluate the patient's description of the occurrence, frequency, and intensity of anginal pain. Be aware of any adverse reactions indicating that his drug dosage should be increased or decreased or that he needs a different drug entirely.

Percutaneous transluminal coronary angioplasty

When assessing and planning interventions for the patient who has undergone PTCA, focus on postprocedure care and on preventing complications. The patient's condition after PTCA determines how much care he'll need.

Postprocedure care. Most patients are connected to a cardiac monitor after the test. You'll need to watch them for signs of myocardial ischemia for at least 4 hours. Isoenzymes are also drawn when the patient returns to his room. After surgery, check the catheter site frequently for bleeding and bruising. Because heparin's effects aren't reversed at the end of the procedure, bleeding can be a serious problem. Remind the patient to keep his leg flat for several hours and to stay in bed. After the catheter is removed, apply a pressure dressing until every sign of bleeding has subsided. Assess circulation often by checking for warmth and distal pulses.

Also watch for chest pain, shortness of breath, and mental status changes, which can signal a complication. Monitor vital signs carefully, paying special attention to heart rate and rhythm. Check for increased ectopy and report any unusual findings to the doctor. If the patient develops chest pain shortly after the procedure, the doctor will order a basic acute coronary care protocol, including a 12-lead ECG to substantiate ischemia, vasodilator or other drug therapy to relieve pain, and serial cardiac enzyme tests to determine the extent of myocardial damage. Continued pain indicates a sudden decrease in blood flow from reocclusion of the dilated artery and warrants another angiogram or angioplasty. So you'll also need to assess the patient's emotional status and offer support, especially if the PTCA wasn't successful.

Complications. You'll need to monitor the patient's drug therapy and instruct him about any medications he'll be taking after discharge. Most doctors prescribe a daily dose of aspirin to be taken indefinitely to reduce platelet activity. They may also prescribe dipyridamole for 6 months and a vasodilator, such as a calcium channel blocker or nitrate, for a short time to help prevent vasospasm in the affected arterial segment.

CABG surgery

Assessing and planning interventions for the patient who's undergone CABG surgery focuses on postoperative care and prevention of complications.

Most patients undergoing CABG surgery return to the CCU immediately after the procedure. So postoperative care in the first few hours resembles recovery room care. CABG surgery can affect all body systems, making postoperative care challenging. (See *Postoperative complications of CABG surgery,* page 84.)

When caring for postoperative CABG patients, monitor heart rate and rhythm carefully. Within 48 hours after open-heart surgery, about 50% of all patients experience some cardiac rhythm disturbance.

As many as 90% of patients have a notable decrease in left ventricular ejection fraction and cardiac index 2 hours after CABG surgery. So watch for signs of transient left ventricular dysfunction, a common complication. Also watch for reduced cardiac output, another common complication.

Of all the complications occurring after thoracic and cardiac surgery, respiratory complications (atelectasis) and behavioral changes are the most common.

Atelectasis. Oxygen and carbon dioxide gas exchange is commonly affected postoperatively because extracorporeal perfusion can injure alveolar-capillary membranes and cause increased interstitial lung water levels.

Low postoperative hemoglobin levels can also diminish gas exchange by decreasing the red blood cells' oxygen-carrying capacity. In addition, anesthesia's effects, sedation, pain, and immobility can cause hypoventilation and intensify atelectasis.

Behavioral changes. A few patients also suffer strokes or transient motor deficits after CPBP surgery. A more common problem is behavioral changes, ranging from slight confusion to actual psychosis or postcardiotomy delirium (PCD). PCD usually appears about 24 hours after surgery and clears up 24 to 48 hours after transfer from the CCU. Patients most inclined to have PCD are elderly patients and those with severe preoperative cardiac problems, a history of psychiatric problems, sleep deprivation, or long stays in the CCU.

Postoperative complications of CABG surgery

Complications	Causes
Transient motor deficits	Altered cerebral blood flow
Stroke	Cerebral particulate emboli (especially fat emboli) and air emboli
Cerebral hemorrhage	Systemic heparinization
Hemorrhage	Dilution, absorption, and destruction of coagulation factors in CPBP circuit; heparin rebound after neutralization with protamine; platelet counts reduced by 30% and platelet function impaired for 3 to 5 days
Hypernatremia	Decreased urinary excretion of sodium, most marked on second postoperative day
Hyperkalemia	Defective intracellular transport of glucose and potassium
Hypocalcemia	Dilution of serum calcium and intracellular calcium shifts
Hypomagnesemia	Dilution of serum magnesium and intracellular magnesium shifts; magnesium losses in urine
Hypokalemia	Dilution of serum potassium; intracellular potassium shifts; large potassium losses in urine; use of potassium cardioplegia
Hyponatremia	Dilution of serum sodium
Elevated systemic vascular resistance	Catecholamine release
Risk of steroid inadequacy	Decreased adrenocorticotropic hormone levels and decreased cortisol response during CPBP surgery
Ketoacidosis; hyperosmolar hyperglycemic non-ketotic acidosis	Elevated blood glucose levels and depressed insulin response
Hypertension	Elevated renin, angiotensin, and aldosterone levels

Complications	Causes
Intravascular hypovolemia	Decreased intravascular volume
Interstitial edema	Increased extravascular fluid
Total body hypervolemia	Increased total body water
Gastrointestinal bleeding	Catecholamine release and "stress response"; coagulation defects
Acute pancreatitis	Complement activation
Intestinal ischemia or infarction	Emboli to intestinal vasculature; low perfusion state
Perioperative myocardial infarction	Emboli; inadequate perfusion; inadequate myocardial cooling and ventricular fibrillation
Low postoperative cardiac output	Release of capillary-damaging enzymes; lowered colloid osmatic pressure; high coronary perfusion pressures; distention of the left ventricle
Myocardial injury	Reperfusion injury
Postoperative infections	Decreased complement and immunoglobulin levels for up to 1 week; exposure to multiple pathogen sources
A total body inflammatory reaction (postperfusion syndrome)	Release of complement anaphylatoxins
Atelectasis	Alterations of ventilatory patterns during bypass; complement activation, air, and particulate emboli contributing to alveolar-capillary membrane damage; hemodilution, decreased colloid osmotic pressure, and interstitial pulmonary edema
Renal failure	Damage to red blood cells with release of hemoglobin; decreased renal blood flow and decreased glomerular filtration rate; microemboli to renal vasculature

Because of these potential problems, you'll need to center your nursing care on pinpointing signs of neurologic function abnormalities. You'll also need to reorient the patient to time, place, and person; ensure periods of uninterrupted sleep; encourage family visits; and provide familiar objects, such as a radio and pictures from home. These interventions should curtail postoperative psychiatric complications.

CABG surgery patients are usually hospitalized in the CCU for only 2 to 3 days; then they're usually transferred to an intermediate care unit. Most patients are glad to leave the bright lights and hectic atmosphere of the CCU, but if the transfer takes place at night or is so abrupt that the patient hasn't been prepared, he may feel anxious or insecure. So reassure him by emphasizing that a doctor will visit him daily, that he'll have access to monitoring equipment, and that the staff in the new unit is highly experienced and familiar with his case. Also stress that he's being transferred because his condition is improving. Be sure to notify the family of the patient's transfer so they won't be shocked by an empty bed. Once the patient is transferred to the intermediate care unit, you should begin more intensive patient teaching.

Other complications. Infection can also occur postoperatively, so follow sterile procedures meticulously when handling invasive lines and incisions, and watch closely for signs of infection. Although few patients suffer acute renal failure after cardiopulmonary bypass, you'll still need to monitor fluid intake and output, blood urea nitrogen levels, and serum creatinine levels carefully. Also assess your patient for possible emboli, which can occur in numerous sites after cardiopulmonary bypass. Also monitor for gastrointestinal complications. Check the patient for postoperative ileus, return of bowel sounds, and effective gastric decompression.

Patient teaching
Both the nurse and the doctor are legally responsible for providing patient teaching before discharge. Your teaching will be strengthened if your patient trusts you, so let him know that you care about his well-being both in and out of the hospital, and listen to his concerns attentively. But even if the time you can

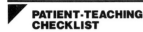

PATIENT-TEACHING CHECKLIST

Angina pectoris

If your patient has angina, be sure to cover the following points in your teaching.

Reduce risk factors
☐ Stop smoking.
☐ Avoid foods high in saturated fat and cholesterol.
☐ Decrease sodium intake and take prescribed medication if you're hypertensive.
☐ Lose weight if you're overweight.
☐ Learn to cope with stress by changing your life-style.

Exercise regularly
☐ Avoid activities that cause angina, dyspnea, or fatigue.
☐ Start a progressive exercise program, keeping activity below angina level.
☐ Avoid heavy lifting or other isometric activity.

Avoid trigger activities
☐ Avoid emotional upsets, severe fatigue, stressful situations, exposure to extreme temperatures, and caffeine-containing beverages.
☐ Don't overeat.

Treat angina when it occurs
☐ Always carry nitroglycerin.
☐ Stop activity and put nitroglycerin under your tongue at the first sign of angina. Then rest. Take one tablet every 5 minutes up to three tablets until pain is relieved. To avoid pain, take nitroglycerin prophylactically. If angina continues, call the doctor.

spend with the patient is too limited to develop a trusting nurse-patient relationship, be sure to provide appropriate teaching.

Your teaching environment should be calm, quiet, and as distraction-free as possible. Be sure to include family members or other caregivers in your sessions to ensure continuity of care after discharge. Group and individual cardiac rehabilitation programs also include patient and family teaching, so encourage your patient and his family to attend. Visual aids, films, pamphlets, charts, and models can make your teaching come alive and provide a valuable resource for your patient to study at home. To help you formulate a teaching plan, first assess the patient's level of knowledge about his disease.

Your teaching plan for the patient with angina should include information on the following: risk factor modification, lifestyle changes, medical treatments, and avoiding and relieving angina attacks. Also instruct the family on how to obtain emergency medical care (for example, how to call the local emergency medical services), on when to contact the doctor, and on the importance of keeping follow-up appointments.

If your patient has had PTCA or CABG surgery, be sure he understands that these procedures are only palliative; they don't cure CAD, and they must be combined with risk-factor modification and life-style changes. So review risk factors with your patient and discuss ways that he can change his life-style and lower his chance of having an angina attack. Also discuss medication dosage and administration. If your patient's being discharged with several medications, you might write each one on an index card, including both the generic and trade name, dosage, administration route, and adverse effects. Be sure to document your patient teaching and the patient's response in his medical record. (See *Patient-teaching checklist: Angina pectoris.*)

Discharge planning

Discharge planning for the patient with angina should reinforce your patient teaching. And, like patient teaching, it should begin at the very beginning of the patient's hospitalization. For example, if the patient needs help from social services or needs other home care services, make referrals as soon as his diagnosis is made. Also be sure to include family members in discharge planning. They should know what medications the patient's taking and why he's taking them, and at least one close family member should be encouraged to take a class in cardiopulmonary resuscitation.

When doing discharge planning, consider the patient's response to his treatment. If he feels his care is too complicated, he may become noncompliant and need repeated hospitalizations to control his angina. So make every effort to help him understand his medication schedule and life-style changes before discharge.

Patients with angina, including those with successful physical recovery, commonly experience such psychological problems as anxiety, depression, denial, and dependence. Anxiety and depression may keep them from making adequate life-style adjustments—for example, they may fear resuming sexual intercourse or stop social activities.

Depression, the most common emotional problem during recovery, can imitate physical illness by causing fatigue, insomnia, memory loss, headache, and vague chest pain. Overprotective families can add to the problem. Although most patients recover from depression, some end up invalids, afraid to return to their former life-styles, retiring early, and withdrawing from social life.

How can you help patients avoid or overcome psychosocial complications? Education, counseling, and physical activity are the keys. Rehabilitation for angina patients means altering their life-style and regaining the capacity to meet life's demands. Your job is to provide the necessary skills, techniques, and knowledge.

Case study: Part 5

Recovering from a successful PTCA, Carl Neimann was in surprisingly good spirits and was anxious to return to his work. Because the angina hadn't recurred and the ECG showed no signs of myocardial ischemia, he was scheduled to be discharged. According to the discharge plan, Mr. Neimann was taught how to live with his condition, how to prevent or reduce the anginal episodes, how to follow the prescribed diet and drug therapy, and how to meet the recommended exercise requirements and life-style changes that would help halt the progression of the disease. Mr. Neimann agreed to continue the cardiac rehabilitation program as an outpatient. He also promised to stick with his low-sodium, low-cholesterol diet and to enter a quit smoking program.

Chapter 3
Myocardial infarction

Each year, about 1½ million people suffer acute myocardial infarction (AMI). This deadly cardiac crisis causes one of every four deaths in the United States, about 500,000 hospitalizations each year for confirmed AMI, and at least as many for suspected AMI. More than 60% of AMI deaths occur within the first hour after infarction, usually as the result of dysrhythmias (most often ventricular fibrillation); 10% of deaths occur during hospitalization and another 10% occur during the first year after AMI. The annual economic burden of myocardial infarction (MI) may run as high as $50 billion.

AMI can strike any patient in any unit—not just the cardiac care unit—at any time. So you must be ready to assess and intervene quickly, to anticipate your patient's needs or possible complications, and to provide nursing care that promotes both short- and long-term recovery. Providing such care challenges your nursing skills in many ways. The patient may or may not have complications. His treatment may range from standard therapies with oxygen, analgesics, and antiarrhythmic drugs to coronary bypass graft surgery. The patient and his family will probably need your help to overcome the anxiety that usually attends AMI. And he'll require careful discharge planning, especially now that so many AMI patients leave the hospital only 3 days after receiving thrombolytic therapy.

Case study: Part 1

"Nurse," said the patient, grimacing and clutching his chest, "I have a bad case of indigestion. I feel nauseated." Tom Ingold, a 32-year-old third baseman for a minor-league team, was embarrassed to be in the emergency department (ED) for what he thought was just a stomachache. But his fiancee insisted that he go, even though it meant he'd miss morning practice.

The ED triage nurse quickly assessed the man standing before her. His pale, diaphoretic skin, anxious expression, and chief complaint told her she didn't have a moment to waste. She wheeled Mr. Ingold into the cardiac monitoring treatment room, where she helped him undress and get settled in bed while taking his history. Then she administered oxygen via nasal cannula at 3 liters/minute and attached a cardiac monitor. The ECG showed sinus tachycardia with ST-segment elevation in lead II.

The ED doctor ordered an I.V. infusion of dextrose 5% in water (D_5W) at a keep-vein-open rate, a 12-lead ECG stat, blood work (including cardiac enzyme analysis), and a portable chest X-ray.

Causes and characteristics

MI is a condition of ischemia and injury that results from occlusion of one or more coronary arteries, usually related to coronary artery atherosclerosis. The resulting myocardial tissue destruction, caused by blocked myocardial blood supply, significantly alters cardiodynamics, decreasing cardiac output. Compensatory mechanisms intensify oxygen demand, destroying more myocardial tissue. The patient's prognosis depends on the extent of tissue involved, the tissue's remaining contractility, and the effectiveness of the tissue's inflammatory response. (See *How an AMI develops*.)

In patients with atherosclerosis, plaque narrows the blood vessel lumen of the coronary arterial tree, reducing the heart's blood supply; pieces of plaque can break off, blocking blood supply further. In such patients, thrombosis, coronary artery spasm, and platelet aggregation—either alone or in concert—can also cause AMI.

Thrombosis. Thrombosis usually acts as the main precipitating event in AMI by abruptly blocking blood flow to the heart. Thrombosis can result from rupture of atherosclerotic plaque, hemorrhage into the plaque, and intimal erosion over the fibrous cap. Plaque rupture favors thrombosis by allowing platelet aggregation at sites of denuded collagen, by stimulating release of tissue thromboplastin, and by mechanically obstructing the vascular lumen.

Coronary artery spasm. A result of atherosclerosis, coronary artery spasm seems to stimulate thrombosis and platelet

How an AMI develops

• Injury to the coronary artery's intimal lining increases endothelial cell membrane permeability. The arterial lumen narrows as platelets, white blood cells, fibrin, and lipids adhere to the injury site.
• Collateral circulation helps maintain myocardial perfusion distal to the obstruction.
• Stress creates a greater myocardial oxygen demand than collateral vessels can supply. Myocardial metabolism, normally aerobic, shifts to anaerobic, producing lactic acid, which stimulates pain receptors.
• Oxygen deficit causes myocardial cell death, leading to decreased contractility, stroke volume, and blood pressure. Hypotension stimulates baroreceptors, triggering release of epinephrine and norepinephrine. These catecholamines boost the heart rate and peripheral vasoconstriction, intensifying myocardial oxygen demand.
• Damaged cell membranes in the infarcted area spill their contents into the systemic vascular circulation.

aggregation. According to some experts, thrombi release vaso-constrictors that trigger sustained coronary artery spasm, preventing inflow and favoring more thrombosis.

Platelet aggregation. Blood flow turbulence at a stenotic area favors platelet adhesion and aggregation. Tissue damage also triggers platelet aggregation as part of the normal response to injury. When that response occurs in an injured vessel, the resulting platelet clump can block blood flow, causing ischemia and tissue necrosis.

In patients without atherosclerosis, causes of MI include coronary artery embolization, congenital abnormalities, inflammatory processes, viral infections, and cocaine abuse (see *Non-atherosclerotic causes of AMI*). Cocaine abuse can also cause AMI by increasing heart rate and blood pressure; by diminishing coronary artery blood flow, either through vasospasm or thrombosis; and, with high cocaine doses, by damaging heart muscle directly.

Predisposing factors

Experts have identified severe exertion, emotional stress, and trauma as factors that seem clearly linked to MI.

Severe exertion. Often coupled with fatigue and emotional stress, severe exertion may trigger an MI by increasing myocardial oxygen consumption while narrowing coronary arteries. An AMI that follows exertion seems more common among patients with no history of angina.

Emotional stress. Studies reveal that upsetting life events commonly precede and may trigger an AMI.

Trauma. Severe trauma may trigger an MI through myocardial contusion, hemorrhage, or coronary artery damage.

MIs appear to follow a circadian pattern, occurring most commonly between 6 a.m. and noon, with peak incidence between 10 a.m. and 11 a.m. This circadian pattern may be linked to higher plasma levels of catecholamines and cortisol, and to platelet aggregation, which peak in the early morning hours.

Other factors. The following factors may also precipitate AMI: surgical procedures that cause acute blood loss, neurologic disturbances (such as transient ischemic attacks or cerebrovas-

Nonatherosclerotic causes of AMI

Arteritis
• Luetic lesions
• Granulomatous lesions (Takayasu's disease)
• Polyarteritis nodosa
• Mucocutaneous lymph node (Kawasaki) syndrome
• Disseminated lupus erythematosus
• Rheumatoid arthritis
• Ankylosing spondylitis

Trauma to coronary arteries
• Laceration
• Thrombosis
• Iatrogenic injury

Coronary mural thickening
• Mucopolysaccharidosis (Hurler syndrome)
• Homocystinuria
• Fabry's disease
• Amyloidosis
• Juvenile intimal sclerosis (idiopathic arterial calcification of infancy)
• Intimal hyperplasia associated with contraceptive use or the postpartum period
• Pseudoxanthoma elasticum
• Radiation-induced coronary fibrosis

Luminal narrowing by other mechanisms
• Coronary artery spasm (Prinzmetal's angina with normal coronary arteries)
• Spasm after nitroglycerin withdrawal
• Dissection of the aorta
• Dissection of the coronary artery
• Mucocutaneous lymph node (Kawasaki) syndrome

Coronary emboli
• Infective endocarditis
• Mitral valve prolapse
• Mural thrombus from left atrium or left ventricle
• Prosthetic valve embolus
• Cardiac myxoma

Cardiopulmonary bypass graft surgery and coronary arteriography
• Paradoxical embolus
• Papillary fibroelastoma of the aortic valve—fixed embolus

Congenital anomalies
• Left coronary from pulmonary artery

• Left coronary artery from anterior sinus of Valsalva
• Coronary arteriovenous and arteriocameral fistulas
• Coronary artery aneurysm

Disproportion of myocardial oxygen supply and demand
• Aortic stenosis (all forms)
• Incomplete differentiation of aortic valve
• Aortic insufficiency
• Carbon monoxide poisoning
• Thyrotoxicosis
• Prolonged hypotension

Hematologic abnormalities
• Polycythemia vera
• Thrombocytosis
• Disseminated intravascular coagulation
• Hypercoagulability
• Thrombocytopenic purpura

Miscellaneous causes
• Cocaine abuse
• Myocardial contusion

cular accidents [CVAs]), respiratory infections, hypoxemia, pulmonary embolism, hypoglycemia, ergot alkaloid poisoning, serum sickness, allergy, and wasp stings. In patients with Prinzmetal's angina, AMI may result from recurring coronary artery spasm.

Pathophysiology
Infarction usually develops distal to a totally occluded coronary artery. Necrosis begins in the subendocardium and extends to-

ward the epicardium. According to experts, the extent of necrosis depends on the duration of ischemia, which must last from 25 minutes to several hours to kill myocardial cells. It also depends on how quickly the occlusion developed; which artery is occluded and how much myocardial tissue is supplied by that artery; the amount of collateral flow available to ischemic cells; and the presence, site, and severity of any coronary artery spasm.

Myocardial changes. Within 6 hours after the onset of MI, the affected myocardium appears pale, bluish, and slightly swollen. Within 18 to 36 hours, it appears tan or reddish purple, with a serofibrinous exudate on the epicardium in transmural infarcts. After 48 hours, it turns gray. Neutrophilic infiltration creates fine yellow lines that spread throughout the infarct.

During the next 8 to 10 days, the infarcted cardiac wall becomes thinner as mononuclear cells remove necrotic tissue. A cross-section of the infarct looks yellow with a surrounding band of reddish purple granulation tissue that spreads through the necrotic tissue by 3 to 4 weeks. Over the next 2 to 3 months, the infarcted area acquires a gelatinous, ground-glass, gray appearance and eventually changes into a shrunken scar that slowly whitens. The endocardium below the infarct becomes thicker, gray, and opaque.

Psychophysiologic responses. During AMI, the release of catecholamines causes psychological, mechanical, electrical, and metabolic changes. The primary psychological changes (anxiety, loss of control, and fear of death) drive the other psychophysiologic factors. The resulting mechanical changes (vasoconstriction and increased contractility) raise blood pressure and increase cardiac output and myocardial oxygen consumption. Electrical changes accelerate conduction velocity and heart rate. Metabolic changes (fuel mobilization due to glycogenesis and lipolysis; inhibition of insulin release; and changing use of myocardial substrate) raise levels of serum glucose and free fatty acids. Together, these four types of psychophysiologic responses can undermine the patient's ability to cope with his illness and augment damage to the ischemic myocardium.

Types of infarcts. Myocardial infarcts are commonly classified as transmural or nontransmural. Usually identified by location in the left ventricle (anterior, lateral, inferior, or posterior), transmural infarcts cause necrosis through the full thickness of the ventricular wall. Because such infarcts usually produce Q waves on the ECG, they are also known as Q-wave infarcts.

Nontransmural infarcts arise in the superficial regions of the ventricular inner lining and have three subclassifications: subendocardial (producing necrosis on the subendocardial surface); subepicardial (producing necrosis on the epicardial layer); and intramural (producing necrosis in isolated sections of the myocardium). Seldom producing Q waves, they are often known as non-Q-wave infarcts.

Once considered less serious, nontransmural infarcts are now known to cause as much damage as transmural infarcts or more. Both types require aggressive treatment, as appropriate for the patient's clinical signs and symptoms.

Site of infarction. The site of coronary artery occlusion determines the site of infarction (see *Coronary arteries and infarction sites,* page 94). Although most MIs affect the left ventricle and interventricular septum, about one-third to two-thirds of patients with an inferior infarct also show some right ventricle involvement. Autopsies reveal isolated right ventricular infarction in 3% to 5% of MI patients, usually in those with chronic lung disease and right ventricular hypertrophy. However, right ventricular infarction occurs less commonly than atheroma frequency would predict, possibly because of lower oxygen demands in the right ventricle and because the right ventricle has a large collateral system and a thin wall that allows this chamber to derive some nutrition from the blood it contains.

Most transmural infarcts occur distal to a totally occluded coronary artery. Anterior infarcts tend to be larger and cause a greater degree of left ventricular impairment than inferior infarcts. Atrial infarction, which may appear with left ventricular infarction, can rupture the atrial wall. More common in the right than the left side, this infarction occurs more commonly in the atrial appendages than in the lateral or posterior atrial walls. Right atrial infarction commonly appears with obstructive sinus node artery disease and atrial dysrhythmias. (See *Right ventricular and atrial MI,* page 95.)

Coronary arteries and infarction sites

The primary area of infarction and the resulting structural damage will depend on which of the major coronary arteries are occluded and how well the collateral circulation perfuses the affected area.

Development of collateral circulation is stimulated by coronary artery disease, possibly through the release of vasodilators. It is particularly well developed in patients with 75% or more reduction in the coronary lumen. Nearly 40% of AMI patients develop collateral circulation during recovery.

Collateral circulation appears to reduce myocardial necrosis in patients with coronary occlusion. In patients with extensive collateral vessel development, the collateral vessels can perfuse the area when total occlusion is present as long as no stress is placed on the heart.

The chart below correlates the major areas and structures supplied by the coronary arteries with the areas of infarction associated with obstruction of these arteries.

ANTERIOR VIEW

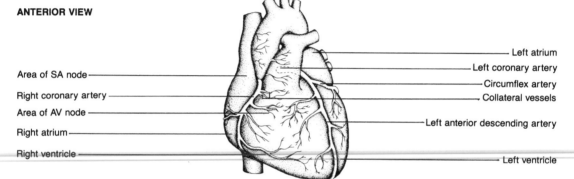

Area of SA node
Right coronary artery
Area of AV node
Right atrium
Right ventricle

Left atrium
Left coronary artery
Circumflex artery
Collateral vessels
Left anterior descending artery
Left ventricle

Coronary artery	Major areas and structures supplied	Primary area of infarction
Right coronary	Sinoatrial (SA) node (55%) Atrioventricular (AV) node (90%) Bundle of His Right atrium and right ventricle Inferior surface of left ventricle Posterior one-third of septum Posteroinferior division of left bundle	Inferior wall Inferoposterior wall Right ventricle
Left main	Massive left ventricular area	Left ventricle
Left anterior descending	Anterior wall of left ventricle Anterior two-thirds of septum Bundle of His Right bundle branch Anterosuperior division of left bundle branch Posteroinferior division of left bundle branch	Anterior wall Septal wall Anterolateral wall Inferoapical wall Apical wall
Left circumflex	SA node (45%) AV node (10%) Inferior surface of left ventricle Lateral wall of left ventricle Left atrium Posteroinferior division of left bundle branch	Lateral wall Inferolateral wall Posterior wall Inferoposterior wall

Signs and symptoms

AMI typically produces characteristic signs and symptoms that clearly suggest its presence even before confirmation by laboratory tests.

Pain. About 80% of AMI patients experience chest pain, which probably arises from nerve endings in the ischemic or injured myocardium. Referred pain may result from the spatial and temporal excitation patterns of afferent sympathetic nerves and vagal afferent fibers.

In most patients with MI, pain is severe and sometimes intolerable. Unlike anginal pain, which lasts for only 3 to 5 minutes, MI pain usually lasts for more than 30 minutes. It is often described as constricting, crushing, oppressing, compressing, choking, or viselike; less often, as stabbing, knifelike, boring, or burning. The acute pain can be relieved by opiates (particularly morphine), but a soreness, pressure, or dull ache may persist for several hours or longer despite intensive analgesic treatment.

Usually retrosternal, MI pain commonly spreads to both sides of the anterior chest, although it favors the left side. Pain can radiate down the ulnar side of the left arm and produce a tingling sensation in the left wrist, hand, and fingers. Some patients with substernal or precordial pain report only a dull ache or numbness of the wrists. Others report pain in the shoulders, arms, neck, jaw, and intrascapular area, again favoring the left side.

In some patients, MI pain may begin in the epigastrium and mimic various abdominal disorders. Commonly, the patient may think he has indigestion and treat himself with antacids.

Associated symptoms. In approximately half of MI patients, particularly those with inferior MI, the acute phase of MI is associated with nausea and vomiting. In a few, chest pain occurs with diarrhea or a violent urge to evacuate the bowels. Many patients experience profound weakness, dizziness, palpitations, cold perspiration, and a sense of impending doom. A few patients with inferior MI report intractable hiccups. Elderly patients commonly experience chest tightness, overwhelming weakness, diaphoresis, vomiting, and diarrhea.

Right ventricular and atrial MI

Right ventricular MI can arise independently but is usually associated with an inferior or posterior left ventricular MI, because the right coronary artery and its posterior descending branch perfuse these areas.

Suspect right ventricular MI when your patient shows signs and symptoms of unexplained right ventricular failure: neck vein distention, increased right atrial pressure, or right ventricular S_3 or S_4. Hemodynamic pressures (increased CVP with low pulmonary artery pressures) and radionuclide imaging may aid diagnosis. The 12-lead ECG rarely diagnoses right ventricular infarction because its leads orient to the left ventricle.

In caring for a patient with right ventricular MI, administer fluids first, as ordered, to maintain or improve left ventricular filling and optimize cardiac output. Avoid diuretics, which reduce right ventricular filling pressures by decreasing circulating blood volume.

Atrial MI may occur with left ventricular MI or obstructive disease of the sinus node artery. Commonly accompanied by atrial dysrhythmias, an atrial MI usually occurs on the right side, in the atrial appendages. An atrial MI can result in atrial wall rupture.

ECG evidence of an atrial MI includes depressed or elevated PR intervals, altered P-wave configurations, and ectopic atrial rhythms, such as atrial fibrillation, atrial flutter, or wandering pacemaker.

Treatment of right ventricular and atrial MI focuses on relieving symptoms and preventing complications.

Case study: Part 2

Tom Ingold's pain began suddenly at breakfast 2 hours before he came to the ED. His history revealed that he has been a one-pack-per-day smoker for the past 15 years, eats a diet high in cholesterol, and has a family history of coronary artery disease—his father died 3 years ago with an MI. He has no known history of coronary disease, is moderately overweight, takes no medications, and has no allergies.

During her assessment, the nurse found Mr. Ingold in acute distress, complaining of a crushing pain and nausea. His color was gray and ashen and he was diaphoretic. His blood pressure was 146/90 mm Hg, his pulse rate was 114 beats/minute and irregular, and his respiratory rate was 20 breaths/minute. Chest auscultation revealed muffled heart sounds, S_4, and normal breath sounds. The cardiac monitor showed sinus tachycardia. The ST-segment elevation in leads II, III, and aV_F confirmed the ED doctor's suspicion that Mr. Ingold was having an MI.

The nurse sensed that Mr. Ingold was extremely upset about his admission to the ED. He insisted that he was there only because his fiancee is such a worrier and insisted that he come. He stated that if it were up to him, he would not have come. After all, he had relieved similar episodes in the past with nothing more than an antacid. But he did admit that past episodes were less intense than this one. When speaking to Mr. Ingold's fiancee, the nurse found out that their wedding was scheduled in 3 weeks.

Assessment and diagnosis

Assessment findings vary with the location and severity of the infarct. But MI usually produces an obvious condition of acutely distressing illness, severely abnormal findings on physical examination, and confirming abnormalities in the results of various diagnostic tests.

The patient looks acutely ill and displays severe discomfort. His skin appears normal or gray and ashen, and feels moist, warm, or cool. The patient may clutch his chest and appear anxious, restless, or apprehensive.

Physical examination

The patient with MI shows abnormal vital signs, abnormal heart and breath sounds, and neck vein distention.

Vital signs. About 40% of patients with anterior infarction and 25% of those with inferior infarction show signs of *sym-*

pathetic stimulation (elevated blood pressure and rapid and irregular heart rate). Such sympathetic overactivity may result from pain, anxiety, or stimulation by substances released from infarcted cells. Such patients show an elevated respiratory rate related to pain and anxiety. When these factors return to normal, the respiratory rate should return to normal. Ventricular failure keeps the respiratory rate high.

About 30% of patients with anterior infarction and 65% of those with inferior infarction show *parasympathetic overactivity* (bradycardia and hypotension). Administration of atropine and fluids will reverse such hypotension.

In AMI patients who appear normotensive with a rapid and regular pulse rate (sinus tachycardia at 100 to 110 beats/minute), you may see a small decline in systolic pressure and a rise in diastolic pressure resulting from reduced stroke volume accompanying tachycardia. Patients in cardiogenic shock show low systolic pressure (less than 90 mm Hg), but low blood pressure doesn't always mean shock. Patients with inferior infarction may have low systolic pressure without peripheral manifestations of hypoperfusion.

About 24 to 48 hours after infarction, the patient may develop a fever as a nonspecific response to tissue necrosis. Such fever usually resolves by the 7th or 8th day after infarction.

Heart sounds. Auscultation reveals abnormal heart sounds. Reduced ventricular contractility may muffle heart sounds, which will return to normal as healing occurs. An S_4 sound usually means ischemic heart disease; it indicates decreased left ventricular compliance and reflects elevations in left ventricular end-diastolic pressure. An S_3 may occur in patients with extensive infarctions or with transmural anterior infarcts. Remember, these patients have a greater risk of death in the immediate postinfarction period. Systolic murmurs, resulting from acute mitral regurgitation, may occur in patients with papillary muscle dysfunction. A pericardial friction rub is audible in about 20% of AMI patients. Chest palpation may reveal a precordial pulse.

Breath sounds. Auscultation may reveal moist bibasilar crackles in AMI patients with left ventricular failure. In other AMI patients, breath sounds may be normal.

Neck veins. The height and contour of the jugular venous pulse reflect right atrial and right ventricular diastolic pressures.

Recognizing atypical onset of AMI

About 20% to 60% of nonfatal AMIs pass unnoticed until routine ECG or postmortem studies reveal them. They occur most commonly in patients without previous angina and in those who are diabetic or hypertensive. Half of these AMIs are truly silent; the patient recalls no symptoms whatsoever. The rest cause symptoms that the patient recognizes when asked the right questions.

Atypical onset of AMI may include congestive heart failure; angina without a severe attack; atypical pain location; central nervous system effects, resembling stroke, that follow reduced cardiac output in a patient with cerebral arteriosclerosis; apprehension and nervousness; sudden mania or psychosis; syncope; overwhelming weakness; acute indigestion; and peripheral embolism.

In AMI patients, the usually normal (or only slightly elevated) diastolic pressures make the jugular venous pulse appear normal. But right ventricular infarction may cause jugular venous distention. Cardiogenic shock commonly elevates jugular venous pressure. Hypovolemia may depress left ventricular performance in patients with flat neck veins.

Diagnostic tests and results

In most patients with AMI, the patient's signs and symptoms and history suggest the diagnosis; the 12-lead ECG and cardiac enzyme analysis usually confirm it. (See *AMI: Diagnostic profile*, page 103.) Because ventricular fibrillation is 15 times more likely during the first hour after onset of AMI symptoms than during the next 12 hours, treatment should not await diagnostic test confirmation. Suspected AMI requires quick actions to prevent sudden death. (See *Recognizing atypical onset of AMI*, at left, and *12-lead ECG: A closer look*.)

12-lead ECG. Abnormal Q waves and characteristic progression of ST-segment and T-wave changes on the ECG definitely identify a transmural AMI. (See *Telltale ECG findings: The three I's of transmural MI*, page 101.) ST-segment elevation appears first, followed by T-wave inversion with the appearance of Q waves, which can show up from several days to a week after infarction. However, many factors can influence the accuracy of the ECG. The extent of injury, the age and location of the infarct, conduction defects, previous infarcts or acute pericarditis, electrolyte changes, and cardioactive drugs can all interfere with the ECG's ability to diagnose and locate the infarct. (See *Identifying the site of MI*, page 102.)

Cardiac enzyme analysis. Because AMI damages cell membranes, releasing enzymes and isoenzymes (molecularly distinct subtypes) into the plasma, measuring them is an important part of the diagnostic workup for AMI. Enzyme molecular size, regional myocardial blood flow, lymph flow, and the concentration gradient among interstitial fluid, lymph, and blood all influence the blood level of the enzymes. Cardiac enzyme tests typically measure the following enzymes.

Creatine phosphokinase (CPK), an enzyme that influences energy production and storage, occurs in three forms: CPK-MB

12-lead ECG: A closer look

The 12-lead ECG shows the heart's electrical activity from 12 different angles. The chart belows lists each lead with corresponding direction of electrical potential and view of the heart. The normal ECG waveforms for each of the 12 leads appear at right.

Views of the heart (left ventricle) reflected on the 12-lead ECG	Leads	Direction of electrical potential	View of heart	Waveform
	Standard limb leads (bipolar)			
	I	Between left arm (positive) and right arm (negative)	Lateral wall	
	II	Between left leg (positive) and right arm (negative)	Inferior wall	
	III	Between left leg (positive) and left arm (negative)	Inferior wall	
	Augmented limb leads (unipolar)			
	aV$_R$	Right arm to heart	Provides no specific view	
	aV$_L$	Left arm to heart	Lateral wall	
	aV$_F$	Left foot to heart	Inferior wall	
	Precordial, or chest, leads (unipolar)			
	V$_1$	Fourth intercostal space, right sternal border, to heart	Anteroseptal wall	
	V$_2$	Fourth intercostal space, left sternal border, to heart	Anteroseptal wall	
	V$_3$	Midway between V$_2$ and V$_4$ to heart	Anterior wall	

(continued)

12-lead ECG: A closer look (continued)

Views of the heart (left ventricle) reflected on the 12-lead ECG	Leads	Direction of electrical potential	View of heart	Waveform
	Precordial, or chest, leads (unipolar)			
	V₄	Fifth intercostal space, midclavicular line, to heart	Anterior wall	V₄
	V₅	Fifth intercostal space, anterior axillary line, to heart	Lateral wall	V₅
	V₆	Fifth intercostal space, midaxillary line, to heart	Lateral wall	V₆

(in the heart), CPK-BB (in the brain), and CPK-MM (in skeletal muscle). Elevated CPK-MB levels most reliably indicate AMI. Levels rise about 4 to 8 hours after infarction and peak at 18 to 24 hours. CPK-MB levels may peak earlier—around 12 hours after infarction—in patients who've undergone reperfusion and in those with early spontaneous thrombolysis. Elevated CPK-MB levels may persist for 72 hours but usually return to normal 3 to 4 days after infarction. (Normal CPK-MB levels range from undetectable to 7 units/liter. Total CPK values range from 23 to 99 units/liter in men and from 15 to 57 units/liter in women.) Elevated total CPK levels may also result from skeletal muscle disease or trauma, defibrillation, acute alcohol intoxication, diabetes, vigorous exercise, seizures, I.M. injections, pulmonary embolism, or central nervous system disorders.

Lactic dehydrogenase (LDH), which catalyzes the conversion of lactate to pyruvate, can help confirm AMI a day or more after infarction, when LDH levels begin to rise. LDH levels peak in 3 to 6 days and return to normal in 8 to 14 days. (Normal LDH values range from 48 to 115 units/liter.)

LDH includes five organ-specific isoenzymes. LDH₁ activity usually increases before total LDH levels rise—around 8 to 24

Telltale ECG findings: The three I's of transmural MI

Ischemia, injury, and infarction produce characteristic ECG changes, as explained below.

• Ischemia temporarily interrupts blood supply to myocardial tissue but usually doesn't cause cell death.

ECG changes: T-wave inversion resulting from altered tissue repolarization. Depressed ST segment may also be seen. (See waveform at top right.)

• Injury results from prolonged blood supply interruption, causing further cell injury.

ECG changes: elevated ST segment resulting from altered depolarization. Consider an elevation greater than 1 mm significant. (See middle waveform.)

• Infarction results when failure of perfusion causes myocardial cell death (necrosis).

ECG changes: pathologic Q wave (or QS) resulting from abnormal depolarization or from scar tissue that can't depolarize. Look for Q-wave duration of 0.04 second or more or an amplitude measuring at least a third of the QRS complex.

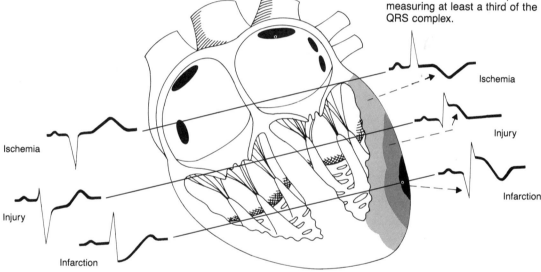

Ischemia

Injury

Infarction

Ischemia

Injury

Infarction

CHANGES ON THE OPPOSITE SIDE (RECIPROCAL CHANGES)

CHANGES ON THE DAMAGED SIDE

hours after infarction. More than 95% of AMI patients show elevations in LDH levels and in the ratio of LDH_1 to total LDH. The ratio of LDH_1 to LDH_2 also rises after infarction. Normally, LDH_2 levels exceed LDH_1 levels; however, about 24 to 48 hours after MI, this pattern reverses. Hemolytic anemia, hemolysis, renal infarction, hyperthyroidism, and stomach carcinoma can also reverse the pattern of LDH levels.

Identifying the site of MI

Use this chart to identify the location of an MI. But remember, myocardial damage may spread to other areas. *Note:* ECG changes occurring in the acute phase of a transmural MI include a pathologic Q wave, ST-segment elevation, and T-wave inversion.

Type of infarction	Affected wall	Leads	Possible ECG changes	Possible coronary artery involved	Possible reciprocal changes
Transmural	Inferior (diaphragmatic)	II, III, aV$_F$	Q, ST, T	Right coronary artery	I, aV$_L$
	Lateral	I, aV$_L$, V$_5$, V$_6$	Q, ST, T	Circumflex, branch of left anterior descending artery	V$_1$, V$_3$
	Anterior	V$_1$, V$_2$, V$_3$, V$_4$, I, aV$_L$	Q, ST, T, loss of R-wave progression	Left coronary artery	II, III, aV$_F$
	Posterior	V$_1$, V$_2$	R greater than S, ST depression, elevated T wave (mirror change); Q wave in V$_6$ may also be seen	Right coronary artery, circumflex	
	Apical	V$_3$, V$_4$, V$_5$, V$_6$	Q, ST, T, loss of R-wave progression		
	Anterolateral	I, aV$_L$, V$_4$, V$_5$, V$_6$	Q, ST, T	Left anterior descending artery, circumflex	II, III, aV$_F$
	Anteroseptal	V$_1$, V$_2$, V$_3$	Q, ST, T, loss of septal R wave in V$_1$	Left anterior descending artery	
Non-transmural	Subendocardial	Any of the above	ST elevation or depression, T for more than 3 days with enzyme changes		
Right ventricular		II, III, aV$_F$	Q waves; ST in right precordial leads; V$_1$, V$_3$, R		
Atrial			Depression or elevation of the PQ segment, alterations in P-wave contour, and abnormal atrial rhythms, including atrial flutter, atrial fibrillation, wandering atrial pacemaker, and AV nodal rhythm.		

The *hydroxybutyric dehydrogenase* (HBD) test measures LDH_2 indirectly. This test, which reflects LDH_1 activity, is simpler and easier to perform than an LDH enzyme fractionation study but is less reliable distinguishing between myocardial and liver damage. (Normal HBD values range from 114 to 290 units/ml. The ratio of LDH to HBD varies from 1:2 to 1.6:1.) Conditions other than AMI that can elevate total LDH levels include anemia, leukemia, liver disease, hepatic congestion, renal disease, neoplasms, pulmonary embolism, myocarditis, skeletal muscle disease, and shock. Hemolysis can also raise LDH levels, so careful collection of the blood specimen is necessary for accurate results.

Aspartate aminotransferase (AST), formerly called SGOT, is an enzyme that concentrates in the heart, liver, skeletal muscle, pancreas, kidneys, and lungs. AST concentration exceeds the normal range approximately 8 to 12 hours after the onset of chest pain, peaks 18 to 36 hours later, and returns to normal within 3 to 4 days. Because many other disorders also elevate AST levels (liver disease, skeletal muscle disease, I.M. injection shock, pericarditis, and pulmonary embolism), many hospitals no longer perform this least sensitive and least specific of the cardiac enzyme tests. (See *Serum enzyme level changes after transmural MI,* page 104.)

Radionuclide studies. These scanning tests help determine the extent of myocardial damage.

Thallium imaging (also known as cold-spot imaging) distinguishes between normal and ischemic or infarcted tissue. Active transport carries the thallium ion into normal cells. But ischemic and infarcted cells, which won't pick up thallium, show up as cold spots on the scan. After an ischemic episode, previously ischemic cells can take up thallium, but infarcted cells remain abnormal.

Thallium imaging proves most useful during treadmill testing by revealing the ischemic area in a patient who exercises to the point of myocardial ischemia. A follow-up scan 3 to 4 hours later, when the ischemic areas have recovered, should show normal thallium uptake.

Technetium pyrophosphate (PYP) scanning (also known as hot-spot imaging and myocardial imaging) helps detect the size, location, and approximate age of an MI that occurred within 7 to 10 days. Infarcted and ischemic cells take up the test isotope,

AMI: Diagnostic profile

12-lead ECG
• T-wave inversion
• ST-segment elevation
• pathologic Q wave in the leads facing the area of myocardial damage

Cardiac enzyme analysis
• CPK elevation within 4 to 8 hours after MI onset
• CPK-MB elevation within 4 to 8 hours after MI onset
• LDH elevation within 24 to 48 hours after MI onset
• LDH_1 elevation within 8 to 24 hours after MI onset
• LDH_1/LDH_2 ratio>1 within 24 to 48 hours after MI onset
• AST (SGOT) elevation within 8 to 12 hours after MI onset

Serum enzyme level changes after transmural MI

The graph below shows how serum enzyme levels may change after a transmural MI.

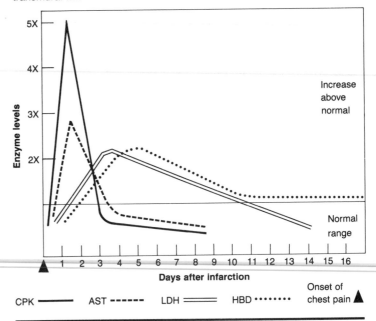

whereas normal cells don't. The results are graded as four degrees of uptake: A diffuse uptake, graded +1 or +2, appears with subendocardial infarction or severe angina pectoris; the more serious +3 and +4 grades indicate transmural infarction. This scan will not detect an infarct that's smaller than 3 g and sometimes will fail to show subendocardial infarctions; it may show old infarcts as hot spots, falsely indicating a new infarction. (See *Comparing hot-spot and cold-spot imaging.*)

PYP scanning must be timed carefully because it remains negative for the first 12 hours after AMI. Uptake peaks around 36 hours and begins to fade at 4 days. This scan localizes all types of infarcts because it includes views from three positions—anterior, left anterior oblique, and lateral; it may be used when standard enzyme analyses and ECGs fail to confirm AMI. This test proves most useful in patients with complete left bundle

Comparing hot-spot and cold-spot imaging

The information below tells how these diagnostic tests for MI differ.

Test	Purpose	Reliability	Disadvantages
Technetium pyrophosphate scanning (hot-spot imaging)	• To detect irreversibly infarcted myocardium • To identify MI type, location, and size • To help confirm MI when the ECG can't; the patient has a complete left bundle branch block; enzyme tests prove unreliable (for example, after cardiac surgery); or pacemaker activity distorts MI changes	This test can detect MI 12 hours to 6 days later. Peak uptake occurs after about 36 hours. Scan is usually negative 7 to 10 days after MI.	Other abnormal conditions may appear as hot spots (for example, ventricular aneurysms, tumors, or other myocardial damage).
Thallium scanning (cold-spot imaging)	• To differentiate ischemic from normal or infarcted myocardium, especially when used in conjunction with treadmill testing • To evaluate blood flow through coronary arteries • To identify high-risk MI patients	This test can detect MI in its first few hours.	Results are less specific and harder to interpret. Poorly perfused areas, electrodes, breast implants, and such conditions as sarcoidosis, cardiac contusion, and coronary spasm appear as cold spots. Tests can't distinguish old from new MIs.

branch block, an old MI on the ECG, or pacemaker activity that distorts infarction changes. It also helps locate right ventricular infarction, assess cardiac trauma after a chest injury, and determine whether an infarction has occurred after cardiac resuscitation.

Multiple-gated acquisition (MUGA) scanning, also called radionuclide ventriculography, assesses cardiac function (ejection fraction), analyzes wall motion abnormalities in infarcted tissue, and helps detect ventricular aneurysms. MUGA scanning shows lower radionuclide ejection fractions in anterior infarctions than in inferior infarctions.

Magnetic resonance imaging (MRI) localizes and sizes the infarcted area, assesses ischemia severity, and may even allow early MI detection. Safe and noninvasive, this increasingly useful tool may also assess tissue perfusion, ventricular chamber size, and segmental wall motion; pinpoint areas of endangered myocardium; and identify myocardial edema, fibrosis, wall thinning, hypertrophy, and the temporal transition from ischemia to infarction. The major disadvantage of MRI is that it may require moving the patient.

Positron emission tomography (PET) measures the extent of MI by assessing myocardial blood flow and metabolism. PET can detect both infarcted and ischemic areas.

Echocardiography. This test estimates the extent of damage, identifies wall motion abnormalities, and detects intracardiac thrombi. Two-dimensional echocardiograms help distinguish old from new infarcts. When done on the day of hospital admission, this test helps predict the patient's short-term clinical course.

Cardiac catheterization and angiography. This test visualizes occlusion in the coronary vessels. After an acute left ventricular infarction, it may reveal elevations in left ventricular end-diastolic pressure and volume and a reduction in the ejection fraction. Left ventriculography may reveal hypokinesia (reduced wall motion), akinesia (absent wall motion), or dyskinesia (paradoxical wall bulging during systole).

After right ventricular infarction, catheterization of the right and left ventricles may reveal increased right atrial pressure. In pure right ventricular infarctions, left-sided diastolic pressure and pulse pressure in the right ventricle and pulmonary artery may decrease.

Chest X-ray. Radiographic studies can't diagnose MI, but they may reveal other problems or complications, such as congestive heart failure, left ventricular failure, cardiomegaly, and ventricular aneurysm. Done on admission, chest X-rays establish a clinical baseline for evaluating the patient's progress and response to treatment.

Other laboratory tests. Laboratory studies that aid diagnosis include a complete blood count, including white blood cell (WBC) count and hematocrit, and an erythrocyte sedimentation rate (ESR). Hemodynamic monitoring may also be required, especially for the patient with complications.

The *WBC count* rises within about 2 hours after the onset of chest pain, in response to tissue necrosis or increased secretion of adrenal glucocorticoids. The WBC count usually peaks 2 to 4 days after MI (at between $12 \times 10^3/mm^3$ and $15 \times 10^3/mm^3$) and returns to normal a week later. The percentage of polymorphonuclear leukocytes also rises with MI, and the differential count shifts to band forms.

Hematocrit rises, reflecting hemoconcentration the first few days after MI.

The *ESR* may peak 4 or 5 days after MI and stay high for weeks. (Serum concentrations of copper and nickel parallel ESR elevations.)

Other laboratory tests may reveal elevated myoglobin levels in the blood and urine; hyperglycemia; and decreased serum zinc, iron, and magnesium levels.

Case study: Part 3

Mr. Ingold was given I.V. morphine to relieve his continuing chest pain and anxiety. Because the onset of chest pain began less than 6 hours ago, the doctor ordered alteplase, a thrombolytic agent, after determining that the patient had no contraindications to thrombolytic therapy. The nurse administered the first hour's dose of alteplase, then performed a 12-lead ECG. The results showed a decrease in the height of the elevated ST segment in leads II, III, and aV_F. Once Mr. Ingold's pain began to subside, he was transferred to the cardiac care unit (CCU) for continuing thrombolytic therapy and continuous cardiac monitoring for reperfusion dysrhythmias.

By the time Mr. Ingold arrived in the CCU, his pain was gone. He was already asking to get out of bed, go to the family waiting room, and smoke a cigarette. He told the admitting CCU nurse that he believed he had been right all along—it was only indigestion. The nurses agreed that an important factor in his cardiac rehabilitation program would be to get him to accept his medical diagnosis.

Over the next 2 days, Mr. Ingold continued to improve. The thrombolytic therapy was completed and his oxygen was discontinued. He remained pain-free and his continuous cardiac monitoring showed sinus tachycardia with occasional premature ventricular contractions (PVCs). By the third day, his PVCs had stopped and his heart rate and rhythm returned to normal sinus rhythm. He was transferred to the intermediate care unit.

Treatment options

Treatment focuses on relieving the patient's pain and anxiety and preventing further damage by improving tissue oxygenation, reducing myocardial oxygen consumption, and maintaining cardiac output. The urgency of this life-threatening condition requires that interventions be performed swiftly, but without alarming the patient. Remember, the patient's emotional condition can profoundly affect his treatment responses and the risk of complications.

Specific interventions depend on the patient's clinical signs and symptoms and on the presence of complications. The patient will probably enter a CCU for continuous ECG and hemodynamic monitoring. Initially, he'll need bed rest and an I.V. line (usually with D_5W to keep the vein open) for delivering medication.

Relieving pain and anxiety

AMI pain stimulates the sympathetic nervous system, producing potentially damaging effects: a rise in blood pressure; increased heart rate and contractility, which increase the myocardial work load and metabolic demands; and excessive catecholamine release, which increases ventricular irritability and potentiates dysrhythmias. To control pain and prevent sympathetic overactivity, treatment requires oxygen therapy; drug therapy with opiates, nitrates, or other drugs; and holistic care.

Oxygen therapy. Most AMI patients suffer hypoxemia from perfusion abnormalities, pulmonary congestion from left ventricular failure, and preexisting pulmonary disease, among other factors. These patients need supplemental oxygen (100% oxygen delivered by nasal cannula or mask at 2 to 4 liters/minute) for the first 24 to 48 hours, unless arterial blood gas analysis clearly shows that the patient is not hypoxemic.

Opiate analgesics. The analgesic of choice for relieving pain, morphine reduces anxiety, relieves restlessness, diminishes autonomic nervous activity, and reduces the heart's metabolic demands. Expect to administer an initial 4- to 8-mg dose of I.V. morphine sulfate, followed by 2- to 8-mg doses repeated at 5- to 15-minute intervals until pain stops or the patient shows signs of toxicity (hypotension, respiratory depression, or severe vomiting).

The patient who develops respiratory depression may need 0.1 mg to 0.2 mg of I.V. naloxone, which can be repeated if respiration doesn't improve in 15 minutes. The patient who experiences nausea and vomiting will need a phenothiazine antiemetic, such as promethazine, to prevent the circulatory stress of vomiting. The patient who is hypersensitive to morphine may receive 50- to 150-mg doses of I.V. meperidine. I.V. administration of these analgesics allows better absorption and prevents misleading elevation of serum enzyme levels, which may occur with I.M. injection.

Nitrates. The normotensive patient may receive nitrates to ease chest pain. Give a sublingual nitroglycerin tablet and watch for relief of pain or hemodynamic change. If all goes well, you can administer further nitrates, but be careful to monitor vital signs. Avoid long-acting nitrates in the early stages of AMI.

If the patient's chest pain wanes and waxes for a prolonged period, I.V. nitroglycerin may be indicated, but it requires careful monitoring of blood pressure. I.V. nitroglycerin causes vasodilatation, which decreases both preload and afterload, reducing myocardial oxygen consumption and demand. Such treatment may begin with a dose of 10 to 20 mcg/minute, increased by 5 mcg/minute every 3 to 5 minutes until pain stops. Excessive nitroglycerin will cause hypotension or severe headaches.

Use nitrates cautiously in patients with inferior wall infarction because even small doses may produce sudden hypotension and bradycardia. And watch patients with suspected right ventricular MI, who may be particularly sensitive to the vasodilatory effects of nitrates and may develop sudden hypotension from inadequate right ventricular filling.

Other drugs. Calcium channel blockers and beta-adrenergic blocking agents may also relieve pain. Beta-adrenergic blocking agents may limit infarct size and relieve pain by reducing ischemia. Because beta blockers improve heart rate and blood pressure, expect to administer them to patients with sinus tachycardia and hypertension. Many hospitals follow this protocol for administering beta blockers:
• Exclude patients with heart failure, hypotension, bradycardia, or heart block.
• Give metoprolol in three 5-mg boluses.
• Observe the patient for 2 to 5 minutes after each bolus.
• Give no more drug if the heart rate falls below 60 beats/minute or if systolic pressure falls below 100 mm Hg.
• If hemodynamic functions remain stable for 6 to 8 hours, begin oral metoprolol therapy with a 50-mg dose for 1 day.

• Advance the dose to 100 mg/day if the patient tolerates the lower dose.

Anxiolytic agents. To relieve severe anxiety and provide sedation, the patient may need diazepam or phenobarbital.

Holistic care. Consider that nonpharmacologic methods also help control pain. Teach relaxation techniques, meditation, imagery, and proper breathing. To take advantage of the placebo effect, tell your patient how much better his medications will make him feel. And frequently remind him of real time; pain can distort the patient's sense of time, making a few minutes seem like hours and magnifying his pain.

Preventing myocardial damage

Treatment to prevent further myocardial damage focuses on limiting the size of the infarct and reducing myocardial ischemia. Methods to achieve this include drug therapy and myocardial reperfusion techniques (percutaneous transluminal coronary angioplasty [PTCA], coronary artery bypass graft [CABG] surgery, and the intra-aortic balloon pump [IABP]).

Drug therapy. Thrombolytic agents, nitrates, beta-adrenergic blockers, calcium channel blockers, anticoagulants, aspirin, and glucose-insulin-potassium infusions help prevent further myocardial damage.

Thrombolytic agents dissolve thrombi or emboli, digesting their supporting fibrin network (see *Thrombolytic agents,* opposite page, and *How alteplase lyses a coronary thrombus,* page 113). Experts now believe that 90% of transmural MIs result from thrombosis. Thrombolytic therapy allows myocardial reperfusion, improves left ventricular function, and reduces mortality during the critical 4 to 6 hours after symptom onset. After 6 hours, irreversible necrosis makes thrombolytic therapy useless, except for the stuttering infarct, which waxes and wanes over several hours. (See *Problems of reperfusion,* page 114.)

Indications for thrombolytic therapy include:
• persistent anginal chest pain of at least 30 minutes' duration
• ST-segment elevation of at least 1 mm in two contiguous leads
• MI within the first 4 to 6 hours of symptom onset, except for stuttering infarct, which allows a longer time limit.

Thrombolytic agents

The timely use of thrombolytic agents after MI can restore myocardial perfusion and prevent extensive necrosis.

Drug	Indications, route, and dosage	Special considerations
alteplase (recombinant alteplase, tissue plasminogen activator) Activase	**Lysis of coronary artery thrombi after AMI** *Adults (over 65 kg):* 60-mg I.V. bolus in the first hour, with 6- to 10-mg I.V. bolus over first 1 to 2 minutes; then 20 mg/hour for another 2 hours for a total dose of 100 mg. *Adults (65 kg or less):* 1.25 mg/kg with 60% given in the first hour (10% of the first hour's dose given over the first 1 to 2 minutes).	• Expect to begin alteplase infusion within 6 hours after MI onset. • Expect to give heparin during or after alteplase as part of treatment regimen. • Prepare solution with sterile water for injection. Do not mix other drugs with alteplase. Use 18G needle for preparing solution—aim water stream at lyophilized cake. Expect a slight foaming to occur. Do not use in absence of vacuum. • You may dilute drug with normal saline solution or dextrose 5% in water (D_5W). Reconstituted or diluted solutions remain stable for up to 8 hours at room temperature. • Expect altered results in coagulation and fibrinolytic tests. Aprotinin (150 to 200 units/ml) in the blood sample may attenuate this effect. • Monitor for bleeding. Excessive I.V. dose can cause bleeding from punctures and recent wounds, and in GI, GU, and intracranial sites. Stop infusion if you observe signs or symptoms of bleeding. Avoid I.M. injections, venipuncture, and arterial puncture during therapy. Use pressure dressings or ice packs on recent puncture sites to prevent bleeding. If arterial puncture is necessary, choose a compressible site and apply pressure for 30 minutes afterward. Concomitant use of platelet antagonists (aspirin, dipyridamole) increases bleeding risk. • Monitor ECG for transient dysrhythmias (sinus bradycardia, ventricular tachycardia, accelerated idioventricular rhythm, ventricular premature depolarizations) associated with reperfusion after coronary thrombolysis. Keep antiarrhythmics at hand. • Monitor for urticaria, nausea, vomiting, hypersensitivity reactions, and fever.
anistreplase (APSAC) Eminase	**Lysis of coronary artery thrombi after AMI** *Adults:* 30 U I.V. over 2 to 5 minutes, administered by direct injection.	• Anistreplase is derived from human plasma. No cases of hepatitis or HIV infection have been reported to date. The manufacturing process is designed to purify the plasma used in the preparation of the drug. • Reconstitute the drug by slowly adding 5 ml of sterile water for injection. Direct the stream against the side of the vial, not at the drug itself. Gently roll the vial to mix the dry powder and water. In order to avoid excessive foaming, don't shake the vial. The reconstituted solution should be colorless to pale yellow. Inspect for particulate matter. • Do not mix the drug with other medications; do not dilute the solution after reconstitution. If the drug is not administered within 30 minutes of reconstituting, discard the vial.
streptokinase Kabikinase, Streptase	**Lysis of coronary artery thrombi after AMI** *Adults:* Intracoronary loading dose of 15,000 to 20,000 IU via coronary catheter, then a maintenance dose of 2,000 to 4,000 IU/minute for 60 minutes as an infusion; or 1,500,000 IU by I.V. infusion over 60 minutes.	• Streptokinase increases thrombin time, activated partial thromboplastin time (APTT), and prothrombin time (PT). It sometimes reduces hematocrit moderately. • Reconstitute vial with 5 ml normal saline solution, and further dilute to 45 ml; roll gently to mix. (Do not shake.) Use immediately; refrigerate remainder and discard after 24 hours. Store powder at room temperature.

(continued)

Thrombolytic agents *(continued)*

Drug	Indications, route, and dosage	Special considerations
streptokinase Kabikinase, Streptase *(continued)*		• Rate of I.V. infusion depends on thrombin time and streptokinase resistance; higher loading dose may be necessary in patients with recent streptococcal infection or streptokinase treatment. • Monitor for spontaneous bleeding, prolonged systemic hypocoagulability, bleeding or oozing from percutaneous trauma site; transient blood pressure lowering or elevation; reperfusion atrial or ventricular dysrhythmias; periorbital edema; bleeding gums; nausea; urticaria; ecchymosis; phlebitis at injection site; hypersensitivity; fever; musculoskeletal pain; minor breathing difficulty; bronchospasm; angioneurotic edema; and hematuria. • Do not stop therapy for minor allergic reactions treatable with antihistamines or corticosteroids. About one-third of patients show slight fever or chills, which you should treat with acetaminophen, not aspirin or other salicylates. • If minor bleeding proves controllable with pressure, do not lower dose, to make more plasminogen available for conversion to plasmin. • Streptokinase antibodies can persist for 6 months or longer after initial dose, so urokinase may be appropriate if further thrombolytic therapy becomes necessary. • Using streptokinase with anticoagulants may cause hemorrhage. You may need to stop anticoagulant therapy before starting streptokinase. • To prevent increased bleeding risk, don't use streptokinase with aspirin, indomethacin, phenylbutazone, or other platelet-affecting drugs. • Aminocaproic acid inhibits streptokinase-induced plasminogen activation.
urokinase Abbokinase, Abbokinase Open-Cath	**Coronary artery thrombosis** *Adults:* 6,000 IU/minute of urokinase intra-arterial D_5W via coronary artery catheter until artery opens maximally, usually within 15 to 30 minutes. Drug administration may prove necessary for up to 2 hours. Average total dose amounts to 500,000 IU.	• Urokinase increases thrombin time, APTT, and PT and sometimes reduces hematocrit levels. • To reconstitute I.V. solution, add 5.2 ml sterile water for injection; dilute further with normal saline injection or D_5W before infusion. Don't use bacteriostatic water, which contains preservatives. A catheter-clearing product is available in a Univial, containing 5,000 IU urokinase with the proper diluent. Discard unused portion; product contains no preservatives. • Monitor for spontaneous bleeding, prolonged systemic hypocoagulability, bleeding or oozing from percutaneous trauma sites, low hematocrit; transient lowering or elevation of blood pressure; reperfusion atrial or ventricular dysrhythmias; periorbital edema; bleeding gums; nausea; urticaria; ecchymosis; phlebitis at injection site; hypersensitivity; anaphylaxis; musculoskeletal pain; bronchospasm; and hematuria. • Concomitant use with anticoagulants may cause hemorrhage; stop anticoagulant and allow effects to diminish. You may need to reverse effects of oral anticoagulant therapy before starting urokinase. • To prevent bleeding, don't use urokinase with aspirin, indomethacin, phenylbutazone, or other drugs that affect platelet activity. • Aminocaproic acid inhibits urokinase-induced plasminogen activation.

How alteplase lyses a coronary thrombus

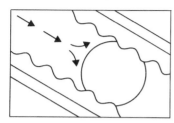

1. When a blood thrombus becomes lodged in a coronary artery, it cuts off the flow of blood to the heart, causing a myocardial infarction.

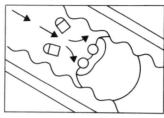

3. Alteplase speeds the action of plasminogen, accelerating its change into clot-dissolving plasmin and the thrombus disintegrates within 45 minutes.

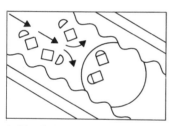

2. After being injected into a vein, the drug alteplase rushes to the thrombus to aid a natural substance, plasminogen, which begins the process that dissolves fibrin clots.

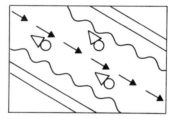

4. With blood flow restored, plasmin is inactivated by another natural substance, alpha$_2$-antiplasmin, preventing the breakup of vital blood components.

Key: ◖ = alteplase   □ = plasminogen   △ = alpha$_2$-antiplasmin   ○ = plasmin

Contraindications for thrombolytic therapy include:
• active bleeding
• history of CVA
• intracranial neoplasm, arteriovenous malformation, or aneurysm
• presence or history of bleeding diathesis
• recent prolonged cardiopulmonary resuscitation

Problems of reperfusion

Reperfusion may relieve ischemia by delivering oxygen to ischemic muscle; it may prevent cell death, depending on the severity and duration of ischemia. The earlier blood flow resumes, the better the recovery.

Collateral vessels may help restore left ventricular function after reperfusion. Their importance is probably greatest in patients whose reperfusion takes place more than an hour after MI.

Some studies suggest (but don't prove) that reperfusion, although necessary to salvage ischemic myocardium, may actually damage cells not irreversibly injured by:

• increasing cell swelling, which may interfere with blood flow at the microvascular level, leading to a hemorrhagic infarct. Thrombolytic reperfusion appears more likely to produce a hemorrhagic infarct than mechanical reperfusion; such hemorrhage doesn't appear to extend the original infarct.

• by allowing oxygen-derived free radicals, possibly with leukocyte mediation, to damage myocardial cells. Future improvements of reperfusion therapy may include drugs to scavenge free radicals and reduce leukocyte activation.

• by altering cardiac rhythm. Accelerated idioventricular rhythm and ventricular tachycardia commonly follow successful reperfusion. Patients with inferior infarcts show transient sinus bradycardia, often with hypotension. Premature ventricular contractions also commonly accompany reperfusion; but these dysrhythmias are common in MI and may not reflect the effect of reperfusion.

• recent surgery or trauma (intracranial or intraspinal within 2 months; major thoracicoabdominal or pelvic within 10 days)
• uncontrolled hypertension (180/110 mm Hg or higher).

Relative contraindications for thrombolytic therapy include:
• acute pericarditis
• age over 70
• diabetic hemorrhagic retinopathy or other hemorrhagic ophthalmic conditions
• gastrointestinal bleeding within previous 10 days (an absolute contraindication at some hospitals)
• high risk of intracavitary left ventricular thrombus, as in mitral stenosis with atrial fibrillation
• menstruation
• oral anticoagulant therapy
• pregnancy
• recent (within 10 days) obstetric delivery, organ biopsy, or puncture of noncompressible vessels
• subacute bacterial endocarditis.

Keep in mind that thrombolytic agents increase the risk of bleeding, both internally and superficially. To minimize this risk, limit venipunctures and patient handling and avoid I.M. injections. Obtain vascular access before beginning thrombolytic therapy, and then only in compressible sites. If arterial puncture proves necessary, choose an arm vessel accessible to manual compression. After arterial puncture, apply pressure for at least 30 minutes, then apply a pressure dressing and check the site frequently for bleeding. Also avoid venous or arterial catheter placement in noncompressible sites, such as the internal jugular or subclavian vein.

Thrombolysis will occur, if at all, within 30 to 45 minutes of treatment, producing sudden relief of chest pain, regression of ECG abnormalities, and the appearance of reperfusion dysrhythmias. Failure to reperfuse may mandate emergency coronary angiography and mechanical revascularization, which must begin within 4 to 6 hours of symptom onset.

Thrombolytic agents lyse thrombi but don't decrease blood vessel stenosis. Without intervention (such as PTCA or CABG) to open the vessel, it will probably reocclude.

Nitrates dilate blood vessels, decreasing oxygen consumption and demand by decreasing preload. Some studies suggest that I.V. nitroglycerin may limit infarct size. While the evidence remains inconclusive, I.V. nitroglycerin given a few hours after chest pain begins may lower the risk of congestive heart failure (CHF), infarct enlargement, and sudden death.

Expect to administer one or two 0.3-mg nitroglycerin tablets to patients who present with chest pain. However, patients with established AMI should not receive the drug routinely, and patients with hypotension should not receive I.V. nitroglycerin. I.V. nitroglycerin can help lower preload and afterload in patients with pump failure, pulmonary edema, or continuing ischemia.

Titrate the I.V. nitroglycerin dosage to prevent reflex tachycardia or systemic arterial hypotension (systolic pressure equal to or less than 95 mm Hg). With continuous infusion, watch for alcohol intoxication. (I.V. nitroglycerin solutions contain ethanol.) Also monitor for methemoglobinemia, which can cause lethargy and headache and reduce the blood's oxygen-carrying capacity.

Beta-adrenergic blockers reduce myocardial oxygen consumption by reducing the cardiac index, stroke index, heart rate, blood pressure, and tension-time index. By lowering circulating levels of free fatty acids, beta blockers also decrease the risk of dysrhythmias.

Indications for beta blockers include:
• development of AMI while the patient is already receiving these drugs
• persistent or recurrent ischemic pain
• progressive or recurring elevations of serum enzyme levels, suggesting extension of the infarct
• tachydysrhythmias refractory to lidocaine and procainamide soon after onset of infarction.

Contraindications for treatment with beta blockers include:
• adverse reactions to these drugs
• heart failure or heart block
• history of bronchial asthma.

However, beta blockers may be prescribed for patients with relative contraindications, such as mild asthma, mild bradycardia, mild heart failure, and first-degree heart block. Such patients will need a trial dose with a very short-acting beta blocker to ensure their ability to tolerate therapy.

In AMI patients who have not received beta blockers in the preceding 24 hours, expect to use 15 mg of I.V. metoprolol (the only agent approved for I.V. use) divided into three equal doses given at 2- to 5-minute intervals. Monitor the patient's heart rate and arterial pressure, and record an ECG strip after each injection. Stop the infusion if any of the following events occur:
• second- or third-degree atrioventricular (AV) block or a PR interval lasting beyond 0.24 second
• crackles extending more than one-third of the way up the lung fields
• wheezes detected on auscultation
• ventricular heart rate below 50 beats/minute
• systolic arterial pressure less than 95 mm Hg
• pulmonary artery wedge pressure greater than 20 mm Hg.

Oral administration of metoprolol (50 mg twice daily) usually follows the I.V. dose by 6 to 8 hours. The oral dose increases to 100 mg twice daily if the patient tolerates the lower dose. The heart rate should stay between 50 and 65 beats/minute, and systolic pressure should remain above 95 mm Hg in patients without heart failure, wheezing, or advanced AV block.

Calcium channel blockers, including nifedipine (Adalat, Procardia) and verapamil (Calan, Isoptin), have questionable value in the early stage of acute transmural MI. But diltiazem (Cardizem) may prevent reinfarction and improve the chance of survival in patients with non-Q-wave infarction. Diltiazem seems to reduce subsequent cardiac events in patients *without* left ventricular failure, but it appears harmful in patients *with* left ventricular dysfunction. Calcium channel blockers may relieve angina or reduce the risk of coronary spasm; they may also reduce hypertension uncontrolled by beta blockers and nitrate therapy. Alone or with beta blockers, they may limit reperfusion injury and become a useful adjunct in reperfusion therapies.

Anticoagulants are used routinely in many hospitals. For example, heparin is commonly used to maintain activated partial thromboplastin time at 1½ to 2 times normal; after about 3 days, antiplatelet medication may be substituted for the anticoagulant.

Evidence that anticoagulants prevent reocclusion remains inconclusive. Anticoagulants don't seem to reduce the incidence of reinfarction, limit infarct size, or reduce mortality after AMI. In fact, hemorrhage during thrombolysis may actually stem from heparin treatment. Nevertheless, because of the hazard of CVAs and pulmonary emboli, heparinization remains a part of the standard treatment for AMI and unstable angina.

An echocardiogram before discharge indicates whether anticoagulant therapy should continue. If the test shows a left ventricular thrombus, the patient will need warfarin treatment for about 3 months. Warfarin may also prove necessary for patients with apical wall motion abnormalities, depending on the patient's risk-benefit profile.

Aspirin use remains controversial for AMI patients. The Food and Drug Administration has approved the use of one 325-mg aspirin tablet daily to reduce the risk of death and reinfarction, but actual clinical use varies. Available evidence suggests that aspirin could play a wider role during the acute phase of MI. In one group of patients, streptokinase and aspirin, started within 5 hours of AMI onset, reduced mortality at 5 weeks by 50% to 60%. Aspirin alone reduced mortality by 21%.

Glucose-insulin-potassium infusion counteracts ischemic biochemical changes, decreases infarct size, and enhances survival. The infusion increases the glucose transport into myocardial cells, providing needed fuel. It also enhances potassium entry, restoring ionic gradients and reducing ventricular dysrhythmias. A solution of 300 g of glucose, 50 units of insulin, and 80 mEq of potassium in 1,000 ml of water, given at a rate of 1.5 ml/kg/hour, lowers free fatty acid concentration, improves ventricular performance, and decreases the frequency of ventricular premature beats. This therapy is most effective within 6 hours after MI onset.

Other pharmacologic treatments are also being studied for effectiveness in preventing myocardial damage after AMI (see *Promising research: Investigational protocols in AMI,* page 118).

Myocardial reperfusion. Several special techniques are now used to restore and support myocardial perfusion.

PTCA may be required to produce myocardial reperfusion. This wire-guided balloon angioplasty replaces thrombolytic ther-

▶ PROMISING RESEARCH

Investigational protocols in AMI

The following agents are being studied for their ability to prevent further myocardial damage after AMI.

Hyaluronidase
This enzyme depolymerizes mucopolysaccharides. It may increase nutrient diffusion to the ischemic zone and inhibit edema in infarcted myocardium. Studies suggest that hyaluronidase may reduce infarct size if given earlier than 9 hours after AMI onset.

Corticosteroids and nonsteroidal anti-inflammatory drugs
Corticosteroids may protect ischemic myocardium by decreasing the inflammatory response to injury and enhancing collateral flow to ischemic myocardium, among other mechanisms. However, studies have yielded conflicting results. In one, a single dose of methylprednisolone decreased infarct size; in another, multiple doses of the same drug increased infarct size. Methylprednisolone has also caused persistent elevation of plasma CPK-MB levels. Some experts suspect that it may stimulate ventricular rupture and increase mortality. High steroid doses appear to impair healing and cause thinning of the scar. Experts now believe that multiple high doses of corticosteroids, begun several hours after ischemic injury, cause more harm than good.

Unlike aspirin, ibuprofen and indomethacin also cause thinning of the scar. They may also impair coronary blood flow by increasing coronary vascular resistance. Experts now recommend that these drugs be avoided in early AMI.

apy when thrombolysis fails or when severe residual stenosis remains after successful thrombolysis. PTCA requires an experienced catheterization team and special facilities. Its other disadvantages include the risk of vessel injury, occlusions, spasm, and subintimal hematoma.

CABG may be used to limit infarct size; however, it can succeed only when revascularization occurs with the first 4 to 5 hours after onset of AMI. (Necrosis occurs at about 6 hours.) Emergency use of CABG requires that the appropriate medical staff, laboratory, and operating room be available during the critical period.

IABP, also called intra-aortic balloon counterpulsation, may help hemodynamically unstable patients who need circulatory

PROMISING RESEARCH

Free radical scavengers

Investigators are studying oxygen-derived free radical scavengers, such as superoxide dismutase, for their potential to reduce necrosis and improve myocardial function after severe ischemia.

Oxygen-derived free radicals contain an odd number of electrons, making them chemically reactive. Abundant in ischemic tissue, they may worsen injury, especially during reperfusion, by causing cell membrane peroxidation or by acting on the mitochondria and sarcoplasmic reticulum.

The three main types of oxygen-derived free radicals are the superoxide anion, hydrogen peroxide, and the hydroxyl radical. Severe ischemia increases their production by dissociating electron transport; by activating phospholipase, which enhances arachidonic acid metabolism, a producer of oxygen radicals, and converting the normal myocardial enzyme xanthine hydrogenase to the radical-producing xanthine oxidase; and by activating complement, which enhances the accumulation of radical-releasing neutrophils.

Oxygen-derived free radical scavengers seem to preserve mitochondrial function, and they prevent the loss of calcium sequestration by the sarcoplasmic reticulum. They enhance myocardial recovery after transient ischemia. Their use may prove particularly important during reperfusion, because the reintroduction of oxygen into ischemic tissue causes a burst of free radical production.

support for diagnostic studies to assess lesions; patients in cardiogenic shock who don't respond to medical management; and patients with persistent ischemic pain that doesn't respond to treatment with 100% oxygen, beta blockers, nitrates, and calcium channel blockers. (See *Promising research: Free radical scavengers.*)

Case study: Part 4

On arriving at the intermediate care unit, Mr. Ingold was pain-free and seemed to be cooperative. However, talking with him confirmed that he still was not accepting his disease. He still referred to his disorder as indigestion even though he willingly participated in his rehabilitation program. Noting this, the nurses called a conference with the doctor, Mr. Ingold, and his fiancee. They discussed his diagnosis and prognosis with him, considering his

Case study: Part 4 *(continued)*

prognosis both with and without compliance. After the discussion, Mr. Ingold agreed to enter a treatment contract with the team to continue in the cardiac rehabilitation program and even agreed to begin a stop-smoking program.

By the 7th hospital day, telemetry cardiac monitoring, repeat 12-lead ECG, blood studies, and cardiac enzyme analysis showed no significant changes, and radionuclide scanning revealed only minor areas of myocardial injury.

Nursing management

After initial treatment, nursing care of the patient with AMI emphasizes guiding physical activity and diet to reduce myocardial oxygen demand and avoid cardiac stimulation, continuing assessment to prevent or promptly detect complications, providing interventions to minimize emotional stress, patient teaching, and preparing the patient for discharge and rehabilitation.

Guiding physical activity and diet

Guide the patient's activity to reduce cardiac work load and prevent recurrence of symptoms. For the patient with uncomplicated AMI on bed rest for 24 to 36 hours, plan leg exercises, such as ankle, plantar, and dorsiflexion. Provide a bedside commode and, as ordered, administer 100 to 300 mg of docusate sodium (Colace) to prevent constipation and help the patient avoid straining. Encourage the male patient to use a urinal; allow him to stand if he can't void lying down. After the first 24 to 48 hours, he can begin 30 minutes of chair rest twice daily. On the 4th or 5th day, the patient may ambulate in his room. After 5 days, the patient may take a tub bath or shower if he has no dysrhythmias, heart failure, or recurring chest pain. For the patient with complications, start physical activity even more slowly, as appropriate for his condition.

To reduce the risk of nausea and vomiting, AMI patients need a liquid diet for the first 24 hours. Thereafter, they may receive a 1,500-calorie, salt-free, low-fat, soft diet. Withhold beverages containing caffeine, which acts as a cardiac stimulant. However, if your patient is used to drinking four or five cups of coffee daily, abrupt caffeine withdrawal may prove dangerous.

Also restrict large amounts of ice cold beverages; however, recent evidence suggests that a glass or less of iced water doesn't harm the patient.

The AMI patient must have adequate sleep, which lowers the heart rate and myocardial oxygen consumption. Sleep deprivation increases myocardial oxygen consumption and the rate of dysrhythmias and may even precipitate myocardial ischemia. Unfortunately, AMI patients, particularly those who are acutely ill, often suffer loss of sleep because of interruptions for treatments and procedures and because of the lights and activity of the CCU. To benefit from sleep, the patient must complete the normal 60- to 90-minute sleep cycle; therefore, plan nursing procedures and schedule tests to allow the patient as much uninterrupted sleep as possible.

Preventing complications

Several potentially life-threatening complications are commonly associated with AMI: dysrhythmia, heart failure, cardiogenic shock, right ventricular infarction, rupture of the papillary muscle, rupture of the left ventricular free wall, ventricular aneurysm, rupture of the interventricular septum, pericarditis, pericardial effusion, left ventricular thrombus and arterial embolism, and postinfarction ischemia and extension. Recognizing them early can save the patient's life by allowing prompt intervention.

Dysrhythmia. In about 72% to 96% of AMI patients, dysrhythmias require vigorous treatment when they impair hemodynamics, increase myocardial oxygen demand, or predispose the patient to ventricular tachycardia, other ventricular dysrhythmias, or asystole. All forms of bradycardia and tachycardia may reduce cardiac output in AMI patients. (See *Recognizing dysrhythmias and conduction disturbances,* pages 122 to 124.)

Heart failure. This complication claims the lives of about 20% of hospitalized AMI patients. Ischemia and infarction cause some degree of left ventricular dysfunction in all AMI patients. Such impairment seems mild and resolves quickly in some patients, particularly those with small non-Q-wave infarctions; however, about 50% of AMI patients have significant, but transient, left ventricular failure.

(Text continues on page 124.)

Recognizing dysrhythmias and conduction disturbances

Patients with AMI are at greatest risk of dysrhythmias during the first 24 hours after infarction. Most deaths that occur within the first 2 hours after AMI onset result from dysrhythmias. The information below describes common dysrhythmias and conduction disturbances and their significance in the AMI patient.

Ventricular dysrhythmias

The most common rhythm disturbances after AMI, ventricular dysrhythmias appear in two phases: early and late. Early-phase dysrhythmias usually occur within the first 12 to 48 hours after infarction, probably from the immediate effects of ischemia on ventricular muscle. The disparity between injured and healthy tissue allows the reentry mechanism to produce ventricular extrasystoles, tachycardia, and fibrillation. Late-phase ventricular dysrhythmias probably result from enhanced automaticity of ventricular cells.

Learn to identify AMI patients at increased risk for life-threatening ventricular dysrhythmias to institute preventive measures. Expect dysrhythmias in elderly patients and patients with:
• Parkinson's disease, peptic ulcer, diabetes, or pulmonary disorders
• congestive heart failure (CHF), hypertension, angina, or palpitations
• transmural rather than subendocardial infarctions
• anterior infarctions.

Lidocaine may prevent primary ventricular fibrillation, but its prophylactic use remains controversial. Some experts point out that the drug is costly, that it poses a risk of hepatotoxicity and neuro-

logic effects, and that primary ventricular fibrillation is not common and can occur despite lidocaine; some suggest that close monitoring makes prophylaxis inappropriate. However, warning dysrhythmias may correlate poorly with ventricular fibrillation, because they occur as often in patients who don't develop ventricular fibrillation as in those who do and they may be absent in patients who do develop it.

Some experts recommend that prophylactic lidocaine be given to transmural AMI patients during the first 24 to 48 hours after infarction. AMI patients who should not receive prophylactic lidocaine routinely include:
• patients over age 70 who have a low incidence of ventricular fibrillation and a high incidence of adverse reactions to lidocaine
• patients with cardiogenic shock, severe CHF, heart block, or sinus bradycardia.

If an elderly patient is receiving prophylactic lidocaine, monitor him closely for central nervous system disturbances stemming from decreased drug clearance. Expect to give prophylactic lidocaine in an initial infusion of 50 mg repeated three to four times at 5-minute intervals, followed by a maintenance infusion of 2 mg/minute for 24 to 48 hours.

Premature ventricular contractions (PVCs). These dysrhythmias occur almost invariably in AMI patients. Frequent PVCs (more than five per minute), PVCs with multiform configuration, early coupling (the "R-on-T" phenomenon), and repetitive patterns in the form of couplets or salvos may warn of ventricular fibrillation. However, these pat-

terns appear in as many patients who don't develop fibrillation as in those who do.

Frequent PVCs occurring very soon after AMI onset, particularly during the first hour, may depend primarily on reentry rather than on increased automaticity. At this time, lidocaine, which impairs conduction in ventricular myocardium and diminishes automaticity, may prove less effective than it would later. Augmented sympathoadrenal stimulation often contributes to PVCs occurring with sinus tachycardia at the very inception of infarction. Beta-adrenoceptor blockade may control these PVCs. Early administration of an I.V. beta blocker also reduces the incidence of ventricular fibrillation in evolving MI.

Ventricular tachycardia. This dysrhythmia consists of three or more consecutive ventricular ectopic beats occurring at a frequency exceeding 120 beats/minute. It occurs in about 10% to 40% of AMI patients. Ventricular tachycardia in the first 24 hours commonly results from PVCs occurring late in the cardiac cycle. and is transient and benign. Ventricular tachycardia that occurs late in the course of AMI is more common in patients with transmural infarction and left ventricular dysfunction, is sustained, usually induces marked hemodynamic deterioration, and is associated with a relatively high hospital mortality (40% to 50%).

Hypokalemia increases the risk of all types of ventricular tachycardia. Rapid identification and treatment is necessary after admission for AMI. Throughout hospitalization, ensure that the patient's serum potassium level remains consistently above 4 mEq/liter. Prompt intervention to

Recognizing dysrhythmias and conduction disturbances *(continued)*

stop ventricular tachycardia is essential to prevent its deleterious effect on pump function and to keep it from deteriorating into ventricular fibrillation.

Ventricular fibrillation. The leading cause of sudden death after AMI, ventricular fibrillation occurs in 4% to 18% of AMI patients in cardiac care units. It has the same incidence in patients with anterior and inferior Q-wave infarctions but appears rarely in patients with non-Q-wave infarctions.

Ventricular fibrillation may occur in one of two phases.

• Primary (early) ventricular fibrillation, accounting for more than 80% of all instances of this dysrhythmia, occurs suddenly and unexpectedly in patients with no or few signs or symptoms of left ventricular failure. About 60% of these episodes occur within 4 hours and 80% within 12 hours of AMI onset.

• Secondary (late) ventricular fibrillation occurs as the final phase of a progressively downhill course with left ventricular failure and cardiogenic shock. Late ventricular fibrillation usually occurs 1 to 6 weeks after AMI. Patients with intraventricular conduction defects, anterior wall infarction, persistent sinus tachycardia, atrial flutter, early fibrillation, or right ventricular infarction requiring ventricular pacing are all at risk for late ventricular fibrillation.

Sinus dysrhythmias
Sinus bradycardia. Occurring commonly during the early phases of an AMI, sinus bradycardia occurs more commonly after inferior wall infarction, possibly as a result of decreased blood flow to the sinoatrial (SA) node. Enhanced vagal stimula-

tion may also play a role. Sinus bradycardia may be a protective mechanism, because the decreased rate of SA node discharge reduces myocardial oxygen needs after AMI. But it can also prove harmful by creating conditions favorable for PVCs, ventricular tachycardia, and ventricular fibrillation.

Sinus tachycardia. About a third of AMI patients (mainly those with an anterior infarct) develop sinus tachycardia. Its causes vary but related factors include pain, anxiety, hypovolemia, vasoactive medications, left ventricular failure, and right ventricular infarction. It's associated with transient hypertension or hypotension and augmented sympathetic activity. Sinus tachycardia increases myocardial oxygen consumption and decreases diastolic filling time and coronary artery perfusion time.

Atrial dysrhythmias
Premature atrial contractions (PACs). PACs occur in up to half of all AMI patients. They may result from atrial distention secondary to increases in left ventricular diastolic pressure, from pericarditis with its associated atrial epicarditis, or from ischemic injury to the atria and sinus node (uncommon).

Atrial flutter. This least common of the atrial dysrhythmias occurs in only 1% to 3% of AMI patients. It is usually associated with 2:1 atrioventricular (AV) block. Usually transient, atrial flutter typically results from augmented sympathetic stimulation of the atria, often in patients with left ventricular failure or pulmonary emboli. Atrial flutter often

intensifies hemodynamic deterioration.

Atrial fibrillation. Far more common than flutter, atrial fibrillation occurs in 10% to 15% of AMI patients. Usually transient, it tends to occur in patients with left ventricular failure and in those with pericarditis or ischemic atrial injury. It occurs more commonly after anterior than inferior infarction and appears to result largely from left atrial ischemia. Increased ventricular rate and loss of the atrial contribution to left ventricular filling (the atrial kick) significantly reduce cardiac output. More common during the first 24 hours after infarction, both atrial flutter and fibrillation are associated with higher mortality, particularly in patients with anterior wall infarctions.

Junctional rhythms
Also known as accelerated junctional rhythms, these dysrhythmias appear in patients with a slow sinus rate and an inferior infarction. Usually transient, they occur during the first 48 hours after infarction.

Paroxysmal junctional tachycardia. Uncommon in AMI, this dysrhythmia occurs in only 1% to 2% of patients. It usually produces heart rates between 160 and 220 beats/minute. It may cause a loss of atrial kick, decreasing cardiac output and producing hemodynamic impairment.

Supraventricular rhythms
Paroxysmal supraventricular tachycardia. This dysrhythmia occurs in 2% to 5% of AMI patients. Its damaging effects stem from elevated myocardial oxygen consumption

(continued)

Recognizing dysrhythmias and conduction disturbances *(continued)*

and impaired ventricular performance that results from the rapid ventricular rate. Both transient and recurrent, it is associated with a higher mortality.

Conduction disturbances
First-degree AV block. This disturbance occurs in 4% to 14% of AMI patients. It may progress to higher degrees of block, especially in patients with inferior infarctions.

Second-degree AV block—Mobitz Type I (Wenckebach). This disturbance occurs in about 4% to 10% of AMI patients, commonly in those with inferior infarctions. Usually transient, it seldom persists beyond 72 hours after infarction.

Second-degree AV block—Mobitz Type II. This disturbance occurs in only about 1% of AMI patients. Associated with anterior infarctions, it commonly pro-

gresses suddenly (if it occurs at all) to complete AV block.

Complete (third-degree) AV block (complete heart block). This develops in 5% to 8% of AMI patients. In patients with an inferior infarct, complete AV block usually develops gradually, progressing from first-degree to Mobitz Type I block. In patients with an anterior infarct, complete AV block commonly occurs suddenly, 12 to 24 hours after infarct onset, although it usually follows intraventricular block and often a Mobitz Type II pattern (not first-degree or Mobitz Type I) AV block.

Intraventricular block
A block within one or more of the three subdivisions of the His-Purkinje system (the right bundle and the anterior and posterior divisions of the left bundle), intra-

ventricular block occurs in 10% to 20% of AMI patients.

Intraventricular blocks, such as right bundle branch block, commonly lead to complete AV block. And intraventricular conduction defects, particularly right bundle branch block, account for most instances of late ventricular fibrillation. However, the high rate of mortality in these patients occurs even without AV block and appears related to cardiac failure and massive infarction rather than to the conduction disturbance.

Complete bundle branch block (either left or right), the combination of right bundle branch block and left anterior divisional (fascicular) block, and any of the various forms of trifascicular block are more commonly associated with anterior infarction than with inferoposterior infarction.

The severity of heart failure correlates with the extent of myocardial damage, so expect it in patients with larger (mainly anterior) transmural infarcts or preexisting myocardial damage from a previous MI. Even mild heart failure can exacerbate myocardial ischemia, so stay alert for signs of pump failure and intervene quickly.

Heart failure after AMI differs from that in chronic CHF and requires a different treatment. Heart failure after AMI shows up as decreased ventricular compliance. In this situation, left ventricular filling pressures must be higher than normal to allow normal cardiac output, which becomes sensitive to reduced circulatory volume. For this reason, use diuretics cautiously in AMI patients. In the early stages of heart failure, patients will probably remain normovolemic or hypovolemic with normal cardiac output. However, those with an inferior infarction, especially with right ventricle involvement, may require volume expansion; their catecholamine levels are markedly elevated.

Digitalis preparations (for example, digoxin) may benefit hemodynamically stable patients with mild heart failure. Catecholamines with a short duration of action and half-life can increase contractility; however, because they can exacerbate ischemia, they should be reserved for severe heart failure.

Compensatory responses to heart failure, such as increased peripheral vascular resistance (afterload), can reduce stroke volume, lower cardiac output, compromise peripheral and coronary perfusion, and cause pulmonary congestion. Expect to administer vasodilators to reduce afterload, reduce preload, and relieve pulmonary congestion. Short-acting I.V. agents, such as nitroprusside and nitroglycerin, prove useful in the acute phase because they act rapidly and allow careful dose titration. (See *Hemodynamic profile: Guide to treatment of AMI complications,* pages 126 and 127.)

Cardiogenic shock. Causing the most serious form of heart failure in AMI patients, cardiogenic shock usually follows massive left ventricular damage (40% or more). Cardiogenic shock is associated with systolic pressure less than 80 mm Hg, cardiac index less than 1.8 liters/minute/m², decreased urine output, elevated heart rate, pulmonary artery wedge pressure exceeding 18 mm Hg, pulmonary congestion, and arterial hypoxemia.

In patients with extensive myocardial damage, it causes an 80% to 90% mortality despite aggressive intervention. (See *The downward spiral in AMI,* page 128.) However, it is usually reversible when it's linked to certain treatable complications (such as vagally induced hypotension, intravascular volume depletion, acute right ventricular failure, and such surgically treatable causes as left ventricular aneurysm and rupture of the ventricular septum, papillary muscle, or chordae tendinae).

Treatment of cardiogenic shock includes inotropic agents (such as dopamine and dobutamine) to increase contractility, and vasodilators (such as nitroprusside or nitroglycerin) to reduce afterload impedance and increase forward flow. Dopamine also increases renal blood flow but has a hazardous tendency to increase myocardial oxygen consumption and trigger dys-

Hemodynamic profile: Guide to treatment of AMI complications

Hypotension, hypovolemia
Hemodynamic profile
Pulmonary capillary wedge pressure (PCWP) <15 mm Hg; cardiac output <2.5 liters/minute/m²); systolic blood pressure <90 mm Hg
Management
• Rule out bradydysrhythmias, tachydysrhythmias, and reflex increase in vagal tone (seen with inferior infarction) as causes of hypotension.
• Institute invasive hemodynamic monitoring if not already in place. Assess for hypovolemia by fluid challenge, using a rapid infusion of I.V. normal saline solution (200 ml in 50-ml increments titrated against PCWP) until cardiac output and arterial pressure are normal or PCWP reaches 18 to 20 mm Hg. If raising PCWP fails to restore adequate cardiac output and blood pressure, discontinue infusion and treat for severe heart failure or cardiogenic shock.
Precautions
• Further infusion may worsen pulmonary congestion and precipitate pulmonary edema. Avoid slow I.V. drip infusion, which can precipitate edema without increasing PCWP.

• Avoid diuretics if you suspect hypovolemia (as in right ventricular infarction).

Moderate heart failure with pulmonary congestion and normotension
Hemodynamic and clinical profile
PCWP 18 mm Hg or higher; cardiac output <2.5 liters/minute/m²; normal or slightly elevated blood pressure; systemic vascular resistance of 1,200 dyne/second/cm⁻⁵ or lower
Management
Furosemide in moderate doses (20 to 40 mg) can rapidly relieve pulmonary congestion by an extrarenal venodilating effect. Use furosemide with caution because diuresis may lower volume excessively, leading to compromised cardiac output in the patient with a stiff, noncompliant left ventricle due to ischemia. Assess the patient frequently for warning signs, such as tachycardia or hypotension.
Administer I.V. nitroglycerin in patients with moderate-to-severe heart failure, in those not completely responsive to furosemide, and in those for whom further diuresis might be hazardous. Start I.V. nitroglycerin at 5 to 10 mcg/

minute, and titrate it in 5- to 10-mcg increments every 5 to 10 minutes to a total dosage of 100 to 200 mcg/minute until desired hemodynamic values occur (PCWP of 20 mm Hg or lower), systolic blood pressure falls below 100 mm Hg, or side effects appear.
Monitor PCWP closely because excessive reduction of preload can compromise cardiac output.
Precautions
Avoid vasodilators when systolic blood pressure is at or below 90 mm Hg.

Heart failure with hypertension
Hemodynamic profile
PCWP 18 mm Hg or higher; cardiac output <2.5 liters/minute/m²; systolic BP over 110 mm Hg; systemic vascular resistance above 1,200 dyne/second/cm⁻⁵
Management
Start I.V. nitroprusside, 0.5 mcg/kg/minute, increased in increments of 0.5 to 10 mcg every 5 to 10 minutes with continuous hemodynamic monitoring until arterial systolic blood pressure falls between 95 and 100 mm Hg or side effects occur. If arterial

rhythmias. Vasodilators decrease myocardial oxygen consumption, but nitroprusside may decrease coronary artery perfusion. Be alert for these potential problems when administering any of these drugs.

If drug therapy fails, treatment may include IABP or acute reperfusion, usually with thrombolytic therapy or emergency PTCA. However, reperfusion, which succeeds only during the first 4 to 6 hours after MI onset, is not appropriate for most pressure falls excessively, discontinue the nitroprusside and consider giving an infusion of dobutamine.

Moderate-to-severe heart failure with pulmonary congestion, low cardiac output, and borderline blood pressure
Hemodynamic profile
PCWP 18 mm Hg or higher; cardiac output <2.5 liters/minute/m²); borderline systolic blood pressure (90 to 110 mm Hg)
Management
Heart failure accompanied by systolic blood pressure of 90 to 110 mm Hg may require treatment with either vasodilators or positive inotropic and vasopressor agents. In some patients, a moderately potent vasopressor such as dopamine, added to nitroprusside, will counteract the vasodilator's effect on systemic vascular resistance. Alternatively, start I.V. nitroprusside, 5 to 10 mcg/minute. If the increase in cardiac output is less than 20%, add dobutamine, 5 mcg/kg/minute, increased by 2.5 mcg/kg/minute every 10 minutes up to a maximum of 10 mcg/kg/minute. Reduce the dosage or discontinue dobutamine if hypertension

or excessive tachycardia occurs.

Severe heart failure, preshock state
Hemodynamic profile
PCWP 18 mm Hg or higher; cardiac output< 2.2 liters/minute/m²
Management
Add dobutamine to therapy to augment cardiac output by enhancing cardiac contractility. Dobutamine effectively alleviates pulmonary congestion and lowers left ventricular filling pressure. Titrate the drug to achieve hemodynamic goals without raising the heart rate more than 10% over baseline. Dopamine in low dosages (less than 5 mcg/kg/minute) selectively increases renal blood flow; it may be combined with dobutamine for this purpose.
Precautions
Since high-dose dopamine can elevate left ventricular filling pressure, avoid it when pulmonary congestion and edema are prominent. Use dopamine (and avoid dobutamine) when significant hypotension occurs. Consider an intra-aortic balloon pump (IABP) if heart failure is severe.

Cardiogenic shock (low output state with pulmonary congestion and hypotension)
Hemodynamic profile
Elevation of PCWP (18 mm Hg or higher); severe reduction in cardiac output (<2.2 liters/minute/m²); hypotension; oliguria (urine output <20 ml/hour)
Management
If arterial systolic pressure is 70 to 90 mm Hg, infuse dopamine, starting at 2 to 5 mcg/kg/minute, to establish adequate blood pressure and increase cardiac contractility. When arterial pressure remains stable at 100 to 110 mm Hg, add a vasodilator to further enhance cardiac output. If dopamine in moderately large dosages (20 to 30 mcg/kg/minute) can't maintain arterial pressure or if systolic pressure is below 70 mm Hg initially, begin an infusion of norepinephrine bitartrate, titrated to raise systolic pressure to 100 to 110 mm Hg, and then substitute dopamine. Most patients also require circulatory support with an IABP, which should be used in any patient with persistent hypotension and hypoperfusion after a short trial of aggressive medical therapy.

patients with cardiogenic shock, which usually develops 24 to 48 hours after MI onset.

Ventricular-assist devices allow surgical bypass of severely obstructed vessels, which may improve left ventricular function. Left ventricular bypass, an experimental technique that drastically reduces left ventricular oxygen demand, may prove more effective than IABP in improving patient survival.

The downward spiral in AMI

Patients who die of cardiogenic shock usually enter severe hemodynamic decline 12 to 24 hours after onset of AMI. Their underlying pathology seems to involve a steady encroachment of necrosis into the ischemic zone around infarcted areas. Ischemia spreads into previously healthy tissue. Because this encroachment occurs over hours or days, increasing myocardial blood flow or reducing oxygen demand in the early stages of AMI may help salvage border zones and prevent or reverse cardiogenic shock.

• In the early phase of AMI, severe ischemia and necrosis cause a sudden loss of contractility and decreased ventricular compliance. Reperfusion can relieve occlusion, preventing progression as a result of ischemia and necrosis.

• Cardiac output drops, stimulating compensatory sympathetic activity, which in turn causes vasoconstriction in an attempt to defend peripheral perfusion.

• The compensatory sympathetic response increases afterload, increasing cardiac work load and decreasing output. Increased work load worsens ischemia and further reduces contractility. Arterial vasodilators may improve cardiac output by decreasing vasoconstriction. Positive inotropic agents improve contractility but can worsen ischemia and are commonly used only in severe failure.

• To maintain cardiac output, end-diastolic volume and pressure increase, elevating left ventricular filling pressure. Loss of ventricular compliance and vasoconstriction contribute to increased filling pressure.

• Blood pools in the pulmonary circulation, with varying degrees of congestion and edema. Diuretics and vasodilators can reduce this congestion and edema by reducing left ventricular filling pressure.

• Loss of compliance and elevated left ventricular filling pressure increase diastolic wall tension, increasing myocardial oxygen demand. At the same time, increased wall tension may increase subendocardial coronary blood flow impedance, reducing myocardial oxygen supply.

• Cardiac output and coronary perfusion continue to fall until a state of irreversible decline and shock occurs. Vasopressors can be used to increase perfusion of vital organs. Circulatory support and emergency revascularization are necessary to prevent further progression.

• Blood pressure falls, worsening ischemia and coronary hypoperfusion and precipitating organ failure and circulatory collapse.

Right ventricular infarction. About 5% of AMI patients suffer right ventricular infarction. Half of them develop shock or a shocklike syndrome of low cardiac output, hypotension, or both. Right ventricular infarction almost always follows inferior or inferoposterior infarction.

Signs of right ventricular infarction include elevated jugular venous pressure with distention (absent in some patients in the early phase), Kussmaul's sign (paradoxical increase in jugular venous pressure with inspiration), bradycardia, arterial hypotension, and pulsus paradoxus. You may hear a right, but not a left, S_3 or S_4. Lung fields may sound clear. Crackles and chest X-ray abnormalities are absent unless left ventricular infarction is extensive. Dehydrated patients may not show elevated jugular venous pressure or Kussmaul's sign. Rarely, tricuspid regurgitation and severe hypoxemia result from right-to-left interatrial shunting.

ECG findings after right ventricular infarction include ST-segment elevation in the right-sided precordial leads (V_{4R} to V_{6R}), transient ST-segment elevation in lead V_1, and ST-segment elevation of 1 mm or more in lead V_{4R}. Hemodynamic monitoring reveals a low cardiac index and a disproportionate elevation of right atrial pressure (10 to 28 mm Hg) compared to pulmonary capillary wedge pressure (PCWP). Two-dimensional echocardiography confirms this complication, showing dilatation and hypokinesia of the right ventricle and the absence of significant pericardial effusion and tamponade. MUGA scanning can also show right ventricular hypocontractility and diminished ejection fraction.

In patients with right ventricular infarction, shock stems from inadequate left ventricular filling and output. Appropriate treatment includes infusion of an I.V. crystalloid (or colloid for profound hypotension) to expand volume until hypotension disappears, right atrial pressure reaches 10 to 12 mm Hg, or PCWP rises to 15 to 20 mm Hg. Because excessive volume infusion may cause acute right ventricular failure or pulmonary edema, monitor fluid therapy carefully. Avoid diuretics, which would decrease right ventricular filling pressure and, in turn, decrease blood pressure and cardiac output.

If volume infusion increases right-sided pressures without increasing left ventricular filling pressure or cardiac output, treatment may include inotropic agents. Vasodilator use is controversial. Temporary transvenous atrial or atrioventricular pacing may prove helpful in patients with sinus node dysfunction or AV block.

Good management of right ventricular infarction requires special attention to hemodynamic measurements of right atrial pressure and PCWP, which help determine the appropriate volume status and left ventricular filling.

Rupture of the papillary muscle. This complication, usually involving the posterior medial papillary muscle, occurs within the first several days of hospitalization and causes mitral regurgitation with pulmonary congestion and a loud pansystolic murmur. Increasingly severe heart failure may occur. A pulmonary artery catheter may show large *V* waves on the PCWP tracing, elevated left ventricular filling pressure, and high central pulmonary artery oxygen saturation. Suspected rupture requires immediate echocardiography to confirm the diagnosis.

Patients with papillary muscle rupture require emergency mitral valve replacement. Before surgery, IABP and vasodilators, such as I.V. nitroprusside, may decrease regurgitation temporarily and encourage forward flow by decreasing left ventricular ejection resistance.

Rupture of the left ventricular free wall. This complication kills about 10% of hospitalized MI patients, usually from cardiac tamponade and hemopericardium. Such rupture usually follows expansion of the infarct and results from a distinct tear in the myocardial wall at the junction of infarct and normal myocardium or in a dissecting hematoma that perforates a necrotic myocardial area.

An acute tear can cause instant death. A slow and incomplete tear can cause late rupture or a false aneurysm. In either case, the patient's survival depends on quick recognition of the rupture, hemodynamic stabilization, and immediate surgical repair. Symptoms include sudden profound right ventricular failure with shock, leading to electromechanical dissociation. Immediate pericardiocentesis will confirm the diagnosis and temporarily relieve pericardial tamponade. In a stable patient, echocardiography may be performed to confirm tamponade.

Free wall rupture occurs more often in women than in men, in elderly patients, and in hypertensive patients. Such rupture usually follows transmural infarction of at least 20% of the left ventricle, and commonly involves the anterior or lateral wall in the terminal distribution area of the left anterior descending coronary artery. Free wall rupture usually occurs between days 3 and 6 but can occur as late as 3 weeks after MI.

Ventricular aneurysm. About 12% to 15% of patients with transmural MI develop a true ventricular aneurysm. A weak, thin-walled outpouching that bulges with each systolic contraction, such an aneurysm results from intraventricular tension that stretches the infarcted heart muscle. Over time, the aneurysm becomes more fibrotic and steals some of the left ventricular stroke volume during each systole.

Ventricular aneurysms range from 1 to 8 cm in diameter. They occur four times more often at the apex and in the anterior wall than in the inferoposterior wall and are associated with persistent ST-segment elevations on the ECG. They are confirmed by two-dimensional echocardiography and radionuclide angiography. Left ventricular aneurysms increase mortality sixfold, usually causing sudden death, probably from ventricular tachydysrhythmias. Complications of left ventricular aneurysms include mural thrombi adhering to the aneurysmal wall, systemic emboli, CHF, angina pectoris, and ventricular dysrhythmias. Ventricular aneurysms usually require aneurysmectomy.

False (pseudo) aneurysms may stem from incomplete rupture of the left ventricular wall when a thrombus seals the rupture and a hematoma develops. Their tendency to rupture makes them dangerous.

Rupture of the interventricular septum. This complication occurs in about 2% of AMI patients, usually between days 2 and 5 after MI. It occurs after both anterior and inferior infarctions and leads to cardiogenic shock in more than half of the patients who develop it.

Diagnostic signs and symptoms include sudden clinical deterioration with pulmonary congestion, low cardiac output, and hypotension; and, in some patients, a new systolic murmur at the left lower sternal border radiating to the cardiac apex, and a parasternal systolic thrill (in 50% of the patients). The confirming diagnostic findings are left-to-right shunting, demonstrated by oximetry as a step-up in venous oxygen saturation (increase in partial pressure of oxygen greater than 10%) in right ventricular samples compared to right atrial blood samples, and high central pulmonary artery oxygen saturation despite decreased systemic flow. Two-dimensional echocardiography, Doppler ultrasonography, and MUGA scanning confirm this diagnosis.

Treatment with nitroprusside reduces left ventricular afterload, improves cardiac output, and reduces left-to-right shunting. IABP reduces shunt flow by reducing left ventricular afterload. Placing an umbrella-shaped catheter in the ruptured septum also seems to stabilize critically ill patients until corrective surgery can be performed. Surgical repair within 48 hours of diagnosis reduces mortality from nearly 100% to about 50%.

Pericarditis. Within 2 to 4 days after infarction, about 15% of patients develop early pericarditis as an inflammatory response to transmural damage. Late pericarditis (Dressler's syndrome or postmyocardial infarction syndrome) develops as a delayed autoimmune response.

Signs and symptoms of early pericarditis include a transient pericardial friction rub and positional chest pain that worsens with inspiration. The ECG shows diffuse ST-segment elevation during the acute phase and T-wave inversion, but no abnormal Q waves. Pericarditis occurs most commonly in men, among patients with transmural (Q wave) infarctions, and in those with CHF. Treatment for early pericarditis includes anti-inflammatory drugs, such as aspirin, nonsteroidal anti-inflammatory drugs, and steroids. Watch for signs of cardiac tamponade in patients with early pericarditis who receive anticoagulants.

Signs and symptoms of late pericarditis include persistent fever between 101° and 102° F (38.3° and 38.9° C), leukocytosis, malaise, positional dull chest pain that intensifies with inspiration, and pericardial friction rubs. Treatment for late percarditis also includes anti-inflammatory agents. Reassure the patient that this condition resolves spontaneously over time and should require no further treatment.

Pericardial effusion. Occurring in about 25% of all MI patients, most commonly in those with anterior MI, larger infarcts, or CHF, pericardial effusion doesn't cause clinical problems. Effusion may accompany pericarditis and may take months to resorb.

Left ventricular thrombi and arterial emboli. Mural thrombi are common, especially with large infarcts; most appear in the left ventricular apex, but they may overlie both ventricles with extensive transmural infarction. Mural thrombi are also common in patients with a ventricular aneurysm or a pseudoaneurysm and in those receiving beta blockers. In about 50% of patients with mural thrombi, detached fragments produce systemic arterial emboli.

Echocardiography can detect mural thrombi. Treatment includes prophylactic anticoagulant and antiplatelet therapy. Early ambulation also helps prevent systemic emboli.

Postinfarction ischemia and extension. Some patients develop angina within the first 10 days after AMI. Rest, nitroglycerin, beta blockers, and calcium channel blockers control such pain in most, but not all, patients. When anginal pain is accompanied by ST-T wave changes in the area where Q waves appeared, it may stem from coronary spasm, occlusion of a previously patent vessel, or reocclusion of a recanalized one. Such angina, whether transient or persistent, is linked to higher short- and long-term mortality. Most patients with postinfarction angina need cardiac catheterization and coronary angiography to evaluate surgical revascularization.

Exercise stress tests, particularly with thallium imaging, help confirm ischemia as the cause of postinfarction angina; however, these tests should be avoided when the pain is persistent, accompanies ECG changes, or occurs at rest or with minimal activity. PET may detect a hyperperfused myocardium.

About 10% of AMI patients have extension of the infarct during the first 10 days. Different from postinfarction angina, pain resulting from such extension is more severe and prolonged, with persistent ECG changes—ST-T wave changes, QRS changes, or both. Serum shows recurring CPK-MB level elevation after the initial peak. Infarct extension is most likely to develop in obese women; in patients with nontransmural infarct, diabetes mellitus, or an earlier MI; and in patients whose CPK-MB curve peaks earlier than 15 hours after onset.

Other complications. Hiccups may accompany inferior wall MI. Nausea and vomiting can occur in the acute phase or in later phases from analgesics and other drugs. Act promptly to relieve vomiting, which can cause dysrhythmias.

Abdominal distention, constipation, and fecal impaction may result from lack of exercise, decreased dietary roughage, drug therapy, or potassium depletion after diuresis. In a patient with peptic ulcer, stress can trigger GI hemorrhage.

Controlling emotional stressors

AMI understandably triggers anxiety, denial, anger, and depression in the patient and family. Loss of control imposes enormous stress, especially on patients who are used to being in charge. In such patients (those with what's commonly called a Type A personality), loss of control can be a more significant factor than the disease itself—especially in early stages, when they are still denying their illness. Depending on the severity of the illness, the patient may show any or all of the following psychological responses.

Anxiety. Anxiety is probably most severe during the first 24 to 48 hours of hospitalization. During this period, spend as much time as you can with the patient and family to reassure them, answer their questions, and let them express their concerns. The anxious patient may show the following coping mechanisms:
• isolation or repression, by seeming unconcerned about his condition
• displacement, by complaining about unimportant matters, such as food or noises
• projection, by talking about his family's anxieties and focusing on other problems unrelated to his illness
• rationalization, by blaming the MI on indigestion rather than on his life-style
• hallucinations, delusions, delirium, agitation, or mania.

Transferring the patient from the CCU to the intermediate care unit can cause a form of separation anxiety. To reduce this stress, prepare the patient for transfer, make the transfer during the day, and help the patient become acquainted with his new surroundings. Watch for cardiovascular signs and dysrhythmias, which occur most often during the 2 hours after transfer, and be ready to intervene promptly.

Denial. The patient may ignore his illness and avoid discussing it. Such denial usually lasts for 24 to 48 hours after admission but may last longer. The patient may verbalize or act out his denial by becoming angry and confrontational, refusing to cooperate with treatment, getting out of bed, or exercising to see whether the pain recurs.

Anger. Anger is common but patients deny it, believing that they should control it. Try to recognize repressed anger and help the patient use it positively, following these steps:
• Tell the patient that anger is a normal response to AMI, and accept it yourself. Don't try to joke him out of it.
• Help the patient identify and express the causes of his anger.
• Find constructive outlets for the patient's anger. You may need to modify your care plan to incorporate outlets that help him deal with his anger.

Depression. Depression usually sets in about 48 hours after admission. It can cause chest pain, dysrhythmias, and increased blood pressure. Ask the patient about his feelings, and let him know that depression is a normal response to AMI. Help him take responsibility for some of his own care, which will increase his sense of control and ease his depression. For example, you might let him have some input into how his day is organized.

Abnormal behaviors. In some patients, the emotional stress of AMI triggers aggression, confusion, or fearful behavior. The following behaviors may also follow AMI:
• Aggressive sexual behavior may occur during the first 24 to 48 hours after admission. Try to find out what need or anxiety the patient is expressing through his sexual aggressiveness. Tell him if his behavior makes you uncomfortable.
• ICU psychosis leaves the patient confused, with personality changes. Fear of death, loss of control, sleep deprivation, fear of hospital equipment, drugs, hypotension, impaired cerebral blood flow, and isolation from family can all trigger ICU psychosis. To prevent ICU psychosis, provide frequent orientation to time and place, and try to have the patient transferred to the intermediate care unit as soon as possible.
• Cardiac cripple syndrome is evident in patients who resist resuming normal daily activities from fear of death or disability and probably from loss of self-esteem or control. Because this syndrome commonly appears only after discharge, encourage the patient and family to discuss their concerns with the rehabilitation team.

Patient teaching

Teaching should begin in the CCU if the patient seems ready and able to learn. Try to include the family as well as the patient when you explain:
• the CCU's purpose and routine, hospital equipment and noises, and the need for restrictive visiting hours and frequent monitoring
• treatment medications, procedures, and diagnostic tests
• when to report and how to treat chest pain
• gradual progression of physical activity, including sexual activity
• when the patient can resume sexual activity
• coronary artery disease (CAD) risk factors and life-style modifications to change them, including stress management.

The AMI patient needs the same teaching as the CAD and angina patient. The cardiac rehabilitation team commonly provides such instruction, both in and out of the hospital.

Discharge planning

Discharge may occur as early as 6 or 7 days after admission for AMI, or it may occur after 10 days, when the patient has become fully ambulatory. Usually, patients with complications remain hospitalized until several days after they stabilize.

Begin discharge planning as soon as the patient enters the hospital. Include patient teaching, covering physical activity, risk factor modification, and drug regimens. Encourage the patient to continue cardiac rehabilitation (which usually begins during hospitalization) after he leaves the hospital.

Case study: Part 5

Mr. Ingold was discharged 8 days after admission. He and his fiancee were planning to go ahead with their wedding in 2 weeks, but he was unable to return to his starting position at third base with his baseball team. Participation in the cardiac rehabilitation program would increase his chances of returning to baseball but not guarantee it. Mr. Ingold now understood that he might have to accept a future without baseball and he was very depressed about it. Baseball was always such a big part of his life. The hope of returning to it would motivate him to cooperate fully with his cardiac rehabilitation program.

CHAPTER 4
Congestive heart failure

Congestive heart failure (CHF) can occur in any patient at any time and is surely among the clinical problems you encounter most often. Virtually any patient—the postpartum mother with a congenital heart defect, a patient with severe viral infection, an orthopedic patient with a cardiac history—may develop CHF if an increased hemodynamic burden or decreased myocardial oxygenation impairs the heart's ability to pump adequately.

Early identification of CHF is the key to reducing morbidity and mortality. But the wide variations in presenting symptoms—from ill-defined malaise to severe breathlessness and tachycardia—challenge your diagnostic skills. Moreover, after diagnosis, drastically fluctuating heart function can require swift adjustments of therapy.

Essential for timely and accurate assessment, hemodynamic monitoring techniques provide continuous data on cardiac output, venous oxygen saturation, and other important indicators of cardiac function. Such data, when coupled with a thorough understanding of the cardiac output cycle and the frequent assessment of symptoms, can reliably indicate cardiac status and alert you to sudden reversals of status.

New therapeutic techniques have greatly improved the outlook for CHF patients, but prognosis still depends on the underlying cause and its response to treatment.

Case study: Part 1

Claire Baldwin, a 63-year-old widow with five adult children, suffered an extensive but uncomplicated anterior wall myocardial infarction (MI) 3 weeks after the death of her husband. Cardiac catheterization revealed poor left ventricular function and diffuse, inoperable coronary artery disease (CAD). After 3

Case study: Part 1 *(continued)*

weeks in the hospital, Mrs. Baldwin went to the home of her oldest daughter to recuperate.

During her second week there, she experienced shortness of breath while climbing the stairs, difficulty sleeping in a recumbent position, and increasing fatigue. She complained that she tired easily when playing with her 5-year-old grandson. Concerned about her mother's progressive weakness and sudden swelling in her legs (with weight gain of 6 lb in 2 days), the daughter called Mrs. Baldwin's cardiologist, who suspected acute CHF and who urged her to take her mother to the hospital right away.

The emergency department (ED) staff quickly readmitted Mrs. Baldwin and informed the cardiac care unit (CCU) that she would be transferred there as soon as her condition stabilized. The CCU nurses prepared to resume her care.

Causes and characteristics

Physiologically, heart failure is defined as inadequate cardiac output—the heart cannot pump enough blood to meet the body's metabolic oxygen requirements. Clinically, heart failure is defined according to which side of the heart is most damaged. In *left ventricular failure,* increased pulmonary and venous capillary pressures cause pulmonary symptoms of dyspnea, cough, and orthopnea. In *right ventricular failure,* elevated systemic venous pressure produces dependent edema, jugular vein distention, and sometimes ascites. Because normal heart function depends on both ventricles, failure of one ventricle (if untreated) eventually means failure of the other.

The chain of events leading ultimately to right or left ventricular failure can be set in motion in many ways. Clinicians have grouped these causes of CHF into three classes.

Fundamental causes include biochemical and physiologic mechanisms that interfere with normal cardiac muscle contraction by increasing hemodynamic burden or reducing oxygen delivery to the coronary vessels. (See *Cardiac muscle structure and function.*)

Underlying causes include congenital or acquired structural abnormalities that compromise normal function of the peripheral and coronary vessels, pericardium, myocardium, or cardiac valves and lead to increased hemodynamic burden or insufficient cardiac output.

Cardiac muscle structure and function

Cardiac muscle consists of long, thin cells made up of cylindrical elements called myofibrils. Each myofibril consists of long, thin protein strands arranged in regular repeating units called sarcomeres—the heart muscle's basic contractile unit. Cardiac muscle typically contains these elements:
• *sarcoplasmic reticulum.* This is an extensive intracellular network that regulates calcium concentrations in the cell and plays a key role in cardiac muscle excitation.
• *mitochondria.* These abundant cytoplasmic organelles surround the myofibril sheaths and produce energy in the form of adenosine triphosphate.
• *T tubules.* These are part of the sarcoplasmic reticulum and form a pathway for action potentials. Electrical impulses strike the cell membrane, travel down the T tubules, and cause calcium release.

Sarcomere structure
Under high magnification, myofibril proteins appear as a series of dark and light bands. The diagram to the right of the cross-sectional view shows the dark A bands of myosin and lighter I bands of actin of a single sarcomere. Myosin has thick filaments running the length of the myofibril's A band. Actin, a thinner filament within the I band, extends from each end of the sarcomere. Actin overlaps and connects with myosin, forming dense areas in the A band. Two other proteins, tropomyosin and troponin, together inhibit the interaction of actin and myosin filaments, thereby producing muscle cell relaxation. A thin, dark band known as the Z line marks the boundary between adjacent sarcomeres.

Muscle cell contraction
When a muscle cell receives an electrical impulse, the membrane becomes increasingly permeable to sodium. As sodium ions enter the cell, the membrane becomes depolarized, and calcium moves into the cell through voltage-sensitive calcium channels. Once calcium enters, potassium ions leave the cell, repolarizing the membrane.

Inside the cell, free calcium ions bind to troponin to alter the configuration and function of tropomyosin, the inhibitory protein bound to actin. The binding of troponin and tropomyosin allows actin and myosin to interact and form cross-links of electrochemical activity. As they do, the cardiac muscle shortens and contracts.

During final repolarization, troponin and tropomyosin resume their roles as actin-myosin inhibitors. Actin filaments slide away from each other and from the myosin filaments. The cardiac muscle then lengthens and relaxes.

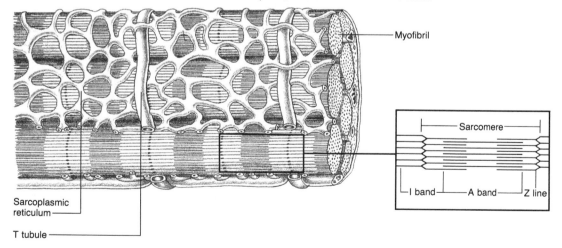

Myofibril

Sarcomere

I band — A band — Z line

Sarcoplasmic reticulum

T tubule

Precipitating causes include specific incidents that lead to heart failure in patients at risk. Such incidents, accounting for nearly 50% of heart failure episodes, include dysrhythmias, systemic infection, pulmonary embolism, stress, and noncompliance with therapy. Asymptomatic patients with silent cardiac defects are also susceptible; activities that strain myocardial capacity or impair ventricular filling can precipitate heart failure.

Understanding cardiac output

Whatever its cause, reduced myocardial blood flow reduces cardiac output. Probably the most important hemodynamic measurement, cardiac output is the amount of blood ejected by the left ventricle into the aorta in 1 minute. This volume typically ranges from 4 to 8 liters/minute. Normally, the heart automatically increases or decreases its output to serve the body's immediate needs. (See *The normal cardiac cycle.*) But in CHF, the normal heart cycle is compromised, and the compensatory mechanisms that maintain sufficient cardiac output eventually break down. (See *Conditions affecting cardiac output,* page 142.)

    Stroke volume. Cardiac output (CO) is the product of stroke volume (SV) and heart rate (HR), as expressed in the formula: $CO = SV \times HR$. The stroke volume, the difference between the volume in the left ventricle at the end of diastole and the volume at the end of systole, measures the milliliters of blood ejected from the left ventricle during a single contraction. Stroke volume is influenced by three factors: preload, afterload, and contractility. (To remember these factors, memorize the initials, P-A-C.) Let's briefly review each.

    Preload. Defined as the ventricular volume plus pressure at the end of diastole, preload determines myocardial fiber length when ventricular contraction begins. Fiber length then determines the force of the contraction and the speed of muscle fiber shortening. Several physiologic factors determine preload: filling pressure, venous return, atrial pressure, and left ventricular end-diastolic pressure. Low cardiac output results if any of these indices are chronically raised or lowered. If preload is low, ventricular volume and pressure are insufficient to fill and stretch

The normal cardiac cycle

The cardiac cycle begins with isovolumetric ventricular contraction. During this phase, the ventricular membranes depolarize and the ventricles contract. This increases ventricular pressure, which closes the mitral and tricuspid valves, preventing the backward flow of ventricular blood. All four valves close momentarily at the end of this phase. In ventricular ejection, the next phase, ventricular pressure exceeds aortic and pulmonary arterial pressure. The aortic and pulmonic valves open to release the ventricular blood.

In the isovolumetric relaxation phase, ventricular pressure drops sharply below that of the aorta and pulmonary artery without a change in volume, and the aortic and pulmonic valves close. *Note:* Atrial diastole occurs now as blood fills the atria.

During the ventricular filling phase, atrial pressure eventually exceeds ventricular pressure, which opens the mitral and tricuspid valves. Blood flows passively into the ventricles. About 80% of ventricular filling occurs now.

Atrial systole, the last phase, coincides with late ventricular diastole, when the atria contract in response to atrial depolarization. This "atrial kick" supplies the ventricles with the remaining 20% of blood. Then the cycle begins again.

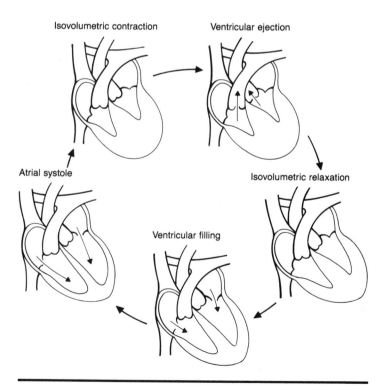

Isovolumetric contraction

Ventricular ejection

Isovolumetric relaxation

Ventricular filling

Atrial systole

Conditions affecting cardiac output

Many physiologic or disease states can affect cardiac output and increase the risk of heart failure. Some examples of conditions that alter preload, afterload, and heart rate, and impair contractility are given below.

Altered preload	Altered afterload	Altered heart rate	Impaired contractility
• *Elevated preload:* damaged left ventricle, where force of systolic contraction is impaired (as in myocardial infarction); hypervolemia; or aortic or mitral regurgitation • *Depressed preload:* hypovolemia, abnormal vasodilation, positive intrathoracic pressure, restrictive cardiomyopathy, or constrictive pericarditis	• *Elevated afterload:* intense vasoconstriction, pulmonic or aortic stenosis, atherosclerosis, systemic or pulmonary hypertension, pulmonary emboli, or increased blood viscosity • *Depressed afterload:* massive vasodilation associated with neurogenic, septic, or anaphylactic shock	• *Tachycardia* from infection, hyperthyroidism, fear, stress, exercise, or pain • *Bradycardia* from MI, dysrhythmias, increased intracranial pressure, or drugs such as digitalis	• *Coronary artery disease* • *Dilated cardiomyopathy*

the myocardial fibers at the end of diastole. High preload overstretches the fibers, making ejection of blood from the ventricle incomplete.

Afterload. To eject its contents into the aorta during systole, the left ventricle must work against considerable resistance. This resistance, or afterload, is influenced by arterial blood pressure, valve characteristics, and ventricular radius and wall thickness. Factors that raise aortic pressure or impede aortic outflow, such as a stenotic aortic valve, atherosclerosis, or elevated hematocrit, cause the ventricle to work harder to open the aortic valve. The increased work load raises myocardial oxygen demand.

Contractility. The ventricle's ability to contract when stimulated depends on several factors:
• initial muscle length—In a relationship known as the *Frank-Starling mechanism,* ventricular muscle fibers lengthen (within limits) in response to increased stretch (generated by preload) to eject larger amounts of blood with greater force.
• chemical composition—Myocardial cells require optimum quantities of calcium, potassium, magnesium, hydrogen, and oxygen for effective contraction.

• sympathetic stimulation—Myocardial contractility is enhanced when catecholamines, released by the adrenal medulla, enhance calcium exchange across cell membranes.

Heart rate. The other major component of cardiac output, heart rate, is primarily influenced by the autonomic nervous system. Parasympathetic nerves release acetylcholine, which depresses sinoatrial (SA) node automaticity, slows conduction through the atrioventricular (AV) junction, and decreases heart rate (for example, in vagus nerve stimulation caused by acute nausea). Sympathetic nerves release norepinephrine, which enhances SA node automaticity, increases AV junction conduction, and increases heart rate (as in exercise, fear, pain, or stress). Heart rate has an inverse relationship with stroke volume. It works this way:

• If stroke volume decreases, heart rate increases to maintain cardiac output; if stroke volume increases, heart rate decreases.
• If heart rate decreases, stroke volume increases; if heart rate increases, stroke volume decreases.

Pathophysiology

Any abnormality that chronically alters cardiac output (preload, afterload, contractility, or heart rate) increases the risk of heart failure. The heart tries to compensate for the reduced cardiac output and manages to sustain adequate circulatory volume for a time. But the heart's compensation mechanisms are limited. Compensation may last during periods of low metabolic oxygen demand, but cardiac output at maximum work load may be increased, normal, or reduced. And when deficient myocardial contraction or hemodynamic burden persists, the compensatory mechanisms eventually fail, resulting in heart failure.

Reduced cardiac output triggers three compensating mechanisms in the heart.

Frank-Starling mechanism (ventricular dilation). Increased preload causes increased stroke work and stroke volume during contraction. In response, the sarcomeres (the functional units of the myocardial cells) lengthen, increasing the overlap between thick and thin myofilaments to enhance contraction. Although increases in preload raise stroke volume, at some point the myocardial fibers stretch beyond their optimum length and stroke volume decreases, causing pulmonary congestion that leads to right ventricular failure.

Increased sympathetic activity. Decreased cardiac output and blood pressure stimulate the adrenergic cardiac nerves and the adrenal medulla to secrete catecholamines, which augment myocardial contraction. Arteriolar vasoconstriction enhances blood flow to the vital organs, while venoconstriction increases venous return to the heart. Increased sympathetic activity also restricts blood flow to the kidneys, which respond by reducing the glomerular filtration rate and increasing tubular reabsorption of salt and water. This renal mechanism, if unchecked, can aggravate congestion and produce overt edema.

Ventricular hypertrophy. Increased muscle mass or diameter of the left ventricle helps the heart pump against increased resistance. However, the increase in ventricular diastolic pressure needed to fill the enlarged ventricle may compromise diastolic coronary blood flow. This limits the oxygen supply to the ventricle, causing ischemia and impaired contractility.

Pathologic changes in CHF

As compensatory mechanisms fail, numerous changes take place in myocardial cells, affecting contractility and pump response to preload and afterload.

Cellular degeneration. Myofibril mitochondria decrease in size but increase in number, and the intercalated disks become thickened and irregular. Sarcoplasmic calcium release slows down, resulting in defective myofibril contraction. Under these deteriorating conditions, the work load becomes acute and excessive. In the early stages of heart failure, mitochondrial metabolism increases. As heart failure progresses, protein synthesis occurs, and more myofilaments form into sarcomeres. But as ventricular pressure increases, the mitochondria become severely edematous and inefficient, and then degenerate. With mitochondrial rupture, the energy-producing metabolic processes of the cells are destroyed. This process occurs in all types of heart failure.

Preload and heart failure. Reduced myocardial contractility decreases force velocity and increases resting fiber length. The more the end-diastolic volume exceeds physiologic limits, the less fiber lengths shorten once the heart has failed. Reduced contractility reduces cardiac output, which leads to compensatory cardiac enlargement. Eventually, however, cardiac enlargement fails to maintain cardiac performance. As the ventricles enlarge, heart-wall tension increases. This drives oxygen consumption up until it exceeds the supply, whereupon the heart dilates and cardiac performance decreases.

Afterload and heart failure. In heart failure, increased afterload reduces stroke volume. As heart failure progresses, more contractility is used to generate tension and less is used for myocardial shortening. Therefore, systolic ventricular pressure rises more slowly than normal, and the ventricle takes longer to overcome resistance before it can eject blood.

Contractility and heart failure. Cardiac norepinephrine is often depleted in heart failure, and cardiac adrenergic stimulation produces a reduced myocardial inotropic response. Because the sympathetic stimulation cannot elevate ventricular performance to normal levels, no improvement in contractility takes place during exercise.

Cardiac and systemic changes

Heart failure usually begins in the left ventricle. When ventricular output begins to fail, baroreceptors in the aorta and other areas cause reflex stimulation of the sympathetic nervous system, which causes vasoconstriction, venoconstriction, and increased contractility and heart rate.

These changes also reduce blood flow to the kidneys. Special cells in renal arterioles detect the decrease and release renin. This stimulates the renin-angiotensin-aldosterone system, leading to vasoconstriction and sodium and water retention. Initially, this compensatory mechanism helps restore cardiac output by increasing blood pressure, augmenting blood volume, and generally improving venous return to the heart. (See *Atrial natriuretic peptide: The heart's hormone,* page 146.) But when heart failure progresses despite compensation, decompensation begins. As the heart beats faster, it demands more oxygen. However, a faster heart rate also shortens diastole, reducing ventricular filling time. As a result, the left ventricle supplies even less oxygenated blood to the coronary arteries.

Atrial natriuretic peptide: The heart's hormone

Atrial natriuretic peptide (ANP), also known as atriopeptin, is a newly discovered cardiac hormone that helps regulate cardiovascular and renal homeostasis. Stored in the heart's atrial cells, ANP selectively but potently modifies blood pressure and fluid and electrolyte balance.

Stored as atriopeptigen, the hormone circulates as ANP, acting through extracellular receptors. It directly affects the kidneys, causing changes in sodium and water metabolism, such as increased urinary sodium excretion, diuresis, aldosterone inhibition, and vasopressin suppression (when vasopressin is elevated as a result of dehydration or hemorrhage).

ANP helps control blood pressure by suppressing elevated serum renin levels and relaxing blood vessels directly, thus reducing vascular resistance.

Although ANP is still under study, evidence suggests that the heart's atria release small amounts of ANP continuously but secrete more during atrial stretch. Basal ANP levels measured by radioimmunoassay range from 10 to 70 pg/ml. ANP levels rise with such diseases as chronic renal failure and congestive heart failure and with conditions causing atrial stretch, such as postural changes, saline solution infusion, use of vasoconstricting agents, high sodium intake, and atrial tachycardia. (Studies of patients with atrial tachycardia suggest that atriopeptin release results from increased cardiac pressures and intravascular volume. In these patients, ANP levels declined when tachycardia stopped.)

Ongoing studies continue to investigate how parenteral ANP affects diuresis, vasodilation, and aldosterone inhibition. Because ANP directly affects the kidneys' glomeruli, it may prove useful in patients with renal injury who become insensitive to tubular diuretics. By leading to substantial water and sodium loss without marked potassium depletion, it may have a clear advantage over conventional diuretics.

As heart failure progresses, peripheral vasoconstriction, which helped protect vital organs during compensation, contributes to decompensation. Vasoconstriction increases vascular resistance in turn, forcing the failing heart to pump even harder.

The renin-angiotensin-aldosterone system may also promote decompensation by overfilling the heart. As compensatory mechanisms eventually fail, volume overload leads to increased ventricular pressure and eventually imposes a self-perpetuating cycle of progressive deterioration. Left ventricular failure progresses from a compensated to a decompensated state; it then leads to right ventricular failure and, ultimately, to CHF.

Types of heart failure

Clinicians recognize several types of heart failure, based on rate of development, degree of output failure, or the physiologic defect that produces the predominant signs and symptoms. These include acute or chronic, low-output or high-output, systolic or diastolic, forward or backward, right or left ventricular failure, and refractory heart failure.

Acute or chronic heart failure. In *chronic heart failure,* inadequate cardiac output develops gradually, as in hypertension, CAD, and cardiomyopathy. In such patients, the compensatory mechanisms have time to partially or completely restore normal output, but conditions that increase oxygen demand (such as exercise, stress, infection, or further myocardial deterioration) can precipitate another episode of heart failure. In *acute heart failure,* impaired ventricular function and oxygen delivery occur suddenly, as in MI, extreme bradycardia, and acute pulmonary emboli. The sudden reduction in perfusion reduces cardiac output and causes symptoms. The body's compensatory mechanisms are not involved.

High-output or low-output heart failure. In *high-output failure,* the increased metabolic oxygen demands brought on by certain diseases and conditions (such as anemia, pregnancy, early septic shock, hyperthyroidism, and pulmonary emphysema) force the heart to increase its output. As a result, heart rate and venous return increase, plasma volume expands, and blood circulates faster than normal. Eventually, the greater metabolic demand overburdens the heart, leading to ventricular dysfunction and inadequate cardiac output. In high-output failure, cardiac output is normal or higher than normal but is insufficient to meet the body's excessive oxygen demands. In *low-output failure,* the heart is unable to meet normal metabolic oxygen demands because of abnormal stroke volume or heart rate.

Systolic or diastolic heart failure. *Systolic failure* refers to abnormalities in contraction during systole, which prevent ventricular ejection of blood. Inadequate forward output reduces systemic pressure and delivery of blood through the arterial system to the vital organs. The resulting ischemia causes decreased urine output and mental confusion. Acute, massive pulmonary embolism or dilated cardiomyopathy produces systolic failure. *Diastolic failure* refers to abnormalities in ventricular filling during diastole resulting from incomplete ventricular relaxation, acute myocardial ischemia, myocardial hypertrophy, or restrictive cardiomyopathy. High ventricular and venous pressures cause both pulmonary and systemic congestion.

Forward or backward heart failure. *Forward failure,* caused by compromised left ventricular function, reduces systemic pressure and delivery of blood through the arterial circulation to vital organs. Angina, decreased urine output, and mental confusion result from ischemia in the corresponding organs. *Backward failure* occurs when the left ventricle fails to eject blood. As ventricular blood backs up into the pulmonary and systemic veins, the volume and pressure in the venous and capillary beds rise. When this increased pulmonary vascular pressure causes hydrostatic pressure to exceed osmotic pressure, fluid moves from the pulmonary capillary beds into the interstitial space, causing congestion. The resulting symptoms include shortness of breath, orthopnea, cough, and auscultatory crackles. Backward failure of the right ventricle produces elevated systemic venous pressures and tissue congestion.

Most patients with CHF have symptoms of both forward and backward heart failure; however, patients with acute failure may develop only one set of symptoms.

Right or left ventricular failure. *Right ventricular failure* causes sequestration of fluid into interstitial spaces. Elevated systemic venous pressure, edema, fatigue, and possibly ascites result. *Left ventricular failure* primarily produces pulmonary effects, including pulmonary capillary hypertension, dyspnea, and fatigue. Although one ventricle is primarily affected, the excessive work load on the functioning heart eventually leads to biventricular (congestive) failure.

Refractory heart failure. This term describes severely diseased heart muscle that does not respond to any treatment.

Case study: Part 2

Mrs. Baldwin had a significant family history of cardiac disease. Her father had died after an MI at age 59, and her mother was hypertensive. The patient had developed hypertension herself 4 years earlier and was taking 50 mg of captopril three times a day. Postmenopausal and moderately overweight, she'd stopped smoking cigarettes after her MI after smoking one pack per day for the past 43 years.

Emergency assessment revealed that the patient was acutely short of breath, had a respiratory rate of 30 breaths/minute, and used accessory neck muscles to breathe. Crackles were audible at both lung bases on inspiration; her chest X-ray showed moderate congestion and Kerley's B lines. Mrs. Baldwin's jugular veins distended approximately 5 cm (2″) from the sternal angle, and her skin was pale, warm, and moist with sluggish capillary refill and obvious clubbing of the fingernails. Suspecting a developing new MI along with CHF, the doctor ordered a 12-lead ECG and cardiac enzyme analysis.

Mrs. Baldwin's blood pressure was 80/50 mm Hg. Sinus tachycardia (140 beats/minute) with occasional premature ventricular contractions (PVCs) was noted on the cardiac monitor. Auscultation revealed a gallop rhythm (S_3). Peripheral pulses were equal and full. The point of maximum impulse was palpable at the fifth intercostal space, on the anterior axillary line, and over a 5-cm area.

When the laboratory report showed normal cardiac enzyme levels and the 12-lead ECG was unchanged from the patient's previous ECG at discharge, the doctor ruled out a new MI. Mrs. Baldwin, he concluded, was experiencing acute CHF.

Three of Mrs. Baldwin's children arrived to join their oldest sister after their mother's condition began to deteriorate. They were having a difficult time accepting her illness, especially since their father had died so recently. The primary nurse spoke with the family and decided to call the hospital counselor to assist the family in this crisis.

Assessment and diagnosis

Obtain a complete health history. This should go beyond the patient's chief complaints, symptoms, and physical signs to include his medical, family, and social history as well; however, collecting data about family and social history may have to be postponed until the crisis has subsided. This information helps you gauge the severity of failure, identify the involved heart chambers, and identify psychological factors that can impair healing.

Signs and symptoms

In most patients with CHF, abnormal findings result from expanding blood volume, congestion of the pulmonary and systemic vascular bed, and excessive sodium and water retention. The classic signs and symptoms of CHF include gradually progressing shortness of breath (dyspnea) and cough, followed by weight gain and edema, fatigue, weakness, and renal and abdominal symptoms. (See *CHF: Signs and symptoms,* page 150.)

CHF: Signs and symptoms

As a rule, expect pulmonary signs and symptoms (especially breathlessness or dyspnea) in left ventricular failure and systemic signs and symptoms (especially peripheral edema) in right ventricular failure. Read the following for details on how signs and symptoms differ.

Left ventricular failure	Right ventricular failure
Elevated blood pressure	Weakness
Fatigue	Hepatomegaly with or without pain
Paroxysmal nocturnal dyspnea, dyspnea on exertion, orthopnea	Ascites
Bronchial wheezing	Dependent pitting peripheral edema, sacral edema
Hypoxia, respiratory acidosis	Jugular vein distention
Crackles	Hepatojugular reflux
Cough with or without frothy pink sputum	Dysrhythmias
Cyanosis or pallor	Elevated central venous or right atrial pressure
Third or fourth heart sound	Nausea, vomiting, anorexia, abdominal distention
Palpitations, dysrhythmias	Weight gain
Elevated pulmonary artery diastolic and pulmonary capillary wedge pressures	
Pulsus alternans	
Nocturia	
Oliguria	

Dyspnea. Transudation of fluid into the interstitial spaces (because hydrostatic pressure exceeds oncotic pressure) increases pulmonary venous pressure, causing pulmonary congestion and impairment of alveolar capillary gas exchange. The patient's lungs become less compliant and airway resistance increases, producing symptoms of breathlessness. In heart failure, the patient's breathing pattern is rapid and shallow, as opposed to the long, deep breaths that are typical of dyspnea in anxiety neurosis. In right ventricular failure, dyspnea is uncommon except when pulmonary disease exists, as in pulmonary hypertension or pulmonary thromboembolic disease.

Several types of dyspnea commonly occur in patients with left ventricular failure: exertional dyspnea, orthopnea, paroxysmal nocturnal dyspnea, and dyspnea at rest.

Exertional dyspnea occurs during increased physical activity. Although dyspnea normally occurs during physical exertion, the progressive shortness of breath while performing an ordinary activity distinguishes dyspnea caused by heart abnormalities from that caused by poor conditioning.

Orthopnea is shortness of breath that occurs only when the patient is in a reclining position. Orthopnea develops suddenly after the patient lies down and disappears when he uses pillows to raise his head above trunk level. The recumbent position causes a sudden increase in venous return. Because this extra volume cannot be managed by the already compromised ventricle, it backs up in the pulmonary system. The number of pillows needed to relieve breathlessness is a measure of the severity of orthopnea. In severe CHF, patients may have to sleep sitting upright in a chair.

Paroxysmal nocturnal dyspnea (PND) is acute shortness of breath that occurs after prolonged recumbency, usually during sleep. Patients often awaken feeling anxious and suffocated, which forces them to sit upright. As blood pools to the periphery, the preload burden on the heart lessens, which usually enables patients to return to sleep within 15 to 20 minutes. Nightmares, restless sleep, or anxiety, which stimulate sympathetic activity, may initiate PND. Other possible physiologic causes include slowed respiratory rate and sympathetic nerve activity during sleep, increased thoracic blood volume upon recumbency, and the slow resorption of interstitial fluid. Cardiac asthma is a common complication of PND. It increases respiratory distress in CHF patients through congestion of the bronchial mucosa.

Dyspnea at rest is the inability to carry out most activities because of breathlessness. Such dyspnea can be so severe that the patient may have difficulty finishing a sentence or climbing a few stairs.

Cough. Lung congestion may initially produce a dry, nonproductive cough that occurs during exercise or while the patient is recumbent. It may accompany noisy breathing. Later, as the lungs absorb more fluid because of the increased pulmonary capillary hydrostatic pressure, the patient may cough up blood-stained sputum.

Weight gain and edema. Increased blood volume, fluid accumulation in the venous system, and systemic congestion produce weight gain and edema. As a result of hypoperfusion to the kidney and the resulting renin-angiotensin system compensatory response, hydrostatic pressure falls below osmotic pressure. These pressure changes favor reabsorption of sodium and water, which raises circulating blood volume, causing weight gain.

The backup of venous blood returning to the heart in right ventricular failure causes fluid accumulation and edema. Fluid accumulates first in the ankles and feet, the dependent portion of the body; it later progresses to the legs, thighs, and even the abdomen (ascites) and upper limbs. The patient may complain that rings, shoes, and belts have become too tight. In a bedridden patient, the sacrum is dependent and is commonly affected first. In advanced CHF, edema may be generalized over the entire body, a condition known as anasarca. Clinically, edema is not usually apparent until 5 to 10 lb (2.3 to 4.5 kg) of excess fluid accumulate.

Fatigue and weakness. Patients may complain of heaviness in the limbs, lassitude, or the inability to function at previous activity levels. Decreased blood flow to the skeletal muscles is partly responsible for the gradual awareness of fatigue and weakness, but the use of diuretics, work of breathing, and general exhaustion from poor sleeping patterns also contribute to fatigue.

Renal and abdominal symptoms. Nocturia results from diminished oxygen demands and work load on the heart during sleep. As renal vessels receive more blood, urine formation increases. In late heart failure, oliguria results from low cardiac output.

As systemic congestion spreads to the abdomen, edema can produce a sense of fullness in the abdomen and may cause anorexia, nausea, and vomiting. If congestion involves the liver, the patient may also complain of tenderness in the right upper quadrant.

Assessment of CHF

Your assessment of the CHF patient will vary, depending on the location of heart failure (left, right, or both), type of heart failure (such as low-output or high-output), and onset (acute or chronic).

General appearance. The patient with mild or moderate CHF may not exhibit any symptoms while at rest; however, on exertion, shortness of breath becomes apparent. (See *Classification of heart disease.*) A patient recovering from a recent episode of severe CHF appears well nourished but acutely ill. In contrast, a chronic patient looks malnourished despite edema and may have visible systolic pulsation of the eyes. A patient with severe heart failure appears anxious, acutely dyspneic, and may look jaundiced, flushed, or cyanotic. In such a patient, decreased blood flow to the extremities produces pallor and coldness due to delayed capillary refill time, and increased adrenergic nervous system activity produces cyanotic digits, diaphoresis with tachycardia, and distended peripheral veins.

Cardiovascular assessment. In the patient with CHF, the *pulse* will often reflect changes in stroke volume. A strong bounding pulse that alternates with a weak, thready one (pulsus alternans) commonly occurs in severe left ventricular failure. In this situation, the pulse rhythm is regular, but the contractions alternate in intensity. The variable pulse reflects changes in contractility and stroke volume.

You'll usually detect *pulsus alternans* while assessing the patient's blood pressure. Auscultations reveal alternately loud and soft Korotkoff sounds or a sudden doubling of the apparent heart rate sometime after the systolic pressure. An elevated pulse rate may also reflect compensatory cardiac effort to overcome inadequate oxygenation and perfusion of peripheral tissue. In patients with moderate CHF, the pulse rate does not usually rise above 100 beats/minute, but patients with severe failure may have tachycardia. Atrial fibrillation, atrial flutter, premature atrial and ventricular contractions, and ventricular tachycardia may also be present.

A *narrowed pulse pressure* may develop in low-output failure as systolic pressure drops in a proportionately greater degree than diastolic pressure. In contrast, blood pressure in high-output failure may be normal or elevated. Elevated blood pressure reflects the hyperdynamic state of high cardiac output and increased metabolic requirements. If you think of systolic pressure as cardiac output and of diastolic pressure as afterload, the trend in blood pressures becomes obvious.

The patient's *blood pressure* may be normal or reduced in low-output failure. Compensatory mechanisms (vasoconstriction,

Classification of heart disease

The following classification system developed by the New York Heart Association describes the severity of heart disease according to the amount of effort required to provoke symptoms. This classification system is useful in comparing groups of patients as well as the same patient at different times.

Class 1
No limitation: The patient tolerates ordinary physical activity without undue fatigue, dyspnea, or palpitations.

Class II
Slight limitation of physical activity: The patient is comfortable at rest, but ordinary physical activity causes fatigue, palpitations, dyspnea, or angina.

Class III
Marked limitation of physical activity: The patient is comfortable at rest, but light activity will lead to symptoms.

Class IV
Inability to carry on any physical activity without discomfort: The patient has symptoms of congestive heart failure even at rest and experiences increased discomfort with any activity.

Assessing for hepatojugular reflux

If you suspect right ventricular failure, assess for hepatojugular reflux. With the patient seated at a 30- to 45-degree angle, compress the abdomen over the liver for approximately 30 seconds while observing for an increase in jugular vein distention (see illustration). The increased blood flow caused by the abdominal compression raises venous pressure, for which patients with right ventricular failure cannot compensate. This action will increase the forward flow of blood to the right atrium, elevating jugular venous pressure and distending jugular veins. A positive finding is reported as hepatojugular reflux.

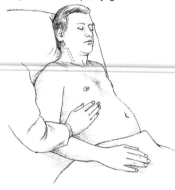

hormonal activation) temporarily maintain blood pressure at normal levels, but when these run their course, blood pressure decreases.

Inspection or palpation of the patient's chest may reveal a *change in the point of maximum impulse* (PMI), the point at which the apical pulse occurs. The PMI results from left ventricular contraction; it is the thrust of the left ventricle against the chest wall. Normally, the PMI is located at the fifth intercostal space and the midclavicular line. In left ventricular failure, it shifts left toward the axillary line. Usually, the greater the shift of the PMI, the greater the damage to the left ventricle.

Auscultation of heart sounds may reveal *a third heart sound* (S_3) in the CHF patient. Usually considered a normal finding in children and in adults under age 30, S_3 is abnormal in adults over age 30. As blood rushes through the open AV (mitral and tricuspid) valves early in diastole, it strikes a distended, damaged, stiff, or incompetent ventricular wall. The sharp acceleration of ventricular inflow that occurs immediately with the early filling phase creates the S_3. The S_3 and tachycardia may produce a rhythm that sounds like a galloping horse. An S_3 gallop is one of the earliest signs of left ventricular failure in adults.

To check for *left ventricular gallop,* listen at the apex of the heart with the patient in the left lateral recumbent position. Sometimes the rhythm is palpable when the patient is in this position. To check for *right ventricular gallop,* listen at the left sternal edge in the fourth or fifth intercostal space with the patient supine. You may detect a fourth heart sound (S_4), caused by decreased ventricular compliance associated with ischemic heart disease, hypertension, cardiomegaly, or advanced age.

Systolic murmurs, caused by mitral or triscuspid regurgitation resulting from ventricular dilatation, are common in heart failure. Such murmurs diminish or disappear when compensation is restored.

Check for *elevated jugular venous pressure,* an important sign of CHF. Because of backward failure and pulmonary hypertension, the patient's right ventricle fails as it struggles to pump against the resistance created by the pulmonary congestion of left ventricular failure. The elevated ventricular and atrial pressures produce congestion in the right atrium, inferior and superior venae cavae, and jugular veins. Normally, jugular veins are not visible more than 3 cm (1¼″) above the sternal angle when the patient is in a 30- to 45-degree position. But with elevated pressures, the jugular veins become visibly distended; the amount of distention usually relates to the degree of venous pressure elevation. Most clinicians consider jugular vein distention of 3 to 5 cm (1¼″ to 2″) as moderate and above 5 cm as severe.

Respiratory assessment. If your patient has left ventricular failure, you'll need to check for signs of pulmonary congestion and increased work of breathing. *Tachypnea, visible shortness of breath,* and the *use of the accessory muscles* in the neck to assist breathing are classic signs.

Auscultation of breath sounds usually reveals *crackles,* caused by air moving across fluid-filled tissue. Fluid within the alveoli produces fine crackles, whereas fluid within the lumens of bronchioles and bronchi produces coarse crackles. Crackles may be heard unilaterally but are usually bilateral.

Abdominal assessment. Physical inspection may detect the systemic congestion and edema characteristic of right ventricular failure. The increased systemic capillary pressure forces fluid into tissues, producing visible enlargement and possibly liver tenderness. Congestive hepatomegaly commonly develops before overt edema, and it may persist after other signs and symptoms have disappeared. Epigastric fullness, dullness in the right upper quadrant, hepatic pulsations, ascites, and splenomegaly may also be present.

Signs of *systemic congestion,* such as an engorged liver, ascites, and edema, are usually late signs of CHF. When performing the abdominal assessment, be sure to also assess for hepatojugular reflux, seen in patients with right ventricular failure. Such reflux is a sign that the right ventricle cannot accommodate increased blood flow without a corresponding rise in venous pressure. (See *Assessing for hepatojugular reflux.*)

Extremities assessment. *Peripheral edema* is the most common symptom of heart failure in patients who are ambulatory. Capillary hydrostatic pressure rises, causing fluid to move out of the capillaries to the interstitial tissues. You should grade and record the severity of peripheral edema on each extremity.

To distinguish between edema of heart failure and lymph-edema, you need to determine the degree of pitting that results from finger compression. Edema from heart failure tends to appear pitted, or indented, whereas edema from lymphedema does not. A scale of $1+$ to $4+$ (with $4+$ the most severe indentation) is used to quantify pitting subjectively: up to $\frac{1}{4}'' = 1+$; $\frac{1}{4}''$ to $\frac{1}{2}'' = 2+$; $\frac{1}{2}''$ to $1'' = 3+$; greater than $1'' = 4+$.

Renal assessment. When reduced blood flow to the kidneys decreases the glomerular filtration rate, expect urine output to be less than fluid intake.

Systemic assessment. In a patient with severe chronic CHF, expect *low-grade fever* and *cardiac cachexia*—a profound state of general ill health and malnutrition. Such fever usually subsides when cardiac output improves, but cachexia may lead to anorexia from hepatic and intestinal congestion and, occasionally, from digitalis intoxication.

Diagnostic tests and results

Diagnostic tests gauge the severity of CHF, help determine treatment options, and provide data about the effectiveness of treatments. Useful diagnostic tests include routine laboratory studies, chest X-ray, radionuclide imaging, and possibly echocardiography, cardiac catheterization, angiography, and myocardial biopsy. Assessing hemodynamic parameters and their trends is also valuable.

Laboratory studies. Although routine blood tests and urinalysis cannot diagnose CHF, they help gauge the effectiveness of treatment and may signal the onset of CHF complications.

Blood tests provide information about renal blood flow, glomerular filtration rate, impaired fibrinogen synthesis, the effects of dietary and drug therapy, and impaired hepatic function. Some common findings from blood testing include:
• moderately elevated blood urea nitrogen and creatinine levels
• low erythrocyte sedimentation rate
• normal serum electrolyte values (except during prolonged sodium restriction, which can lead to hyponatremia, and in prolonged use of kaliuretics or loop diuretics, which can lead to hypokalemia)
• abnormal levels of aspartate aminotransferase (AST), formerly SGOT, and other liver enzymes such as bilirubin
• possible elevated leukocyte count with increased hematocrit.

Urinalysis in CHF commonly reveals proteinuria and high urine specific gravity.

Arterial blood gas (ABG) analyses usually show a low partial pressure of oxygen in arterial blood (PaO_2), normal or decreased partial pressure of carbon dioxide in arterial blood ($PaCO_2$), and mild respiratory alkalosis.

Chest X-ray. The chest X-ray remains the most useful non-invasive diagnostic test in heart failure. Size and shape of the cardiac silhouette reveal the underlying defect in heart failure. Though details of the cardiothoracic ratio and heart volume appear on film, they are not sensitive indicators of increased left ventricular end-diastolic volume.

Analysis of the lung bases indicates the degree of pulmonary edema. With a slightly elevated pulmonary capillary pressure (13 to 17 mm Hg), the vessels to the apexes and bases appear equal in size. At higher pressures (18 to 23 mm Hg), blood vessels leading to the lower lobes constrict while upper lobe vessels dilate. Pulmonary capillary pressures of 30 mm Hg produce interstitial pulmonary edema, which manifests on film as Kerley's lines, blurred central and peripheral vessels, and spindle-shaped accumulations of fluid. Alveolar edema and large pleural effusions from pressures greater than 30 mm Hg may cause a butterfly pattern to appear around the hila. And elevations in systemic venous pressure enlarge the azygos vein and superior vena cava.

Radionuclide imaging tests. Tests like multiple-gated acquisition scanning assess the patient's ejection fraction and wall motion.

Ejection fraction commonly ranges between 60% and 70% (normally, 33% of blood remains in the ventricle). Depressed ejection fraction indicates poor cardiac output and increased probability of decompensation and heart failure. In severe CHF, patients may have ejection fractions as low as 13%. However, ejection fractions that fall below 20% should be verified with other tests of output volumes.

The evaluation of wall-motion abnormalities is an especially useful diagnostic tool in patients who show signs of CHF but have normal ejection fractions. Radionuclide imaging reveals heart movement during the cardiac cycle, which helps identify such wall-motion abnormalities as dyskinesia, hypokinesia, or akinesia. Abnormal, limited, or absent wall motion of the left ventricle indicates a high risk of CHF.

Other diagnostic tests. Echocardiography may reveal enlarged or dilated chambers, valvular defects, impaired contractile properties, and wall-motion abnormalities. Cardiac catheterization and angiography detect any suspected underlying coronary abnormalities and study ventricular function in patients requiring cardiac surgery. Myocardial biopsy identifies underlying myocarditis or cardiac myopathy.

Hemodynamic monitoring

Cardiologists most commonly use a pulmonary artery (PA) catheter to measure hemodynamic parameters, such as intracardiac pressures, cardiac output and cardiac index, systemic vascular resistance, and venous oxygen saturation. (See *Pulmonary artery catheter.*) Catheter transducers sensitive to blood flow and pressure transform hemodynamic data into a waveform, which is displayed on an oscilloscope. (See *Measuring heart pressures,* page 160.)

Intracardiac pressures. To understand intracardiac pressures measured by hemodynamic monitoring catheters, picture the heart and vascular system as a continuous loop with constantly changing pressure gradients that keep the blood moving. Hemodynamic monitoring records the gradients within the vessels and heart chambers. (See *Intracardiac pressures,* page 161, and *Hemodynamic values in CHF,* page 162.) The pressures usually assessed by catheterization include central venous pressure and right atrial pressure; right ventricular pressure; pulmonary artery pressures, including pulmonary artery systolic and diastolic pressures; and pulmonary capillary wedge pressure.

Central venous pressure (CVP) and *right atrial pressure (RAP).* These pressures show right ventricular function and end-diastolic pressure (right ventricular preload). Normal CVP is 6 to 12 cm H_2O. Normal mean RAP ranges from 1 to 6 mm Hg. Increased CVP and RAP may signal right ventricular failure, volume overload, tricuspid valve stenosis or regurgitation, constrictive pericarditis, pulmonary hypertension, cardiac tamponade, or right ventricular infarction. Decreased RAP suggests reduced circulating blood volume.

Pulmonary artery catheter

Also known as the Swan-Ganz catheter, this balloon-tipped, multi-lumen device permits measurement of intracardiac pressures.

Insertion

The doctor inserts the catheter into the patient's internal jugular or subclavian vein. (In some cases, he'll use the basilar vein of the antecubital fossa.) When the catheter reaches the right atrium, the doctor inflates the balloon to help float the catheter through the right ventricle into the pulmonary artery. This permits pulmonary capillary wedge pressure (PCWP) meaurement through an opening at the catheter's tip. Deflated, the catheter rests in the pulmonary artery, taking diastolic and systolic pulmonary artery pressure readings.

Structure and function

Made of pliable radiopaque polyvinylchloride, the catheter may contain two to seven lumens.

The number of lumens determines which functions the catheter can perform. The distal lumen measures pulmonary artery pressures when connected to a transducer and measures PCWP during balloon inflation. This lumen also permits drawing of mixed venous blood samples. The proximal lumen measures right atrial pressure. The balloon inflation lumen inflates the balloon at the distal tip of the catheter for PCWP measurement. The thermistor connector lumen contains temperature-sensitive wires that feed information into a computer for cardiac output calculation. The pacemaker wire lumen, which provides a port for pacemaker electrodes, also allows measurement of mixed venous oxygen saturation when an Opticath catheter is used.

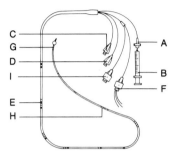

Key
A: Inflation lumen port to wedge balloon
B: Gauge for inflating balloon with 1 to 1.5 ml of air
C: Distal lumen port
D: Proximal lumen port
E: 10-cm markings
F: Pacemaker wire lumen
G: Distal lumen opening
H: Proximal lumen opening
I: Thermistor lumen port

Right ventricular pressure (RVP). In most cases, the doctor measures RVP only when initially inserting a PA catheter. Right ventricular systolic pressure normally equals pulmonary artery systolic pressure; right ventricular end-diastolic pressure, which reflects right ventricular function, equals RAP. Normal systolic pressure ranges from 15 to 25 mm Hg; normal diastolic pressure, from 0 to 8 mm Hg. RVP rises in mitral stenosis or insufficiency, pulmonary disease, hypoxemia, constrictive pericarditis, chronic CHF, atrial and ventricular septal defects, and patent ductus arteriosus.

Pulmonary artery pressures (PAPs). Two components are measured here. Pulmonary artery systolic pressure (PASP) shows right ventricular function and pulmonary circulation pressures. Pulmonary artery diastolic pressure (PADP) reflects left ventricular pressures, specifically left ventricular end-diastolic pressure,

Measuring heart pressures

As the pulmonary artery catheter passes through the right heart chambers to its wedge position, it produces distinctive waveforms showing the catheter's position on the oscilloscope screen.

RIGHT ATRIAL PRESSURE

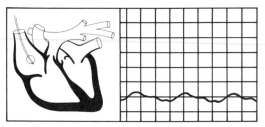

As the tip reaches the right atrium from the superior vena cava, the waveform looks like this.

RIGHT VENTRICULAR PRESSURE

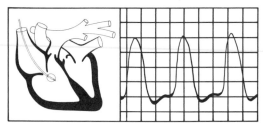

When the catheter tip reaches the right ventricle, the waveform looks like this.

PULMONARY ARTERY PRESSURE

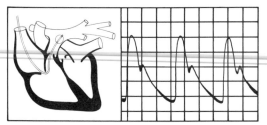

The waveform above indicates that the balloon has floated the catheter tip through the pulmonic valve into the pulmonary artery. The dicrotic notch reflects pulmonic valve closure.

PULMONARY CAPILLARY WEDGE PRESSURE

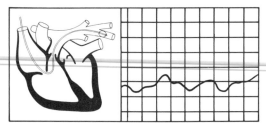

Blood flow in the pulmonary artery then carries the catheter balloon into a smaller pulmonary artery branch. When the vessel becomes too narrow for the balloon to pass through, the balloon wedges there and generates a waveform like this.

assessing left ventricular preload in a patient without significant pulmonary disease. PADP rises in left ventricular failure, increased pulmonary blood flow (left or right shunting, as in atrial or ventricular septal defects), and in any condition that increases pulmonary arteriolar resistance (such as pulmonary hypertension, volume overload, mitral stenosis, or hypoxia).

Pulmonary capillary wedge pressure (PCWP). Upon PA balloon catheter inflation, the catheter migrates to a small peripheral capillary within the pulmonary artery. Inflating the balloon fills the vessel and blocks any influence on the reading by pressures outside the left ventricle. Therefore, this method provides an accurate measure of left ventricular pressures. By effectively blocking off pressures behind the inflated balloon, it is a sensitive indicator of left ventricular pressures. The PCWP measured while the heart is in diastole most closely approximates the pressure present in the left ventricle during end diastole because the mitral valve is open. PCWP reflects left atrial and left ventricular pressures, assessing left ventricular preload, unless the patient has mitral stenosis. Changes in PAP and PCWP reflect changes in left ventricular filling pressure. The mean pressure normally ranges from 6 to 12 mm Hg. PCWP rises in left ventricular failure, mitral stenosis or insufficiency, and pericardial tamponade. PCWP decreases in hypovolemia. *Important:* The balloon must be totally deflated, except when taking a reading. Prolonged wedging may cause pulmonary infarction.

The PCWP measured while the heart is in systole monitors pressure only in the open channel between the balloon and the left atrium because the mitral valve is closed. This measurement most closely approximates left atrial filling pressure.

Cardiac output and cardiac index measurements. *Cardiac output,* the amount of blood ejected from the heart each minute, varies with a patient's weight, height, and body surface area. Adjusting the cardiac output to the patient's size yields a measurement called the *cardiac index.*

The cardiac index normally ranges from 2.5 to 4.2 liters/minute/m². You can calculate it using a nomogram and the formula: cardiac index = cardiac output (liters/minute)/body surface area (m²). But hemodynamic monitors determine cardiac output automatically from the injection of a solution of known temperature and volume through a PA catheter's proximal lumen. This solution mixes with the blood of the superior vena cava or right atrium (depending on the location of the PA catheter). When this mixed blood flows past a thermistor embedded in the PA catheter's distal end, the thermistor detects the temperature of the blood and solution and relays a signal to a computer, which calculates the cardiac output and displays it on a screen.

Systemic vascular resistance (SVR). SVR assesses left ventricular afterload, the resistance the heart works against to eject blood. As the arterioles constrict, SVR increases. You can deter-

Intracardiac pressures

This flowchart illustrates the commonly measured intracardiac pressures and their relationship to cardiopulmonary systems.

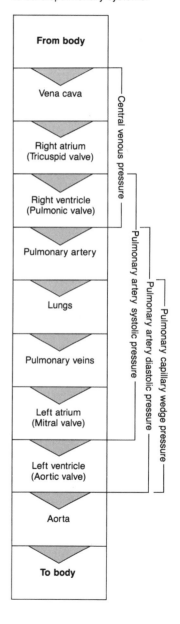

Hemodynamic values in CHF

Measurement	Normal values	Values in CHF
Right atrial pressure	1 to 6 mm Hg	>14 mm Hg
Central venous pressure	6 to 12 cm H_2O	>20 cm H_2O
Pulmonary artery systolic pressure	15 to 25 mm Hg	>35 mm Hg
Pulmonary artery diastolic pressure	0 to 8 mm Hg	>21 mm Hg
Pulmonary artery mean pressure	10 to 20 mm Hg	>23 mm Hg
Pulmonary capillary wedge pressure	6 to 12 mm Hg	>23 mm Hg
Cardiac output	4 to 8 liters/minute	<2 liters/minute
Cardiac index	2.4 to 4.2 liters/minute/m²	<1.8 liters/minute/m²
Systemic vascular resistance	900 to 1,500 dyne/sec/cm^{-5}	>1,800 dyne/sec/cm^{-5}
Venous oxygen saturation	60% to 75%	<52%

mine SVR using the formula: SVR = mean arterial pressure minus right atrial pressure/cardiac output × 80. SVR normally ranges from 900 to 1,500 dyne/second/cm^{-5}. *Note:* Pulmonary vascular resistance reflects right ventricular afterload.

Venous oxygen saturation (SvO_2). SvO_2 estimates the amount of oxygen in venous blood. Tissues normally extract only 25% to 40% of the oxygen from the blood, leaving a 60% to 75% reserve in venous blood that returns to the heart. If cardiac output falls, tissues extract more oxygen, leaving less venous reserve. SvO_2 levels below 60% indicate low cardiac output, and levels above 75% indicate blood shunting from the heart's left to right side. You can measure SvO_2 levels using a fiberoptic oximeter thermodilation PA catheter or from a blood sample drawn from the distal port of the PA catheter. (See *Diagnostic profile in CHF.*)

Case study: Part 3

The doctor immediately prescribed oxygen, 80 mg of furosemide I.V., and 0.25 mg of digoxin I.V. every 6 hours for 24 hours. Within 4 hours, Mrs. Baldwin's condition improved. Her urine output since admission was 2,400 ml, her blood pressure rose slightly to 86/50 mm Hg, her respiratory rate decreased, and her heart rate slowed. Once she was stabilized, the ED team transferred her to the CCU. On admission to the CCU, Mrs. Baldwin still had bibasilar crackles, a pulse rate of 98 beats/minute, a respiratory rate of 22 breaths/minute, and a blood pressure of 115/92 mm Hg. She was no longer using accessory muscles for respiration and her urine output was still increased. She was alert but still anxious and expressed concern for all the worry she was causing her children, who she felt were already suffering enough.

About 24 hours after admission, Mrs. Baldwin took a sudden turn for the worse. She was dyspneic, her skin was cool and clammy, her blood pressure dropped to 50/0 mm Hg, and her pulse was rapid and thready. Auscultation revealed bilateral crackles. The doctor ordered dopamine at an infusion rate of 5 to 10 mg/kg/minute, intermittent positive-pressure inhalation therapy, an ABG analysis, and a 12-lead ECG.

An indwelling (Foley) catheter that was inserted drained 50 ml of urine. The doctor inserted a PA catheter and began to monitor Mrs. Baldwin's pressures. Her PCWP measured 28 mm Hg; cardiac index, 1.8 liters/minute/m²; and SVR, 1,900 dyne/second/cm⁻⁵. Additional furosemide was given along with a 60-mg bolus of amrinone lactate over 3 minutes; sodium nitroprusside I.V. infusion was initiated at 3 mcg/kg/minute.

Despite these intensive interventions, the patient remained in critical condition. The family asked to see their mother because they felt she was so close to death. Even though it was not policy, the staff decided to allow the children to come in one at a time to hold their mother's hand. Before allowing them in, however, a nurse told them what to expect about the treatments being given and how to behave while in the room.

The doctor inserted an intra-aortic balloon pump (IABP) to mechanically assist perfusion and began counterpulsation because pharmacologic intervention didn't produce clinical improvement. The IABP counterpulsations proved effective, and Mrs. Baldwin's condition steadily improved. Her breathing was easier, her urine output improved, and her PAPs stabilized.

Diagnostic profile in CHF

Although CHF presents various clinical signs and symptoms, the following general statements can be made about diagnostic tests.
• CHF patients, except those with high-output failure, exhibit inadequate cardiac output at rest that doesn't improve with exercise. As a result, you can expect to see low venous oxygen saturation (SvO₂) levels because of increased oxygen removal by tissues in most CHF patients.
• In left ventricular failure, you can expect elevated pulmonary artery systolic, pulmonary artery diastolic, pulmonary artery mean, and pulmonary capillary wedge pressures; reduced cardiac output and cardiac index; and reduced SvO₂ levels.
• In left ventricular failure caused by hypertension or afterload defects, expect elevated systemic vascular resistance (SVR).
• In unilateral left ventricular failure, right atrial pressure or central venous pressure (CVP) commonly remains normal until the right ventricle fails. Although the CVP value has limited usefulness alone in unilateral left ventricular failure, combining CVP with urine output readings provides information on patient status. High CVP values and low urine output indicate possible heart failure, whereas low CVP and urine output indicate the need for fluids.
• High-output failure often presents a unique hemodynamic picture. With the increased cardiac ouput and rapid circulation, you can expect elevated or normal cardiac output and cardiac index, high pulmonary artery pressure, very high pulmonary capillary wedge pressure, decreased or normal SVR, normal or increased SvO₂ levels, and elevated CVP.

Treatment options

Treatment of CHF centers on improving cardiac output to increase oxygen delivery and on reducing left ventricular filling pressure to attenuate pulmonary venous and capillary pressures. The medical approach to CHF treatment is fourfold and involves:
• identifying and treating the underlying or precipitating cause
• improving myocardial contractility
• controlling sodium and water retention to maintain optimum preload
• reducing the heart's work load.

As always, treatment is individualized. The treatment plan must take into account the underlying cause and any associated illnesses as well as the patient's age, life-style, occupation, ability to comply with treatment, and physiologic response to therapy. Beginning interventions are usually simple and noninvasive but progress to aggressive and invasive measures, as required to relieve the signs and symptoms of CHF.

Interventions include general supportive measures, drug therapy, use of mechanical devices, and the ultimate treatment, total heart replacement. Several new and investigational therapies have also been developed.

Supportive measures

Supportive measures for the patient with CHF include rest, dietary restrictions, oxygen therapy, and removal of fluids.

Rest. To prevent decompensation, the patient must reduce physical activity and get adequate rest throughout the course of his disease. The severity of the disease determines the activity level. A patient with chronic heart failure typically can exercise just short of provoking symptoms, but one with severe disease must sharply restrict activity. Chair rest is preferable to bed rest because the upright position decreases venous return, which reduces heart rate, pulmonary congestion, heart work load, and the work of breathing.

Dietary restrictions. Dietary sodium restrictions greatly reduce the tendency to retain water. The usual CHF diet limits sodium intake to 3 g/day. As the severity of heart failure progresses, sodium may be restricted to 1 g or less per day.

Restricted water intake is usually not recommended in the long-term management of CHF unless a body sodium deficit or serum sodium dilution exists. However, in acute CHF management, water restriction may also be needed.

Oxygen therapy. Oxygen therapy increases alveolar oxygen concentrations and absorption across the alveolar wall to raise arterial oxygen levels. Patients with mild CHF receive oxygen via nasal cannula, which delivers a concentration of 30% to 40% oxygen at a rate of 6 liters/minute. If the patient's condition deteriorates, he'll receive oxygen according to monitored ABG levels, with oxygen concentrations increased to 40% to 60% with an oxygen mask or to 75% to 100% with specialized equipment.

Oxygen, intermittent positive-pressure breathing (IPPB), and aminophylline may be used together to reduce dyspnea, hypoxia, and pulmonary congestion. IPPB mechanically delivers air to the lungs. This creates a positive intrathoracic pressure, which distends the alveolar spaces, lessens interstitial and alveolar fluid accumulation, and decreases venous return. Aminophylline infusion dilates the bronchioles, decreasing pulmonary venous pressure and increasing contractile force.

Physical removal of fluids. Most CHF patients can eliminate excess fluids through diuresis, but some may need mechanical intervention, such as thoracentesis (for pleural effusion), peritoneal dialysis, hemodialysis, continuous ambulatory peritoneal dialysis, or continuous arteriovenous hemofiltration. Continuous arteriovenous hemofiltration was originally designed for critically ill renal failure patients but is now also used to manage fluid overload in unstable CHF patients.

Phlebotomy or rotating tourniquets are sometimes used to remove or distribute fluids in CHF patients. Phlebotomy decreases preload and the heart's work load. If approximately 500 ml of blood are removed from the venous system, venous return immediately decreases, resulting in improved hemodynamic status and fewer symptoms. Because drug therapy is usually as effective as phlebotomy, this technique is rarely used.

Rotating tourniquets also reduce preload in acute CHF patients by occluding venous return. Tourniquets, blood pressure cuffs, or automatically rotating cuffs applied to the upper and lower limbs decrease preload without affecting the arterial pulse. Though still recommended for treating patients with acute heart failure in mobile intensive care units and emergency departments, rotating tourniquets have not proved more effective than vasodilators in improving patients' clinical or hemodynamic status.

Drug therapy

Drug therapy in CHF commonly includes the use of inotropic drugs, diuretics, and vasodilators to reduce cardiac work load. The goal of treatment is to shift the ventricular function curve to the left. (See *Monitoring ventricular function.*)

Inotropic drugs. The inotropic drugs improve cardiac performance by boosting ventricular contractility. These agents include cardiac glycosides (digitalis, digoxin), nonglycoside inotropic drugs such as sympathomimetics (dopamine, dobutamine), and phosphodiesterase inhibitors (amrinone, milrinone). (See *Inotropic drugs in CHF,* pages 168 and 169.)

Diuretics. Decreasing total plasma volume causes a corresponding decline in preload or venous return to the heart. In the acute or unstable CHF patient, diuretic therapy should produce a negative fluid balance of approximately 700 ml/day or a weight loss of 1 to 2 lb/day. With its fluid burden relieved, the heart can more readily accept and pump an optimum quantity of blood.

Diuretics vary greatly in mechanism and site of action, potency, and adverse effects. Thiazides (such as chlorothiazide, hydrochlorothiazide, chlorthalidone, metalazone, quinethazone, and acetazolamide) and potassium-sparing diuretics (such as spironolactone, amiloride, and triamterene) act on the proximal and distal convoluted tubules to produce more efficient diuresis. Loop diuretics (such as furosemide, bumetanide, and ethacrynic acid) are more potent and interfere with chloride reabsorption at the loop of Henle. They improve cardiac function by decreasing volume load, but they can produce more severe adverse reactions than other diuretics. Excessive use of diuretics may cause dehydration, overcorrecting from volume overload to volume depletion. If diuretics diminish potassium stores, electrolyte imbalance may result. To prevent this life-threatening effect, monitor serum potassium levels and supplement potassium, as needed.

Use extreme care when giving loop diuretics to a patient with severe CHF or renal dysfunction because they may cause metabolic acidosis and hyperkalemia. In many cases, a combi-

Monitoring ventricular function

The ventricular function curve (Starling's curve) reflects the Frank-Starling mechanism: As preload increases, cardiac output increases—until myocardial fibers stretch beyond their optimal length. In other words, increasing preload beyond a certain point decreases stroke volume (cardiac output). Therefore, optimal preload is high enough to obtain optimal stroke volume, but not so high as to overstretch the myocardium and cause pulmonary congestion.

Plotting your patient's curve shows overall cardiac function and allows you to easily monitor therapeutic effectiveness and the patient's clinical trends. Shifting the curve to the left implies a move toward normal ventricular function—clinical improvement. The curve shown below uses the left ventricular stroke work index (LVSWI—cardiac output) and pulmonary capillary wedge pressure (PCWP—preload).

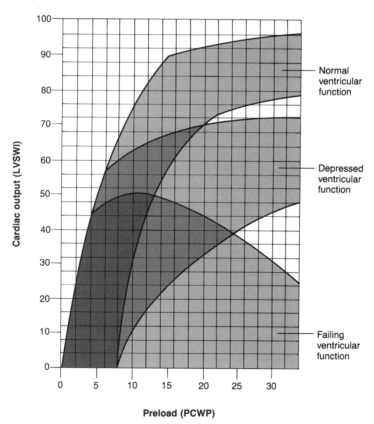

Inotropic drugs in CHF

Drug	Nursing considerations

Cardiac glycosides

digoxin
digitoxin
deslanoside

• Digitalis preparations increase contractility and slow the. heart rate. They may cause diuresis in edematous patients.
• Stay alert for signs and symptoms of digitalis toxicity, which include anorexia, nausea, vomiting, and visual disturbances. If ordered, give Digibind to treat severe digitalis toxicity. If possible, obtain serum digitoxin or digoxin levels before giving Digibind, because after Digibind administration serum digitoxin or digoxin levels rise sharply and don't accurately reflect therapeutic response. Monitor patient for hyperkalemia and hypokalemia.
• Withhold digitalis if patient's heart rate is below 60 beats/ minute. However, many chronic CHF patients have bradycardia in the 50 beats/minute range because they need larger doses of digitalis to remain asymptomatic. For these patients, special apical pulse rate parameters are needed.
• Check for interactions with other medications by monitoring serum digoxin levels. Neomycin, Kaopectate, and some antacids decrease GI digoxin absorption. Antiarrhythmics, such as quinidine and verapamil, can elevate serum digoxin levels.

Nonglycoside inotropic drugs (sympathomimetics)

dopamine
dobutamine

• Adjust dopamine infusion rate carefully to prevent excessive positive inotropic effect, tachycardia, and increased peripheral resistance.
• Effects of dopamine on vascular resistance are dose-dependent. With infusion rates below 2 mcg/kg/minute, drug mainly reduces resistance in renal, mesenteric, and coronary vascular beds. Infusion rates of 2 to 5 mcg/kg/minute exert a positive inotropic effect; cardiac contractility and cardiac output increase, with little change in heart rate and either reduced or unchanged total peripheral resistance. With higher infusion rates (5 to 10 mcg/kg/minute), arterial pressure, peripheral resistance, and heart rate increase and renal blood flow may decline.
• At therapeutic infusion rates of 2.5 to 10 mcg/kg/minute (usually in a concentration of 250 mg/250 ml of dextrose 5% in water), dobutamine reduces both preload and afterload and enhances contractility.
• Dobutamine is usually infused while hemodynamic monitoring is in place; as the desired effects are achieved, the pulmonary capillary wedge pressure (PCWP) should decrease, the cardiac index and cardiac output should increase, and systemic vascular resistance (SVR) should decrease.

Nonglycoside inotropic drugs (phosphodiesterase inhibitors)

amrinone
milrinone

• When giving amrinone, be alert for thrombocytopenia, dysrhythmias, hypotension, nausea, vomiting, hepatotoxicity, and hypersensitivity reactions.

Inotropic drugs in CHF *(continued)*

Drug	Nursing considerations
Nonglycoside inotropic drugs (phosphodiesterase inhibitors)	
amrinone milrinone *(continued)*	• Always give amrinone either as supplied or diluted in normal or half-normal saline solution to a concentration of 1 to 3 mcg/ml. Don't dilute drug with solutions containing dextrose, to avoid a slow chemical reaction. • Amrinone produces acute hemodynamic changes, including increased cardiac output and decreased right atrial pressure, central venous pressure, PCWP, and SVR. • Monitor patient's heart rate and blood pressure during administration of amrinone. If vital signs change, slow or stop infusion. Monitor potassium levels and measure intake and output. • Milrinone is almost 20 times more potent than amrinone and has a duration of action of 3 to 6 hours. Though milrinone produces fewer adverse effects than amrinone, it doesn't arrest progression of CHF. In some patients, it may even worsen the condition.

nation of a thiazide and a loop diuretic will safely promote the required fluid loss.

Vasodilators. These drugs may be used to augment inotropic drugs and diuretics. Vasodilators relax smooth muscle and can directly or indirectly improve the patient's clinical and hemodynamic status. They improve left ventricular function and reduce work load by reducing afterload and preload.

Three types of vasodilators are available: arteriolar dilators, venodilators, and mixed vasodilators. *Arteriolar dilators,* the afterload-reducing agents, act principally on arterioles. They augment stroke volume to reduce symptoms of poor perfusion, and increase renal and cerebral blood flow. Common arteriolar dilators include hydralazine, minoxidil, and the calcium channel blockers (verapamil, diltiazem, and nifedipine). *Venodilators,* primarily the nitrates, directly relax smooth muscles by producing generalized dilatation that affects veins more than arteries. They reduce venous return to the heart. Morphine, a narcotic analgesic, is a commonly used venodilator in acute CHF. It helps reduce venous return by dilating the venous system and slowing the rate of respiration, which decreases the effects of negative intrathoracic pressure on venous return. *Mixed vasodilators* act on both the arterial and venous beds. Their actions are intermediate between those of pure arteriolar dilators and pure venodilators. They improve cardiac output by facilitating ventricular emptying and reducing peripheral vascular resistance, thus decreasing myocardial oxygen demand. Mixed vasodilators include sodium nitroprusside, prazosin, and the angiotensin-converting enzyme inhibitor captopril.

Combination therapy. Combined therapy commonly improves cardiac output and maintains coronary perfusion pressure in patients with refractory CHF. Patients with very low arterial blood pressure (below 100 mm Hg systolic) may require vasopressor therapy to safely administer a parenteral vasodilator. When combinations of glycoside inotropic agents, diuretics, and vasodilators do not control acute symptoms, the doctor usually tries several nonglycoside inotropic agents. The treatment goal is to increase the cardiac index to roughly 2 liters/minute/m^2, to decrease PCWP to 18 to 22 mm Hg (to alleviate pulmonary congestion while maintaining adequate left ventricular filling and stroke volume), and to relieve symptoms. Combined dopamine and sodium nitroprusside therapy is also used to improve ventricular pump performance in these patients.

Mechanical devices

When drug therapy fails to improve cardiac output or maintain arterial blood pressure, mechanical devices are used to support the failing heart until it can function more effectively. Such devices include the IABP, the left ventricular assist device, and the artificial heart.

Intra-aortic balloon pump. Also known as intra-aortic balloon counterpulsation, the IABP mechanically maintains cardiac function. It preserves myocardial tissues, reduces cardiac work load, improves cardiac output, and aids coronary artery blood flow, permitting more oxygen and nutrients to reach the heart and vital organs. (See *How the intra-aortic balloon pump treats CHF.*)

The IABP is most effective in treating patients with cardiogenic shock, pump failure, mechanical MI complications, and unstable angina resistant to medical treatment. It can also help support circulation before heart transplantation. The IABP is

How the intra-aortic balloon pump treats CHF

The intra-aortic balloon is inserted percutaneously through the femoral artery and into the descending aorta, slightly beyond the origin of the left subclavian artery and above the renal artery branches.

The desired effects are achieved through the displacement of blood volume by balloon counterpulsation. The balloon inflates and deflates in synchrony with cardiac events. Inflation, which occurs during diastole, increases aortic pressure and improves coronary artery blood flow and systemic perfusion. Deflation, occurring at the onset of systole, lowers aortic pressure, ventricular resistance, and after-

load. The resulting increase in coronary artery perfusion and decrease in ventricular resistance lead to reduced myocardial oxygen demand and to increased cardiac output.

To provide the most hemodynamic support, the IABP must be set for optimal timing of balloon inflation and deflation. The console determines inflation and deflation cycles according to the patient's arterial pressure waveform or ECG. The balloon is inflated with either helium or carbon dioxide.

IABP therapy usually increases cardiac output by 10% to 20% and elevates arterial diastolic pressure.

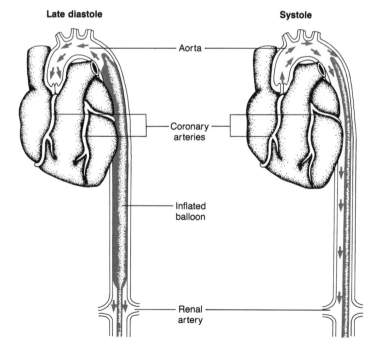

Late diastole   **Systole**

Aorta

Coronary arteries

Inflated balloon

Renal artery

contraindicated in patients with irreversible brain damage, chronic end-stage heart disease, an incompetent aortic valve, an aortic or thoracic aneurysm, or peripheral vascular disease.

Left ventricular assist device (LVAD). The LVAD can be used temporarily to pump the heart's blood. The battery-operated device diverts blood from the ventricular apex to the ascending aorta via surgically implanted outflow and inflow lines. The LVAD almost completely controls stroke volume; thus, it reduces left ventricular work load while maintaining adequate perfusion.

Terminally ill patients, heart transplant candidates, and patients with CHF resulting from recent acute MI commonly benefit from a temporary LVAD. The device allows the failing heart to rest while recovering. Periodic assessments of the patient's unassisted cardiac output and arterial pressure determine when the device can be withdrawn. The LVAD does not remedy inadequate ventricular filling caused by poor right ventricular function unless the condition responds sufficiently to inotropic agents. In this case, a biventricular assist device can be used.

Total artificial heart (TAH). Also known as the biventricular replacement device, the TAH replaces the patient's natural heart, supporting both the systemic and pulmonary circulations. Internally implanted, the TAH consists of two ventricular diaphragms that replace the heart's ventricles and valves. Controlled by one pump, an externally housed pneumatic power unit, drive line, and control system pump air through the device. During systole, pulses of compressed air enter the space between the ventricular diaphragm and base, resulting in ejection of blood to the atrial remnants and outlet connectors attached to the arteries. Several experimental designs include the Penn State and Phoenix hearts and a pump designed by researchers at the University of Akron, which requires no outside air or fluid lines.

Heart transplantation

Because mechanical hearts are still experimental and not sufficiently developed to offer a long-term alternative to a natural heart, transplantation is now the only effective treatment for the severely damaged heart. When protected from rejection, the transplanted heart exhibits normal contractility and contractile reserve and maintains normal cardiac output during rest and exercise. First performed in humans in 1967, heart transplantation is now almost commonplace. But because the donor supply remains limited, approximately one-third of the candidates for such surgery die before a suitable donor heart becomes available. (See *Criteria for heart transplantation.*)

Rejection of the donated organ and risk of infection and nephrotoxicity from pharmacologic immune suppression are the major complications of heart transplantation. Other complications include accelerated coronary atherosclerosis and hypercholesterolemia. Special testing to detect such complications begins postoperatively and must continue periodically throughout the patient's life. Tests used to detect signs of acute rejection include right ventricular endomyocardial biopsy, ECG, and magnetic resonance imaging (MRI). Signs of pending rejection include declining electrocardiographic QRS voltage, atrial dysrhythmia, and an S_3 gallop. MRI scanning reveals edema from rejection. Tests to detect infections occur at 2- to 4-week intervals.

Investigational therapies

Treatment with new mechanical assistance devices, such as the Hemopump, and new surgical techniques, such as cardiomyoplasty and skeletal muscle ventricle, offer new hope to patients who may not respond to other pharmacologic or surgical interventions. (See *Promising research: The Hemopump,* page 174.)

Cardiomyoplasty. For CHF patients with severely damaged hearts unable to withstand bypass surgery or transplantation, cardiomyoplasty holds promise. This technique involves transplanting one of the patient's latissimus dorsi muscles (with thoracodorsal nerves and major blood vessels intact) to the area around the heart with a pacemaker to stimulate contraction of the skeletal muscle in synchrony with myocardial contraction.

Studies of patients treated with cardiomyoplasty show a 15% increase in ejection fraction and a 20% improvement in cardiac output. However, problems persist in gaining uniform pacing of skeletal muscle contraction. Heart muscles need only a single impulse for contraction, whereas skeletal muscles require a series of impulses. Another problem is the 4- to 6-week preparation needed to train skeletal muscles to contract before transplantation can occur or before the muscle is completely ready to augment contraction. This delay, of course, prevents the use of cardiomyoplasty in patients who need immediate treatment.

Criteria for heart transplantation

The patient who is a suitable candidate for heart transplantation:
• has advanced (Class IV) heart disease with a poor prognosis for 1-year survival
• is psychologically stable
• has a history of compliance with medical therapy
• is 54 years old or younger
• has no or limited evidence of systemic diseases.
  The suitable candidate has none of the following conditions that contraindicate heart transplantation:
• pulmonary hypertension
• parenchymal pulmonary disease
• recent pulmonary infarction
• donor-specific cytotoxic antibodies
• active infection
• insulin-dependent diabetes mellitus
• history of coexisting liver or renal disease
• active duodenal ulcer
• drug addiction
• psychosis
• continued excessive consumption of alcohol
• clinically significant cerebral or peripheral vascular disease
• other diseases likely to limit survival or rehabilitation.

The Hemopump

The Hemopump, a mechanical device that assists a failing heart, is unlike any other heart machine ever designed. It consists of a tiny turbine blade, ½" long by ¼" wide, encased in a close-fitting tube. The pump is inserted into the femoral artery and carefully snaked up through the blood vessels into the left ventricle. This miniature pump, linked by a wire-thin cable to a motor outside the body, then assumes most of the heart's work load.

Rotating as fast as 25,000 revolutions/minute, the turbine blade draws blood up from the ventricle, through the tube, and out into the aorta. As the screw turns within the tube, the fluid that is trapped be-tween its vanes is forced to rise. This powerful device can move 6 pints of blood/minute—close enough to the 8 to 10 pints/minute pumped by a healthy heart to support life for several days, even if the patient's heart is barely working.

One fear about the pump was that its whirling blades might destroy blood cells, leading to dangerous clots or hemorrhages. Another was that the body would not be able to tolerate the continuous blood flow and steady blood pressure produced by the turbine pump. However, researchers have found no evidence of such problems in either animals or humans treated with the Hemopump.

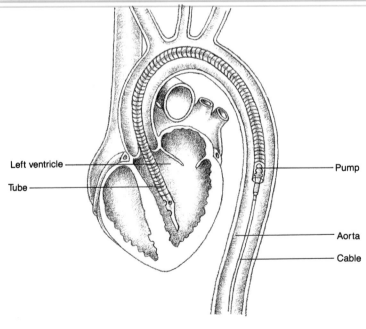

Left ventricle ———

Tube ———

——— Pump

——— Aorta

——— Cable

Skeletal muscle ventricle (SMV). This new technique uses transplanted skeletal muscle to augment ventricular function. In SMV, a sheath of skeletal muscle wrapped around a synthetic bladder is attached to the aorta or another artery. As the bladder fills with blood, it is stimulated to contract in synchrony with the myocardium to boost cardiac output.

Case study: Part 4

After 36 hours on IABP counterpulsation, Mrs. Baldwin's condition stabilized and she was weaned from the device without complication. Her hemodynamic status remained stable, and her vital signs and urine output were adequate. The staff and family were relieved. But the doctor again grew concerned when hemodynamic measurements revealed a ventricular ejection fraction of only 16% and echocardiography showed biventricular enlargement. In light of these findings and the patient's extensive CAD, the doctor decided to discuss the possibility of heart transplantation, a suggestion he knew would stun the Baldwin family. A new heart, he told them, would give Mrs. Baldwin the best possible chance for recovery. And because her health was otherwise good, she was an excellent candidate for the procedure. Mrs. Baldwin and her children told the doctor they needed time to think it over.

Throughout the next few days, the patient's progress continued steadily. Then on the fourth day after admission, she suddenly became acutely dyspneic while talking with her nurse and her daughter. Her blood pressure dropped to 80/50 mm Hg. Her pulmonary artery pressures were elevated, and she became anxious and diaphoretic. She developed loud wheezes and began to cough up pink, frothy sputum. The doctor was notified of her change in condition.

Within minutes, Mrs. Baldwin developed acute pulmonary edema, respiratory arrest, and ventricular fibrillation. A code was called and resuscitative efforts were tried, but Mrs. Baldwin died.

Nursing management

Your patient's clinical condition determines which nursing interventions are needed. In acute CHF, watch for reduced cardiac output, and frequently assess signs and symptoms and hemodynamic parameters. In chronic CHF, focus on the patient's long-term needs and his compliance with treatment procedures.

Complications

Monitor for signs and symptoms of complications, such as pleural effusion, pulmonary edema, and cardiogenic shock.

Responding to pulmonary edema

If your patient's heart failure deteriorates to pulmonary edema, intervene quickly, according to these guidelines.
• Call for help. Notify the doctor at once and gather emergency equipment.
• Assess and ensure airway patency and oxygenation. Maintain proper airway position. Encourage coughing, if it's productive. Suction only if absolutely necessary. Give oxygen by mask or nasal cannula.
• Position the patient to decrease venous return.
• Assess vital signs regularly.
• Start an I.V. infusion. Choose an insertion site unaffected by position changes.
• Attach a cardiac monitor. Observe closely for dysrhythmias.
• Administer medications as ordered. Prepare to give furosemide, morphine, and digoxin I.V., as ordered. Nitroglycerin, nitroprusside, and dobutamine may also be given.
• Prepare rotating tourniquets if needed. This technique decreases venous return to the overloaded heart. *Important:* Don't use this method with a hypotensive patient.
• Calculate strict fluid intake and output. Be prepared to insert an indwelling (Foley) catheter, if ordered, to monitor intake and output.
• Prepare resuscitation equipment.
• Provide emotional support. Maintain a calm, caring attitude. Reassure the patient and his family. Remain with the patient as much as possible and provide the family with a quiet waiting area.

Pleural effusion. In this condition, rising pulmonary venous pressures force fluid out of the pulmonary vascular compartment into the interstitium, alveoli, and finally the pleural space. A small amount of fluid can usually be reabsorbed by the visceral and parietal veins and lymphatics, but as the fluid collects and fills the pleural space, reabsorption may not be possible. A pleural effusion compresses the lung, restricting its expansion and limiting gas exchange. Depending on the severity of the effusion, the patient may manifest acute dyspnea with absent breath sounds over the effusion, asymmetrical chest expansion, and dullness on percussion over the effusion. If the effusion is significant and is causing symptoms, fluid is removed using needle aspiration (thoracentesis).

Pulmonary edema. As left ventricular failure progresses, it leads to extreme pulmonary vessel pressure that forces fluid from the vascular space into the lung interstitium. The resulting pulmonary congestion progresses, depending on the heart's work load and ventricular function. Signs and symptoms of pulmonary edema mimic those of CHF but are more severe, causing the patient to experience air hunger and feelings of suffocation and extreme apprehension. Unable to lie flat without extreme feelings of suffocation, the patient may try to sit upright to improve oxygenation. Expect to see tachypnea and labored breathing. You may hear crackles or wheezes without a stethoscope.

Hypoxia and decreased cardiac output may make the patient restless, pale, ashen, cool, and diaphoretic. His vital signs will depend on the degree of cardiac compromise. Without immediate, effective intervention, pulmonary edema can rapidly lead to marked hypotension, cardiogenic shock, and death. Treatment aims at reducing fluid volume and improving oxygenation. (See *Responding to pulmonary edema.*)

Cardiogenic shock. This life-threatening condition follows severe circulatory failure resulting from impaired pumping ability. It commonly follows an acute MI—especially one that has damaged 40% or more of the left ventricle. Cardiogenic shock may also occur with end-stage cardiomyopathy or a mechanical defect, such as valve rupture, ventricular septal defect, or cardiac tamponade.

Because cardiogenic shock results from a marked decrease in functional ventricular muscle tissue, watch for signs and symptoms of decreased cardiac output, such as restlessness; confusion; diaphoresis; cold, clammy skin; rapid, thready pulse; and diminished urine output. When cardiogenic shock stems from a mechanical defect, the IABP can help stabilize the patient until surgery can correct the defect. But when shock results from extensive myocardial damage, the patient may become dependent on the IABP because existing muscle tissue can't sustain sufficient cardiac output.

Patient teaching in CHF

The patient and family members need to learn about managing CHF. Assess their level of knowledge and willingness to learn. Find a quiet environment to talk with the patient and family, and use visual aids, films, pamphlets, charts, and models, as needed.

Specifically, review the causes of CHF, the signs of deteriorating status, diagnostic tests, and the patient's individual treatment plan. Explain why the patient needs the prescribed rest, dietary restrictions, oxygen therapy, and fluid removal. If the patient is receiving drug therapy, discuss the names, dosage, administration route, and adverse effects of each drug. If the IABP or LVAD is to be used, tell the patient why and what to expect. Plan to use a checklist to help you make your patient teaching consistent and comprehensive. (See *Patient-teaching checklist: Congestive heart failure,* page 178.)

Emphasize that CHF is controllable and that optimal control of the disease comes from the patient's acceptance of life-style restrictions and commitment to comply with treatment. Noncompliance is the leading cause of repeat CHF episodes. Repeated episodes can damage healthy organs and lead to kidney failure, liver cirrhosis, and brain damage. To help educate CHF patients on a continuing basis, some hospitals now offer cardiac rehabilitation programs modified to meet the needs of CHF patients.

Discharge planning

Discharge planning is an important part of nursing care that actually begins with the assessments made during hospital ad-

▶ **PATIENT-TEACHING CHECKLIST**

Congestive heart failure

Teaching the patient about CHF should include instruction about medications, signs and symptoms, activity, and diet.

Medications
Inotropic agents
- [ ] Count pulse rate before taking medication. If pulse rate is less than 60 beats/minute, do not take it.
- [ ] Report yellow halos, loss of appetite, or diarrhea of more than 1 day's duration.

Diuretics
- [ ] Avoid taking them late in the day.
- [ ] Take potassium as prescribed.
- [ ] Report leg cramps or progressive muscle weakness.

Dilators
- [ ] Take at regular intervals to keep blood level constant.
- [ ] Do not try to "catch up" if you miss your dose.
- [ ] Use alcohol sparingly because it may increase drug's hypotensive effect.
- [ ] Report light-headedness or dizziness.
- [ ] Monitor blood pressure trends.

Signs and symptoms
- [ ] 2-lb weight gain from one day to the next
- [ ] Chest pain
- [ ] Increasing fatigue
- [ ] Swelling of fingers or ankles
- [ ] Shortness of breath
- [ ] Pulse rate faster than _____
- [ ] Persistent cough

Activity
- [ ] Moderation is key.
- [ ] Maintain a regular rest pattern.
- [ ] Avoid long working hours.
- [ ] Avoid undue stress.
- [ ] Practice stress management.
- [ ] Increase walking gradually. If fatigue or shortness of breath develops, stop and rest.

Diet
- [ ] Avoid using salt at the table.
- [ ] Avoid condiments, canned goods, lunch meats, and foods high in sodium.
- [ ] Examine food labels for sodium content.

mission. Your detailed assessments of social history, previous life-style, and family considerations help determine the patient's long-term goals and influence your interventions to help achieve these goals.

Patients needing social services or other home care should be referred to the appropriate agencies immediately. Patients using I.V. vasodilators or inotropic agents have typically been monitored in the cardiac care unit because they commonly cannot be weaned from drug therapy without incident. However, recent studies have shown that with good discharge planning and ad-

DISCHARGE PLANNING CHECKLIST

Congestive heart failure

Discharge planning for the patient with CHF must consider the following factors.

Social service
- [ ] Long-term care placement
- [ ] Financial assistance
- [ ] Meal delivery
- [ ] Specialized medical equipment
- [ ] Transportation for follow-up visits

Pharmacy
- [ ] Education about cardiac medications

Diet
- [ ] Education about salt-restricted diet

Home health care
- [ ] Ongoing physical assessments

- [ ] Special equipment care
- [ ] Assistance with activities of daily living

Nursing needs
- [ ] Medication instruction
- [ ] Disease process instruction
- [ ] Low-sodium diet reinforcement
- [ ] Signs and symptoms to report
- [ ] Activity instruction
- [ ] Follow-up instruction

Occupational therapy
- [ ] Career adjustments
- [ ] Life-style adjustments

Cardiac rehabilitation
- [ ] Controlled activity supervision
- [ ] Group support
- [ ] Health education
- [ ] Ongoing physical assessments by nurse

---

equate patient and family teaching, even these drugs may be safely administered at home. Such home care may help provide the compassionate and cost-effective care needed for selected patients with end-stage CHF. (See *Discharge planning checklist: Congestive heart failure* to help you plan your patient's discharge needs.)

Case study: Part 5

Claire Baldwin's case classically demonstrates the special challenges of caring for a patient with acute CHF. The sudden and severe changes in cardiac function that Mrs. Baldwin experienced throughout her hospital stay underscore the need for fast thinking, keen assessment, and continuous monitoring of the patient's response to therapy. For the most part, Mrs. Baldwin's medical treatment and nursing care centered on assessing cardiac output and attempting to boost pump function through the administration of

Case study: Part 5 *(continued)*

drugs and mechanical measures. As commonly occurs, her response to specific measures varied, necessitating a trial-and-error approach aimed at finding the most effective therapeutic combination.

The unpredictable course of CHF kept the patient's family and medical team on an emotional roller coaster. As Mrs. Baldwin alternately improved and deteriorated, the mood of her family and the CCU staff swung from elation to frustration and sorrow. And the family, still trying to cope with the recent death of their father, was now also coping with their mother's imminent death.

After Mrs. Baldwin's death, the nurses held a support session. A formal presentation of her case by the clinical nurse specialist provided additional support. She praised the nurses for their diligent efforts while offering suggestions for improvement in future cases. The death-and-dying counselor made a couple of calls to the family over the next few weeks to help them understand the grieving process. A few months later, Mrs. Baldwin's daughter stopped by to thank the staff for their compassionate care and to let them know what a help they had been to her family in crisis.

CHAPTER 5
Acute respiratory failure

Acute respiratory failure (ARF) commonly follows an acute underlying disease and can strike suddenly, causing up to 50% mortality from respiratory arrest. Nurses caring for patients with ARF must monitor continuously for signs of imminent respiratory arrest. By promptly identifying the onset of ARF, giving appropriate supportive therapy, and watching for signs of progression, they can prevent respiratory arrest or help the patient avoid mechanical ventilation. Expert nursing care of ARF reduces the risk of secondary infection, ensures faster recovery (with shorter, less costly hospitalizations), and increases survival rates.

To provide such effective care, nurses must thoroughly understand the pathophysiology of ARF and its therapies. They must learn the skills they need and keep up with the changing technology of ARF therapy. They must also be prepared to provide appropriate teaching and emotional support to patients and their families, mainly to reduce anxiety arising from ARF and to help at-risk patients recognize the warning signs of recurrence.

This chapter will review the pathophysiology and predisposing factors of ARF; methods of assessment and diagnosis, including arterial blood gas (ABG) analysis; current treatment options, including mechanical ventilation and drug therapy; ethical dilemmas involved in treatment; and nursing management.

Case study: Part 1

As the ambulance crew wheeled William Smith, a 62-year-old retired mechanic, into the treatment room, the emergency department (ED) nurse saw immediately that he was in severe respiratory distress. He had a patent airway but was so short of breath he could only respond with one-word answers. Mr. Smith's breathing was shallow and rapid, at 42 breaths/minute. His mucous membranes and nail beds were cyanotic; he used the accessory mus-

Identifying blood gas sources

Partial pressures of O_2 or CO_2 may be measured from various sources—arterial or venous blood, alveoli, and expired air. To identify the source, a subscript follows the letter P (partial pressure of the gas) and is the first letter or letters of the gas source. A lower case "a" after the "P" (Pa) identifies the source as arterial blood. The specific gas that was measured follows, as in PaO_2. The following abbreviations are commonly used.

Pa: arterial blood
PA: alveolar gas
Pv: venous blood
Pet: end tidal gas
Ptc: transcutaneous

Case study: Part 1 *(continued)*

cles of his intercostal region, neck, and abdomen to inhale; and he pursed his lips when exhaling. The ED nurse rated his degree of dyspnea as 8 on a scale of 1 to 10 (with 1 corresponding to very mild dyspnea and 10 to most severe).

To ease Mr. Smith's breathing, the nurse raised the head of the stretcher to high Fowler's position and gave oxygen at 2 liters/minute by nasal cannula. She continued to assess his respiratory status while obtaining a stat ABG test and notified the ED doctor of the patient's arrival. Mr. Smith's vital signs were stable, with a blood pressure of 142/90 mm Hg and a heart rate of 138 beats/minute.

As the doctor began his physical examination, the laboratory reported Mr. Smith's ABG results as follows: pH, 7.31; partial pressure of carbon dioxide in arterial blood ($PaCO_2$), 64 mm Hg; partial pressure of oxygen in arterial blood (PaO_2), 47 mm Hg; arterial oxygen saturation (SaO_2), 0.78 (78%); bicarbonate (HCO_3^-), 32 mEq/liter (32 mmol/liter). The ED doctor made an initial medical diagnosis of ARF secondary to chronic obstructive pulmonary disease (COPD) and completed a medical history and physical examination.

Causes and characteristics

In ARF, the patient's respiratory system cannot adequately oxygenate arterial blood, remove carbon dioxide (CO_2) from the venous blood, or provide oxygen (O_2) to tissues. This life-threatening condition can occur suddenly, developing in minutes, or it can start slowly, developing over several days.

ARF commonly produces tissue hypoxia, which, if untreated, can cause failure of affected organs. Confirmed by ABG tests, the defining characteristics of ARF (in a patient who is not receiving supplemental O_2) usually include acute dyspnea, a PaO_2 below 50 mm Hg, a $PaCO_2$ over 50 mm Hg, and respiratory acidemia (pH below 7.3). In a patient who is receiving supplemental O_2, PaO_2 readings minimally higher than 50 mm Hg indicate an even more severe respiratory dysfunction. (See *Identifying blood gas sources.*)

Pathophysiology

The two major kinds of pathophysiologic changes producing respiratory failure are ventilatory (also known as hypercapnic) failure and oxygenation (also known as hypoxemic) failure. Each may have myriad causes. (See *Causes of ARF,* page 184.)

Ventilatory (hypercapnic) failure. This condition results from dysfunction of the respiratory pump (consisting of the chest wall, the breathing muscles, and the nerves serving them). When the respiratory pump does not move enough air into the lungs, alveolar hypoventilation results. As the alveoli are inadequately ventilated, their partial pressure of CO_2 rises. The rising level of CO_2 displaces O_2, and the partial pressure of O_2 in the alveoli falls. Blood passing through these alveoli is now exposed to low concentrations of O_2 and high concentrations of CO_2. So, when gas exchange is completed, the PaO_2 decreases and the $PaCO_2$ increases. In this situation, blood-alveolar gas exchange isn't dysfunctional; ABG findings indicate ARF because of ventilatory failure. Supplemental O_2 may correct such hypoxemia, unless the increased $PaCO_2$ results from the patient's inability to breathe; in that case, mechanical ventilation must be used. In ventilatory failure, the primary concern is the patient's ability to breathe.

The defining characteristic of ventilatory respiratory failure is a $PaCO_2$ greater than 50 mm Hg with a pH below 7.30. The presence of acidemia differentiates compensated chronic hyper-capnia (as in COPD) from ARF. The danger to the patient stems not from the hypercapnia, but from the acidemia that it induces; a low pH may cause dysrhythmias and impaired organ function.

Oxygenation (hypoxemic) failure. This condition occurs when blood oxygenation is inadequate because the lungs' alveoli are insufficiently ventilated in relation to the amount of blood flowing through the capillaries—a condition known as ventila-tion-perfusion (V/Q) mismatch. As blood passes through the capillaries, the available O_2 is inadequate to completely oxy-genate the hemoglobin. So blood leaving these capillaries has a very low PaO_2. When it meets blood from capillaries with normal PaO_2, the resulting mixture has a lowered PaO_2.

A V/Q mismatch has a much smaller effect on $PaCO_2$ be-cause of the difference in CO_2 exchange. In oxygenation failure, the decrease in PaO_2 is proportionally larger than the increase

Causes of ARF

The following diseases, disorders, and drugs are associated with development of acute respiratory failure.

VENTILATORY FAILURE

Central nervous system disorders
- Cerebrovascular accident
- Central sleep apnea
- Trauma
- Drug overdose (narcotic, sedative, postanesthesia)
- Guillain-Barré syndrome
- Spinal cord disruption (trauma, tumor)
- Amyotrophic lateral sclerosis

Neuromuscular drugs and disorders
- Neuromuscular blockers (paralytic drugs)
- Myasthenia gravis
- Peripheral neuritis
- Multiple sclerosis
- Myxedema

Thoracic and airway disorders
- Muscular dystrophy
- Obesity
- Kyphoscoliosis
- Trauma (rib fracture, flail chest)
- Pneumothorax
- Pleural effusion
- Airway obstruction
- Obstructive sleep apnea
- Vocal cord paralysis
- Epiglottitis
- Laryngeal edema
- Tracheal stenosis

OXYGENATION FAILURE

Cardiovascular disorders
- Pulmonary edema (acute, chronic)
- Pulmonary embolism
- Fat embolism

Pulmonary disorders
- Infection, pneumonia
- Aspiration
- Asthma
- Chronic obstructive pulmonary disease
- Cystic fibrosis
- Adult respiratory distress syndrome
- Interstitial lung disease
- Atelectasis
- Pulmonary contusion
- Pancreatitis
- Connective tissue diseases

in $PaCO_2$. This unequal change can be identified by an increased A-a gradient (the difference between the alveolar (A) and arterial (a) partial pressures of O_2). The hypoxemia of V/Q mismatch can be corrected by increasing the fraction of inspired oxygen (FIO_2). (See *Calculating the A-a gradient.*)

Another type of oxygenation failure occurs when the membrane that separates the alveoli and capillaries thickens, reducing

Calculating the A-a gradient

The degree of oxygenation failure can be quantified by calculating the difference between the PAO_2 and the PaO_2. This difference in partial pressures of O_2 is called the A-a gradient. When the lungs are functioning normally, the A-a gradient is 5 to 10 mm Hg. It gradually increases with age, remaining normal at 30 mm Hg at age 70. The A-a gradient is calculated by the following formula:

$$(\text{barometric pressure} - 47) \times FIO_2 - (1.25 \times PaCO_2) - PaO_2$$

The first part of the formula calculates the PAO_2. The FIO_2 delivered to the patient must be accurate or the A-a gradient will be increased artificially. The A-a gradient is used to determine if oxygenation failure is also present when ventilatory failure is the primary dysfunction. The A-a gradient compensates for the decrease in PaO_2, which results from an increase in $PaCO_2$. The A-a gradient will be normal if only ventilatory failure is present.

O_2 diffusion from the alveoli to the blood. Under normal conditions, the speed of diffusion is more than adequate, so blood leaving the capillaries is fully oxygenated. But when edema or inflammation thickens the membrane, O_2 cannot cross the membrane fast enough to establish equilibrium between alveolar and arterial O_2 before the blood leaves the capillaries. The resulting hypoxemia can be severe and is remedied only slightly by increasing the FIO_2. (See *Pathways of combined respiratory failure,* page 186.)

ARF almost always results from an underlying disease. A head injury, for example, could shut down the respiratory center of the central nervous system (CNS), preventing the respiratory pump from moving air past an airway obstruction, thus creating alveolar hypoventilation. Respiratory distress may also result from neuromuscular diseases, CNS disorders, a drug overdose, and pneumonia.

In patients with ARF, the underlying cause must be identified so that appropriate interventions can resolve the respiratory failure. Take special care to identify patients with chronic dis-

Pathways of combined respiratory failure

As acute respiratory failure (ARF) develops from either oxygenation or ventilatory failure, it exerts various effects that eventually produce ARF with a combined oxygenation and ventilatory failure.

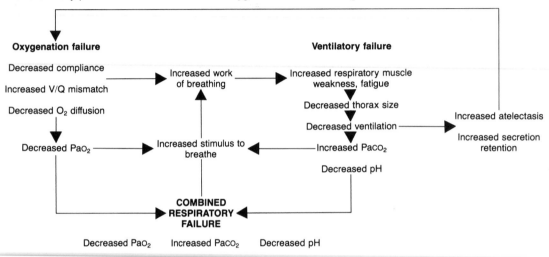

ease—such as COPD—who may experience repeated episodes of ARF. You can prevent, or at least minimize, recurring episodes by teaching these patients about the early warning signs of disorders predisposing to ARF. (See *Pathogenesis of ARF in chronic pulmonary disease.*)

Case study: Part 2

Mr. Smith first learned that he had COPD 6 years before this admission, when he was hospitalized for pneumonia. Although he smoked two to three packs of cigarettes a day for 45 years, he had no symptoms during the first 4 years after his diagnosis of COPD. Two years ago, Mr. Smith was hospitalized again for an exacerbation of COPD. He was discharged on bronchodilator therapy, which included theophylline, 300 mg P.O. every 12 hours, and an albuterol inhaler, as needed. Mr. Smith stopped smoking and returned to work, but increasing fatigue and dyspnea forced his early retirement 6 months later.

During the past year, Mr. Smith became less and less active. He had increasing dyspnea and fatigue and developed a frequent produc-

Pathogenesis of ARF in chronic pulmonary disease

Predisposing factors or injury	Pathogenesis
Acute lung infection	Acute infection increases pulmonary secretions, causing atelectasis and increased work of breathing, which, in turn, causes ventilation-perfusion (V/Q) mismatch.
Heart failure or myocardial infarction	In heart failure and myocardial infarction, increased left ventricular end-diastolic volume causes blood to back up in the lungs, resulting in interstitial edema and decreased compliance. Increased work of breathing follows, triggering the following cycle: Increased work causes increased CO_2 production, which stimulates increased minute ventilation. Eventually, the lungs can't work hard enough to remove excess CO_2, resulting in alveolar hypoventilation.
Pulmonary emboli	Pulmonary emboli may obstruct or impair blood flow to an area of alveoli, causing V/Q mismatch.
Neuromuscular disorders	In neuromuscular disorders, weakening or paralysis of the muscles that control ventilation results in alveolar hypoventilation.
Respiratory depressants	Administration of respiratory depressants, such as sedatives, narcotics, and tranquilizers, causes alveolar hypoventilation. Injudicious administration of oxygen may also cause respiratory depression by dampening the patient's hypoxic drive to breathe.
Abdominal or thoracic injury or surgery	Shallow breathing due to incisional pain or administration of narcotics for pain relief causes respiratory depression and alveolar hypoventilation. Accumulation of secretions due to immobility and shallow breathing causes V/Q mismatch. V/Q mismatch may also occur after pneumonectomy because of hyperperfusion of the remaining lung.

tive cough that was particularly severe on awakening each morning. Recently, he'd begun to cough up more sputum than usual and had become more dependent on his albuterol inhaler.

Two days before admission, his sputum turned yellow. His doctor prescribed ampicillin. Despite the antibiotic, his shortness of breath worsened. He began to purse his lips with each breath, and his cough became so weak that he could not produce any sputum.

After taking Mr. Smith's history, the ED nurse completed a thorough head-to-toe physical examination. Mr. Smith appeared alert, although in acute respiratory distress, and was oriented to person, place, and time. He could follow commands and move all his extremities in full range of motion with fair movement and strength.

His apical pulse was easily audible, with a distinct S_1 and S_2 heart sound as well as an atrial (S_4) and ventricular (S_3) gallop. His heart rate was 128 beats/minute, and his blood pressure was 148/86 mm Hg. Although Mr. Smith was in high Fowler's position, the

Case study: Part 2 *(continued)*

nurse recognized jugular vein distention. He continued to use all of his accessory muscles to breathe and his abdominal muscles for forced expiration. Chest expansion was equal and symmetrical with intercostal retractions, but chest motion was limited and respirations were shallow. His respiratory rate was 32 breaths/minute.

On auscultation, the patient's breath sounds were decreased throughout his lungs, in both the anterior and posterior fields, and almost absent in both lung bases; rhonchi could be heard over the large airways. Further auscultation revealed bowel sounds. Mr. Smith's abdomen was soft and nontender, with a slightly enlarged liver. He experienced no dysuria or pain upon urination. Mild ankle and pedal edema were present, but without skin breakdown. His rectal temperature was 101° F (38.3° C).

A complete blood count (CBC) indicated an elevated white blood cell (WBC) count of 22,000/mm³ (2.2 10⁹/liter) because of an infection. Other laboratory results were as follows: hemoglobin, 15.6 g/dl (156 g/liter); hematocrit, 43.4% (0.43). Mr. Smith's chemistry profile was normal except for an elevated CO_2 level, demonstrating elevated HCO_3^- levels, which reflected compensation for hypercapnia resulting from COPD. His sputum Gram stain indicated a respiratory infection, as demonstrated by gram-positive cocci in pairs and clusters with a few gram-negative bacilli. His theophylline level was within the therapeutic range at 12.6 mcg/ml.

Mr. Smith's chest X-ray indicated his COPD and a respiratory infection, as demonstrated by an increased anteroposterior diameter with a low, flat diaphragm and a right lower lobe infiltrate. His ECG showed that the increased cardiovascular work load imposed by his chronic lung disease was causing right ventricular hypertrophy.

Assessment and diagnosis

Because ARF is not itself a disease but is the potential result of many diseases, effective treatment depends on accurate assessment of the underlying condition. This section will review the steps necessary to build a firm base for an aggressive care plan. An accurate assessment begins with the patient's history, identifies characteristic signs and symptoms, and evaluates the results of appropriate diagnostic tests.

Patient history

A complete patient history is critical for identifying the causes and treatments of ARF. Start by finding out when the patient's breathing difficulty began. If the patient's complaints are vague, you'll need to make the history as detailed as possible to identify the cause of ARF. Once the broad outlines of the history are in place, return to the point at which dyspnea first appeared and ask the patient about any associated signs or symptoms he may have forgotten to mention. Also ask about preexisting contributing factors, such as COPD, neuromuscular disease, or immunosuppression.

To gather information that may contribute to successful follow-up treatment, ask the patient what measures he has used to reduce breathing distress. Also ask about hobbies or occupations that may involve exposure to dust, fumes, or chemicals. Ask him about smoking (see *Determining pack years*), pets, use of prescription and over-the-counter medications, and recent travel patterns.

Signs and symptoms

Expect signs and symptoms that indicate inadequate ventilation, decreased oxygenation, or both, including dyspnea, anxiety, increased or decreased respiratory rate and depth, increased heart rate, respiratory muscle fatigue, abnormal breath sounds, sputum changes, and cyanosis. Assess and evaluate each to determine the type and severity of ARF. (See *Assessment profile: Findings in ARF,* page 190.)

Dyspnea. Ask the patient when he first began feeling short of breath. Identify the associated activity level: Was the patient resting, sitting, or climbing a flight of stairs at the time? Because dyspnea is uncomfortable and frightening, the patient may unwittingly decrease his activity level to avoid it. If he hasn't done this, ask the patient if he has felt fatigued over the last few days. Ask him to rate his dyspnea on a 10-point scale, with 1 to 4 as mild, 5 to 7 as moderate, and 8 to 10 as severe.

Note that the patient with respiratory center depression does not complain of dyspnea, the subjective perception that breathing is difficult. When this center is depressed, it generates no breathing stimulus, and the respiratory muscles remain inactive. Such a patient may not notice that his breathing is inadequate or that he is experiencing ARF.

Anxiety. As the patient focuses on the effort to breathe, and feels that he will become too fatigued to continue the effort, he becomes anxious and stresses already overworked muscles, thereby increasing dyspnea. If the patient is not anxious, he is

Determining pack years

If your patient smokes, you can determine the number of pack years he has smoked by using the following formula: Number of packs smoked per day × number of years the patient has smoked = pack years.

For example, a patient who has smoked two packs of cigarettes per day for 42 years has incurred 84 pack years.

◤ **ASSESSMENT PROFILE**

Findings in ARF

Clinical signs	Expected findings
Respiratory rate	Less than 10 breaths/minute or greater than 20 breaths/minute
Character of respirations	Shallow; abdominal paradox; respiratory alternans with respiratory muscle weakness
Work of breathing	Greatly increased or reduced if respiratory muscle failure has occurred
Dyspnea	Present, varying from mild to severe; absent if respiratory depression caused ARF
Breath sounds	Decreased intensity, poor air movement; possible crackles, rhonchi, or wheezes
Sputum	Increased production with changed color if infection is present
Cyanosis	Absent (if present, more than 5 g of hemoglobin is unsaturated)
Level of consciousness	Variable, from forgetfulness or restlessness to seizures and coma
Heart rate	Tachycardia

not perceiving his dyspnea as severe, possibly because he has experienced it before and knows what to expect, or he is so fatigued or disoriented that he can no longer recognize the dyspnea.

Respiratory rate. Tachypnea (a respiratory rate above 20 breaths/minute) is most commonly associated with dyspnea because of the increased work of breathing. A respiratory rate below 10 breaths/minute may result from a drug overdose or a decreased level of consciousness. Shallow breathing with a decreased or normal respiratory rate strongly suggests ARF. However, shallow breathing at an increased rate may not indicate ARF because the patient is being adequately ventilated.

Be sure to evaluate signs and symptoms of decreased oxygenation as well as ineffective ventilation. Because the brain is particularly sensitive to oxygen deprivation, the effects of inadequate oxygenation progress from fatigue and disorientation to restlessness, agitation, and eventually coma. Oxygenation failure alone increases both the rate and depth of respirations; if ventilatory failure is also present, the rate increases markedly while the depth remains unchanged or becomes shallow.

Respiratory muscle fatigue. As the patient uses more intercostal and abdominal muscles to breathe, the accessory muscles eventually weaken. If they cannot maintain the effort of breathing, ARF will rapidly accelerate to respiratory arrest in only a few seconds or minutes. The adequacy of ventilation is determined by the amount of air entering the chest with each breath, regardless of effort. (See *Assessing respiratory muscle fatigue.*)

Abnormal breath sounds. Wheezing indicates airways narrowed from bronchospasm, cardiac failure, inflammation, or tumor. Rhonchi indicate that secretions are accumulating and impairing ventilation. Crackles resulting from atelectasis or cardiac failure indicate areas of alveoli that are expanding and being ventilated when increased negative pressure is applied to them.

Sputum changes. Increased sputum production results from airway irritation due to dust, pollen, noxious gases, or bacteria. An underlying infection that causes a change in sputum color may be the primary cause of ARF or a secondary complication. Decreased sputum production may indicate that the patient is too weak to cough.

Cyanosis. Although cyanosis results from poorly oxygenated hemoglobin, it may not reliably indicate tissue oxygenation. If hemoglobin levels are low, the hemoglobin may be adequately oxygenated but the patient may not be receiving adequate tissue oxygenation. Conversely, a polycythemic patient who is actually receiving adequate tissue oxygenation may be cyanotic because hemoglobin levels are too high. However, cyanosis that develops after the initial assessment reliably indicates a decreasing level of blood oxygenation.

Laboratory tests

Laboratory tests for confirming ARF include ABG analysis, chest X-rays, pulmonary function tests, ECG, CBC, a blood chemistry profile, and sputum cultures.

ABG analysis. ABG analysis can confirm or rule out ARF. In a normal, healthy individual, values diagnostic of ARF are a PaO_2 below 50 mm Hg, a $PaCO_2$ above 50 mm Hg, and respiratory

Assessing respiratory muscle fatigue

Patients in acute respiratory failure commonly develop respiratory muscle fatigue, a dangerous condition that must be identified and monitored to avoid respiratory muscle failure and subsequent respiratory arrest. To identify respiratory muscle fatigue, use inspection and palpation to reveal the following characteristic signs:
• respiratory rate above the patient's baseline
• development of abdominal paradox, respiratory alternans, or both.

Abdominal paradox is inward displacement of the abdomen that occurs from the decreased abdominal pressure during inspiration. To assess for it, place one hand over the patient's sternum and the other on his abdomen above the umbilicus. As he breathes, observe the relative motion of the rib cage and abdomen. Determine if the change in abdominal pressure is a decrease or an increase in pressure from abdominal muscle contraction.

Respiratory alternans is a cyclic alternation of respiratory movements — abdominal movements for a few breaths followed primarily by chest wall movements. The abdominal pressure also varies with this cycle, increasing when respirations are abdominal and decreasing with chest movement. When this breathing pattern is present, the $PaCO_2$ begins to rise. A simultaneously decreasing respiratory rate indicates that respiratory muscle failure has occurred, with imminent danger of respiratory arrest. It requires immediate intervention.

Interpreting ABG values

Arterial blood gas (ABG) values may be interpreted rapidly by systematically assessing each ABG value, then determining the acid-base balance.

Pao$_2$

The partial pressure of oxygen (O_2) in arterial blood (Pao$_2$) is normally 80 to 100 mm Hg. A Pao$_2$<80 mm Hg on room air is hypoxemia, which means the patient is being insufficiently oxygenated. When the patient receives O_2 therapy, hypoxemia is assumed and the Pao$_2$ assessment reflects how effectively the O_2 corrects the hypoxemia. A Pao$_2$>100 mm Hg means the hypoxemia is being overcorrected.

Hemoglobin

The saturation of hemoglobin is reported as the percentage of arterial oxygen saturation—Sao$_2$. The Sao$_2$ indicates how much O_2 is available to the tissues. Almost all O_2 goes to the tissues bound to hemoglobin. The normal Sao$_2$ is 93% to 97%, which provides adequate tissue oxygenation in nearly all patients. Patients with low hemoglobin levels—below 10 g/dl (100 g/liter)—will not be adequately oxygenated. An Sao$_2$ of 89% to 93% provides adequate oxygenation for most patients but requires frequent assessment because small decreases in Pao$_2$ will spur significant decreases in Sao$_2$. An Sao$_2$ below 89% is adequate except for those patients with chronically low hemoglobin values; an Sao$_2$ below 83% is inadequate in all patients.

Paco$_2$ and blood pH

The partial pressure of carbon dioxide in arterial blood (Paco$_2$) measures the effectiveness of the patient's ventilation. A Paco$_2$ in the normal range of 35 to 45 mm Hg indicates adequate ventilation. A Paco$_2$ above 45 mm Hg indicates alveolar hypoventilation; a Paco$_2$ below 35 mm Hg indicates alveolar hyperventilation.

The blood pH indicates acid-base balance. The normal pH range is 7.35 to 7.45. A pH below 7.35 is acidemia: increased blood acid content or decreased alkaline content. Conversely, a pH above 7.45 is alkalemia: decreased acid content or increased alkaline content. The sources of acid and base are the respiratory and metabolic systems. The respiratory component is Paco$_2$. A Paco$_2$ above 45 mm Hg (hypoventilation) causes increased acid levels, or respiratory acidemia. A Paco$_2$ below 35 mm Hg (hyperventilation) causes decreased acid levels, or respiratory alkalemia. The change in pH is inversely related to the change in Paco$_2$.

Bicarbonate (HCO$_3$$^-$) and blood pH

The normal range of HCO$_3$$^-$ (the metabolic component) is 22 to 28 mEq/liter (22 to 28 mmol/liter). An HCO$_3$$^-$ above 28 mEq/liter (28 mmol/liter) results from decreased metabolic acid levels or increased metabolic base levels and produces metabolic alkalemia. Conversely, an HCO$_3$$^-$ below 22 mEq/liter (22 mmol/liter) results from increased metabolic acid levels or decreased metabolic base

acidemia with a pH below 7.3. These values combined with the patient's characteristic clinical presentation indicate a definitive diagnosis of ARF. Occasionally, signs and symptoms alone may allow diagnosis of ARF. For example, a patient who is breathing minimally after a drug overdose is clearly in respiratory failure. In contrast, a patient in severe respiratory distress with markedly increased work of breathing may have normal ABG levels. Such a patient, though in severe distress, is ventilating adequately. (See *Interpreting ABG values,* above, and *Diagnostic profile: Expected findings in ARF,* page 194.)

levels and produces metabolic acidemia. Changes in pH are directly related to changes in HCO_3^-.

To maintain normal pH when one of the metabolic components becomes abnormal, the other component changes to compensate. For example, respiratory acidemia ($PaCO_2$ above 45 mm Hg) causes compensatory metabolic alkalemia (HCO_3^- above 28 mEq/liter (28 mmol/liter). Metabolic compensation can return the pH to normal in 24 to 48 hours.

However, metabolic compensation is limited to a narrow range and will not overcome the primary disorder. An increase in HCO_3^- levels to compensate for an increase in $PaCO_2$ will not raise the pH above 7.40. In such an instance, the primary acid-base disorder must be identified and corrected.

Predicting pH changes

The primary disorder can be identified by predicting the change in pH expected by each of the components of the acid-base balance. The calculation is as follows:

The midpoint of the normal range of each component is used for prediction. The midpoint of the normal pH range is 7.40; of $PaCO_2$, 40 mm Hg; and of HCO_3^-, 25 mEq/liter (25 mmol/liter).

Rules:
• A change in $PaCO_2$ from 40 mm Hg causes the pH to change in the *opposite* direction from 7.40.
• A change in HCO_3^- from 25 mEq/liter (25 mmol/liter) causes the pH to change in the *same* direction from 7.40.

Steps:
1. Predict the pH change expected from the $PaCO_2$. (Example: A $PaCO_2$ of 50 mm Hg predicts a pH below 7.40.)
2. Predict the pH change expected from the HCO_3^-. (Example: An HCO_3^- of 25 mEq/liter [25 mmol/liter] predicts a pH above 7.40.)
3. In what direction has the pH changed from 7.40? (Example: A pH of 7.32 is less than 7.40.)
4. Compare the *observed* pH change with the *predicted* pH change. The component that predicts the observed change in

pH is the primary disorder. (Example: if the observed pH is 7.32, and the $PaCO_2$ predicts that the pH will be < 7.40, the respiratory component is primary, or respiratory acidemia is present.)
5. Determine if compensation is present. Compare the component predicting a pH change with the actual pH change. If the change is within the normal range, compensation is not present; if it is abnormal, compensation is present. If the pH is abnormal, compensation is partial and the primary disorder is acute; if the pH is normal, compensation is complete and the primary disorder is chronic. (Example: If the pH is 7.36, $PaCO_2$ is 50 mm Hg, and HCO_3^- is 28 mEq/liter [28 mmol/liter], the $PaCO_2$ predicts a pH below 7.40 and respiratory acidemia is present. The HCO_3^- is above its normal range and the pH is within its normal range. Thus, complete compensation is present. These ABG values are interpreted as a completely compensated respiratory acidemia, which is therefore chronic.)

Chest X-rays. Chest X-rays can confirm or rule out lung disorders as causes of ARF. They also identify secondary lung disorders, such as pneumonia, pleural effusion, or pneumothorax. By locating infiltrates within the lungs, chest X-rays help clarify the role and location of infection, inflammation, and atelectasis in ARF. Serial chest X-rays monitor the progression and resolution of ARF. Clear or normal chest X-rays indicate an extrapulmonary source of ARF, such as an airway obstruction, neuromuscular disease, or respiratory center depression.

Expected findings in ARF

Name of test	Normal findings	Expected findings
PaO_2 (breathing room air)	80 to 100 mm Hg	<50 mm Hg
$PaCO_2$	35 to 45 mm Hg	>50 mm Hg
pH	7.35 to 7.45	<7.30
Tidal volume	0.5 liter	<0.5 liter
Vital capacity	4.5 liters	<1.5 liter
Negative inspiratory force	> -75 cm H_2O	< -35 cm H_2O
Chest X-ray	Clear	Clear (with extrapulmonary cause of ARF); infiltrates, atelectasis, pleural effusion (with pulmonary cause of ARF)
White blood cell count	5,000 to 10,000/mm³ (5 to 10 x 10⁹/liter)	>10,000/mm³ when infection is present
Hemoglobin	13 to 18 g/dl (130 to 180 g/liter)	13 to 18 g/dl, but increased if chronic hypoxemia is present
Sputum culture and sensitivity	Normal flora (expectorated); no organisms (tracheal aspirate)	Polymorphonuclear cells and bacteria with infection

Pulmonary function tests. Measuring the ability to ventilate effectively, especially in a patient with neuromuscular disease, helps determine the potential for ventilatory failure. The amount of force generated by respiratory muscles for inspiration is called negative inspiratory force (NIF), maximum inspiratory force, or peak inspiratory pressure. It's measured by having the patient inhale through a closed airway and measuring the resulting negative pressure. To measure the vital capacity (VC), the patient takes as large a breath as possible and exhales through a spirometer to maximal exhalation. A VC of less than 10 ml/kg or an NIF of less than -25 cm H_2O indicates that ARF is likely and ventilatory support may be needed. These ventilatory parameters are measured serially, hourly, or less frequently, depending on the patient's condition.

Other routine tests. An ECG, a CBC, a blood chemistry profile, and sputum studies complete the routine diagnostic workup. The ECG should rule out cardiac disease either causing or resulting from ARF. The CBC reveals infection (increased WBC count) and how much hemoglobin is available for carrying O_2. A patient with an increased hemoglobin level will be able to carry more of a limited O_2 supply to the tissues. When a low hemoglobin level unduly increases the patient's need to breathe, ARF follows.

A blood chemistry profile identifies possible electrolyte abnormalities. This is especially important if respiratory failure has been developing slowly and the patient's fluid intake has been limited. The profile should be analyzed for signs of the underlying cause of ARF—such as the elevated alkaline phosphatase level of acute pancreatitis.

When sputum changes and chest X-rays suggest an infection, a sputum Gram stain and culture should be obtained to guide antibiotic therapy. The sputum sample should be obtained before beginning antibiotic therapy. If necessary, antibiotic therapy can start before test results are complete but should be re-evaluated later according to the test results.

Case study: Part 3

The ED doctor prescribed an albuterol aerosol inhaler for Mr. Smith. When his breathing stabilized, Mr. Smith was admitted to the intensive care unit (ICU) for monitoring and treatment. The admitting doctor increased O_2 to 3 liters/minute by nasal cannula. Repeat ABG results were as follows: pH, 7.32; $Paco_2$, 65 mm Hg; Pao_2, 57 mm Hg; Sao_2, 0.86 (86%); HCO_3^-, 32 mEq/liter (32 mmol/liter).

Pulse oximetry readings showed an Sao_2 between 0.84 and 0.88, acceptable for a patient with COPD. On a cardiac monitor, Mr. Smith's heart rhythm showed as sinus tachycardia at a rate of 128 beats/minute, with two to four unifocal premature ventricular contractions (PVCs) per minute.

The doctor prescribed an aminophylline bolus followed by a constant infusion; methylprednisolone; ceftazidime; and a one-time dose of furosemide.

During the next 24 hours, Mr. Smith's condition did not change significantly. He was able to cough weakly and produce a small amount of yellow sputum. His breath sounds remained diminished, with inspiratory and expiratory wheezes and a few scattered rhonchi. A morning chest X-ray showed a worsening right lower lobe infiltrate. The doctor then prescribed chest physiotherapy, which Mr. Smith toler-

Case study: Part 3 *(continued)*

ated only for short periods. His sputum production increased slightly. Sputum culture and sensitivity test results showed *Streptococcus pneumoniae* resistant to cephalosporins but sensitive to ampicillin, and *Haemophilus influenzae* sensitive to ampicillin and cephalosporins.

Accordingly, antibiotic therapy was changed to 1 g ampicillin. During the next 2 days, Mr. Smith's condition began to improve. His heart rate decreased to 96 beats/minute with only an occasional PVC, and he was afebrile. The doctor noted no jugular vein distention when Mr. Smith sat up at a 45-degree angle and found decreased ankle edema. Mr. Smith's respiratory rate decreased to 28 breaths/minute, and he continued to use accessory chest muscles (but not neck muscles) for breathing. Breath sounds improved, with wheezes present only on expiration and rhonchi present throughout both lungs, but louder on the right side. Mr. Smith now coughed more strongly, and he produced large amounts of thick, yellow sputum. For the first time since admission, he was able to speak in full sentences.

Five days after admission, Mr. Smith's condition was significantly improved. His heart rate was 88 beats/minute, his respiratory rate was 24 breaths/minute, and he had only mildly diminished breath sounds with good air entry, a few scattered rhonchi, and no wheezes. With a stronger cough, Mr. Smith produced thick, greyish yellow sputum. ABG results were as follows on 2 liters/minute of oxygen by nasal cannula: pH, 7.36; $Paco_2$, 55 mm Hg; Pao_2, 63 mm Hg; Sao_2, 0.88 (88%); and HCO_3^-, 32 mEq/liter (32 mmol/liter). A chest X-ray showed that the right lower lobe infiltrate was clearing.

Mr. Smith was transferred to a medical nursing unit. I.V. aminophylline was discontinued after the first oral dose of theophylline. I.V. methylprednisolone was tapered and I.V. ampicillin was continued for 7 days. Mr. Smith could ambulate to the bathroom, but he still had to use accessory muscles and pursed lips to breathe.

After 12 days, the doctor discontinued aerosol treatments and ampicillin and prescribed a synthetic corticosteroid inhaler, beclomethasone. The doctor also resumed Mr. Smith's albuterol inhaler and continued oral theophylline, which measured within the therapeutic range at 17 mcg/ml.

By this time, Mr. Smith could ambulate in the hallway approximately 75' with only slightly increased work of breathing. On auscultation, he had slightly diminished breath sounds with good air entry, a prolonged expiratory phase, and rare rhonchi that cleared with coughing. Mr. Smith's coughing now produced small to moderate amounts of grey sputum. ABG analysis on room air produced the following results: pH, 7.36; $Paco_2$, 52 mm Hg; Pao_2, 52 mm Hg; Sao_2, 0.83 (83%); and HCO_3^-, 32 mEq/liter (32 mmol/liter).

Treatment options

Treatment of ARF and its underlying disease depends on whether ventilatory or oxygenation failure is present and focuses on supporting oxygenation of the body tissues and maintaining an acceptable blood pH.

Supporting oxygenation

Supporting oxygenation involves maintaining a patent airway, administering O_2 in the appropriate quantity and quality, and administering appropriate drug therapy.

   Clearing the airway. When ARF results from partial or complete airway obstruction, opening the airway is the first concern. Such obstruction can result from a foreign body, tracheal stenosis, laryngeal edema, epiglottitis, and a decreased level of consciousness that leads to accumulation of secretions and problems with tongue control. When an obstruction can't be relieved by conservative measures, such as the abdominal thrust or laryngoscopy, emergency cricothyrotomy or tracheotomy is necessary. Securing oropharyngeal and nasopharyngeal airways or side positioning can also be tried before attempting endotracheal intubation. If these measures fail, endotracheal intubation should be performed before airway obstruction becomes complete.

   Administering O_2. O_2 is the single most important therapy for ARF. It's needed when either SaO_2 is less than 0.90 (90%) or the patient has clinical signs of hypoxia. However, several potential problems must be considered:

• Patients who are using the hypoxic drive to stimulate breathing should receive O_2 only in low, well-controlled concentrations. In these patients, low PaO_2 is caused by chronic hypoventilation and CO_2 retention. Giving O_2 alleviates the low PaO_2 and simultaneously removes the breathing stimulus and increases CO_2 retention.

• Suppression of the hypoxic drive may occur unexpectedly in some patients. For example, the stimulus to breathe is strong in patients who have suddenly become acutely hypoxic, and they respond by hyperventilating. If this hyperventilation produces a normal $PaCO_2$, when the PaO_2 is raised with O_2 administration, then ventilation will be depressed; $PaCO_2$ becomes elevated; and significant acidemia results. This may occur when ARF arises from V/Q mismatch, as in patients with pneumonia.

• High concentrations of O_2 are usually toxic to lung tissue. Prolonged therapeutic use of high-concentration O_2 (with an FIO_2 of 0.75) can cause adult respiratory distress syndrome (ARDS). But sometimes high concentrations are needed to treat ARDS. To avoid oxygen toxicity, use the lowest concentration of O_2 that provides acceptable oxygenation. When the oxygenation is dangerously low, high concentrations of O_2 should be used, but they must be reduced as quickly as possible.

• O_2 therapy should be continued until ARF has resolved and the patient's ABG levels on room air are acceptable. Sometimes, after initial O_2 supplementation has eased respiratory muscle fatigue, the patient may feel no further need for treatment. However, if he then increases activity, he'll need more O_2. Therefore, O_2 therapy should be given continuously, even during diagnostic studies. (See *Equipment: Oxygen delivery devices.*)

Providing mechanical ventilation. If O_2 therapy and bronchodilators fail to improve respiration, mechanical ventilation should begin before respiratory muscle failure develops. Physiologic indications include $PaCO_2$ above 50 mm Hg, pH below 7.30, respiratory rate below 6 breaths/minute or above 35 breaths/minute, tidal volume (Vt) below 5 cc/kg, VC below 10 ml/kg, and NIF below − 25 cm H_2O. A high respiratory rate with shallow breaths may mean ineffective ventilation. A high respiratory rate with deep breaths could mean high work of breathing, which cannot be maintained without eventually incurring respiratory muscle fatigue.

The expected course of the underlying disease governs how quickly mechanical ventilation should be applied. If treatment is expected to resolve the underlying disease rapidly, prompt use of mechanical ventilation may not be necessary. But if the underlying disease is expected to worsen, or if treatment will be prolonged, mechanical ventilation should begin at the first signs of ventilatory failure. Note that although mechanical ventilation may prevent respiratory arrest and reduce the severity of organ dysfunction, it may lead to ventilator dependence. Patients with advancing chronic disease may have no hope of being weaned. (See *Ethical dilemma: Deciding about ventilation,* page 200.)

▸ **EQUIPMENT**

Oxygen delivery devices

You can choose from among several devices to provide O_2 therapy for your patient. The choice depends on several factors, including the FIO_2 and the amount of humidity required. Two devices commonly used are the nasal cannula and the Venturi mask.

NASAL CANNULA

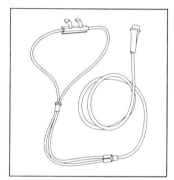

The *nasal cannula* provides comfortable and easy O_2 administration. FIO_2 delivery is determined by the liter per minute (LPM) flow rate set on the flow meter. The higher the flow rate to the cannula, the less room air is entrained during inspiration and the higher the FIO_2 delivered. The flow rate should be monitored carefully; after initial O_2 therapy, the patient's respirations may slow, which will result in a higher FIO_2 being delivered. Slow, shallow breathing delivers a higher FIO_2 than rapid, deep breathing at the same flow rate because of the amount of room air entrained. The O_2 should also be humidified by a bubble (low-humidity) humidifier. The major advantage of using the nasal cannula is that it's well tolerated—if the patient doesn't dislodge the cannula, he'll receive an accurate O_2 dose.

VENTURI MASK

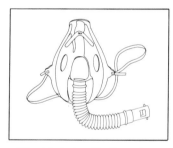

The *Venturi* or *Venti mask* provides a high flow rate with a precise FIO_2. Oxygen flows from a bubble humidifier to the mask through a small orifice and floods the mask with a high flow of oxygen that exceeds the patient's inspiratory flow rate.

Administering drug therapy. Drug therapy may correct the cause of ARF or help prevent disease-related complications. Bronchodilators improve ventilation and aid removal of secretions; antibiotics prevent or treat infection; and steroids reduce airway edema and inflammation. Sodium bicarbonate may be used to correct metabolic acidemia (although it is not the pre-

---

Deciding about ventilation

Deciding to impose treatment with artificial ventilation poses a commonly recurring ethical problem. The doctor is torn between his desire to prolong life and uncertainty about the impact of his efforts on the patient's quality of life. If the nurse is involved, too, she must take steps to help the patient—and protect herself.

Consider a patient who develops acute respiratory failure as a complication of advancing chronic disease. Without mechanical ventilation to support respiration, the disease is usually fatal. But if his respiratory system has been severely damaged, he may become ventilator-dependent with no hope of being successfully weaned, and the treatment becomes merely palliative. In the face of uncertain benefit, should the patient receive mechanical ventilation?

Ideally, the patient should discuss this issue with the doctor before the need for ventilation arises. They should discuss the expected course of the disease and the expected effects of mechanical ventilation. This discussion should include long-term ventilator care at home if the patient is otherwise healthy. In some cases, the doctor, knowing the patient's status, may decide to begin or withhold mechanical ventilation without consulting the patient, considering that his knowledge and responsibilities override the patient's personal autonomy. He may or may not involve the family in his decision.

If the patient chooses ventilation, its economic and social impact should be considered. Prolonged mechanical ventilation, which risks ventilator dependence, may impose an undesirable financial and emotional burden on the patient and his family.

The patient may refuse ventilation, viewing mechanical support as a useless holding action. The patient's family may strongly disagree. In other cases, both the patient and the family may refuse ventilation, even if the patient's clinical status suggests that he may be weanable. This decision is especially difficult for health care professionals to support.

Before deciding about ventilation, the patient may ask the nurse about his disease and about the mechanical ventilation procedure. She must provide him with detailed information to help him make his decision. This conversation should be well documented. If it is not, the nurse may be unable to support the patient's decision in a legally acceptable way. For example, without properly documented statements or input from the family, the doctor is obliged to begin therapy to save the patient's life. This may be contrary to the patient's known, but undocumented, wishes.

---

ferred treatment), and loop diuretics may be used to treat predisposing conditions, such as pulmonary edema or cor pulmonale. The patient's electrolyte and nutritional status may also require administration of electrolytes and nutritional supplements. (See *Drug therapy: Bronchodilators and other drugs in ARF,* pages 202 and 203.)

Experimental therapies
Investigational treatments for ARF include mask continuous positive airway pressure (CPAP) and mechanical ventilation using intermittent positive-pressure ventilation with a mouthpiece or negative pressure ventilation. These treatments aim to reduce or prevent the need for intubation and mechanical ventilation. Re-

cent research includes efforts to develop a temporary artificial lung. (See *Promising research: Intravascular oxygenator.*)

Mask CPAP. In this treatment, CPAP is applied to the patient's face or nose. (See *Equipment: Using mask CPAP,* page 204.) An O_2 blender attached to a continuous high-flow reservoir bag delivers a very high flow of gas with an FIO_2 range of 21% to 100% to a tightly fitting facial or nasal mask. The high flow rate and an adjustable CPAP valve maintain the desired level of CPAP. Mask CPAP can also be provided by attaching a mechanical ventilator in CPAP mode to the mask. Though given by mask, CPAP produces effects that are the same as those provided through endotracheal or tracheostomy tubes. The advantage of mask CPAP is that it doesn't bypass the natural airways' defenses against infection, as tracheal intubation does.

Mask CPAP also effectively treats hypoxemia, which persists with conventional O_2 therapy in patients who have adequate ventilation. In this instance, mask CPAP increases oxygenation before a combined oxygenation and ventilatory failure can occur. The improved oxygenation decreases the work of breathing and avoids respiratory muscle fatigue. Mask CPAP has been successfully used for trauma and postoperative patients who have developed ARF and to prevent the development of ARF. It may be used continuously or intermittently. Intermittent mask CPAP for 1 hour every 4 hours has successfully prevented progression of, and reversed, atelectasis causing ARF.

Facial mask CPAP may make the patient feel uncomfortable or anxious, and he may try to remove the mask. Reassure the patient and use a mask with soft, pliable edges if possible. Positive pressure in the pharynx promotes air swallowing, which can distend the stomach and lead to nausea and vomiting. The patient who vomits may aspirate because his nose and mouth are tightly covered and the mask can't be removed easily. To avoid this risk, the patient who is receiving continuous facial CPAP should have a nasogastric tube connected to suction. The patient who is receiving intermittent facial CPAP must be monitored frequently for gastric distention and nausea. If they develop, discontinue facial CPAP immediately.

Nasal CPAP greatly reduces the possibility of aspiration because it leaves the patient's mouth uncovered. However, if the

(Text continues on page 204.)

▼ PROMISING RESEARCH

Intravascular oxygenator

A new device designed to function temporarily as an artificial lung is being tested as a lifesaving help to patients with respiratory failure. This device, called IVOX, is an intravascular oxygenator; it is expected to provide approximately half the oxygenation of normal breathing, supplementing the impaired lungs and allowing them to rest and possibly recover.

The intravascular oxygenator is made up of hundreds of long, hollow, porous, polypropylene tubes. These tubes, thin as a human hair, allow the exchange of gases, much like the permeable membranes of the alveolar capillaries. Through these tubes, oxygen is pumped into the blood to perfuse and nourish the tissue cells, and carbon dioxide is drawn out. This device is threaded through a vein in the leg or neck into the vena cava.

DRUG THERAPY

Bronchodilators and other drugs in ARF

When the patient's airway has been cleared and his oxygenation stabilized, prescribed drug therapy may include a bronchodilator and possibly other drugs, such as corticosteroids to control airway inflammation, antibiotics to prevent or fight infection, and others as needed.

Bronchodilators
Most important in ARF therapy, these drugs dilate the bronchi and decrease airflow resistance to reduce the work of breathing. Inhaled sympathomimetics are commonly used as bronchodilators in ARF. Although also available in oral forms, inhalants produce fewer adverse effects (which may include tachycardia, dysrhythmias, central nervous system [CNS] stimulation, restlessness, agitation, insomnia, and seizures).

Commonly used sympathomimetics include isoetharine, metaproterenol, and albuterol. They're diluted with normal saline solution and given via a nebulizer. The patient inhales through a mouthpiece on the nebulizer for 15 to 20 minutes, drawing the aerosolized droplets into the bronchi. The resulting bronchodilation begins in about 5 minutes, reaches peak effect in 20 minutes, and lasts 4 to 6 hours. The patient receives the drug every 4 to 6 hours. For the patient in acute respiratory distress, treatments are initially given around the clock. As the patient's breathing improves, nocturnal treatments are stopped to allow adequate rest.

Xanthine derivatives
Anhydrous theophylline and its salts, aminophylline and oxtriphylline, are xanthine derivatives that relax bronchial smooth muscle by reducing the breakdown of cAMP and blocking adenosine receptors. These derivatives contain different amounts of anhydrous theophylline, but all have similar mechanisms of action, half-lives, onsets of action, and peak concentrations.

In the acute phase of ARF, aminophylline is administered I.V. When no theophylline preparation has been used in the past 24 hours, a loading dose of 9 mg/kg (of ideal body weight) of aminophylline is given. If the patient has recently taken theophylline and has a subtherapeutic serum theophylline level, the loading dose can be reduced. Dilute the loading dose and give by constant I.V. infusion over 30 minutes. This rapidly establishes a steady-state therapeutic serum level, usually 10 to 20 mcg; some patients respond to lower levels. Maintain this level with continuous I.V. infusion. Because individual theophylline metabolism varies, check the patient's serum levels 6 to 12 hours after starting the infusion or changing the infusion rate, to ensure adequate levels. Several factors affect the rate of theophylline metabolism: Smoking increases its metabolism; congestive heart failure (CHF), cor pulmonale, and liver disease decrease it.

The usual loading dose of anhydrous theophylline is 5 mg/kg,

given by slow I.V. drip. Reduce this dose by 50% if the patient has received theophylline in the previous 24 hours. The maintenance dose of theophylline should be adjusted according to the following factors: children under age 9, 1 mg/kg/hour; adult smokers and children ages 9 to 16, 0.8 mg/kg/hour; adult nonsmokers, 0.5 mg/kg/hour; patients with CHF or liver disease, 0.2 mg/kg/hour. Dosage adjustment is also needed if aminophylline is used because 79% of the aminophylline dose is theophylline.

As the acute phase of ARF resolves, an oral theophylline preparation is substituted for the I.V. aminophylline infusion. Oral theophylline reaches peak serum levels within 45 minutes. The I.V. infusion can be discontinued as soon as the first oral dose is given.

The interval between doses will depend on whether an extended-release form is used. Extended release provides more stable serum levels, but considerable individual variability still exists. Serum levels should be checked 24 to 48 hours after changing to the oral preparation, to adjust dosage and frequency according to the individual's theophylline metabolism.

Patients receiving theophylline must also be closely monitored for signs of toxicity. Some patients show signs of toxicity with serum levels within the therapeutic range. Others may be symptom-free with serum levels in the toxic range. CNS effects range from headache, irritability, and restlessness to seizures. Tachycardia is one of the earliest toxic effects. Other cardiovascular effects are palpitations, dysrhythmias, and hypotension.

Corticosteroids
Although their use in ARF is controversial, these drugs are used to control inflammation and to stabilize lung capillary membranes. By limiting inflammation within airways, they can reduce airway narrowing, thus reducing the work of breathing and helping to avoid ventilatory failure.

When an inflammatory process (such as asthma, chronic obstructive pulmonary disease, and infection) contributes to ARF, 125 mg of I.V. methylprednisolone is administered every 6 hours. This dose may speed respiratory improvement. After 2 to 3 days, the steroid dose is tapered off. Such tapering may be slow, decreasing the dosage every 2 to 3 days, or rapid, decreasing the dosage daily. When the dosage has been decreased to 40 mg every 6 hours, the administration route is usually changed to oral. As recovery continues, the steroid dose is gradually tapered down to a maintenance dose or is discontinued. When maintenance treatment with steroids is required, as for underlying lung disease, the administration route is changed to inhalation. The inhaled route is preferred because the patient receives the benefit of the steroid with fewer long-term adverse effects.

Antibiotics
Upper respiratory infections and pneumonia in patients with a chronic predisposing disease commonly lead to ARF. Antibiotics are chosen according to the results of culture and sensitivity studies. Culture results may be delayed 2 to 3 days; treatment of infections should begin immediately and be modified later according to test results. The usual community-acquired respiratory infections may be sensitive to penicillins, cephalosporins, erythromycin, and ampicillin. Hospital-acquired infections usually require penicillinase-resistant penicillins, cephalosporins, or aminoglycosides.

During an episode of ARF, another pulmonary infection may develop. Endotracheal intubation and mechanical ventilation carry the greatest risk of introducing pathogens into the airways and causing infection. Oxygen delivery devices and inhalers are also sources of pathogens. Thus, all patients with ARF must be continually monitored for signs and symptoms of infection.

Alkalizers
Sodium bicarbonate may be used to correct metabolic acidemia in ARF. Tissues receiving less oxygen than they need for aerobic metabolism convert to anaerobic metabolism, producing excessive lactic acid with lower pH levels. Sodium bicarbonate must be administered cautiously, because the return to aerobic metabolism metabolizes the lactic acid. Excessive sodium bicar-

bonate levels may induce metabolic alkalemia, which promotes carbon dioxide retention and worsens any existing hypoventilation.

Diuretics
Patients in ARF may need diuretics to treat underlying pulmonary edema or cor pulmonale. Loop diuretics, such as furosemide and bumetanide, are effective but may induce metabolic alkalemia from loss of chloride ion from the kidneys. Less potent acetazolamide works by increasing bicarbonate loss through the kidneys to lower blood bicarbonate and pH levels. The lowered blood pH stimulates increased ventilation to reduce $Paco_2$. However, acetazolamide should be used cautiously if the patient has difficulty tolerating the increased work of breathing.

Nutrients and electrolytes
Treatment of ARF must also prevent respiratory muscle fatigue and promote respiratory muscle strength. Electrolyte abnormalities, such as hypokalemia, hypocalcemia, and hypophosphatemia, must be corrected and adequate nutrition maintained to provide energy for the respiratory muscles. If adequate nutritional support is not in place within 2 to 3 days of the onset of ARF, catabolism will lead to muscle protein breakdown. If the patient's oral intake is inadequate, provide nutrition and electrolyte replacement by nasogastric tube or parenterally.

Using mask CPAP

Continuous positive airway pressure (CPAP) is applied via a tight-fitting nasal mask with the patient's mouth closed. This method, used for patients with sleep apnea, applies positive pressure to the airway to prevent obstruction during inspiration.

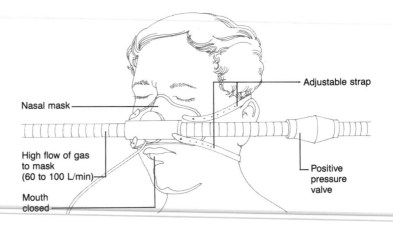

Nasal mask

Adjustable strap

High flow of gas to mask (60 to 100 L/min)

Mouth closed

Positive pressure valve

patient cannot keep his mouth closed, CPAP's benefits are lost. Nocturnal nasal CPAP is effective as a long-term home therapy for obstructive sleep apnea.

Mechanical ventilation. Intermittent positive-pressure ventilation using a mouthpiece (MIPPV) effectively treats chronic ventilatory failure. Patients with respiratory failure from polio, neuromuscular diseases, or COPD have been supported for long periods on MIPPV without needing a tracheostomy. This therapy can be used for short intervals (4 hours) or continuously. When used for a period each day, MIPPV prevents respiratory muscle fatigue, increases spontaneous VC, and reduces $PaCO_2$.

MIPPV requires an alert and cooperative patient. This treatment is applied through a mouthpiece connected to an intermittent positive-pressure ventilator. The patient must keep his lips tightly sealed around the mouthpiece. The ventilator is then set to assist, or augment, the patient's breathing efforts to provide a larger Vt than the patient's spontaneous breaths. The patient must be able to seal his nose to prevent gas from escaping. (Use a nose clip if necessary.) If the patient doesn't breathe spontaneously, the ventilator can be set to provide a number of mandatory breaths each minute. Use of MIPPV in a sleeping patient requires a mouthpiece with a lip seal.

Another method, negative pressure ventilation (NPV), also known as a body ventilator, applies negative pressure to the external chest, expanding it to pull air into the lungs. The Vt obtained is less than that obtained with positive-pressure ventilation, but it may be enough to normalize or reduce $PaCO_2$ to prevent respiratory muscle fatigue. Like MIPPV, NPV may be used for short periods or continuously and for the same chronic respiratory failure conditions. The iron lung is a negative pressure ventilator. Smaller, less cumbersome versions are the chest shell (cuirass) and the Emerson Wrap.

Case study: Part 4

Observing Mr. Smith's severe respiratory distress, the ED nurses identified two nursing diagnoses as their major priorities: *ineffective breathing pattern* and *impaired gas exchange.* They did not choose *ineffective airway clearance* because Mr. Smith showed a patent airway at admission, but they did assess the patency of his airway repeatedly during his stay in the ED.

The ICU and medical unit nurses chose the same two nursing diagnoses for planning Mr. Smith's nursing care. They also identified the following additional nursing diagnoses as the foundation for meeting Mr. Smith's needs during his hospitalization: *ineffective airway clearance, activity intolerance, fluid volume excess, ineffective individual and family coping,* and *knowledge deficit.*

The ED nurses performed continuous assessments of his respiratory rate and depth as well as the quality of his respirations in the first hour after admission. Periodic assessments followed (every 10 to 15 minutes in the ICU and every hour in the medical nursing unit), particularly to note his response to treatment. Because Mr. Smith's ARF was so severe, the nurses performed a complete respiratory assessment every 2 to 4 hours in the ICU and every 4 to 8 hours in the medical nursing unit. They also assessed his breath sounds before and 20 minutes after all respiratory treatments.

To ease Mr. Smith's tachypnea and dyspnea, the nurses encouraged him to assume his position of comfort. He found that high Fowler's position eased his breathing more than any other position.

The nurses sought to avoid intubation and mechanical ventilation. By minimizing his activity, Mr. Smith could focus all his energy

Case study: Part 4 *(continued)*

on breathing. Therefore, the nurses encouraged him to avoid all activity—even speaking—and assisted him with all activities of daily living.

To combat the decreased diffusion of oxygen in his lungs, the nurses administered oxygen as prescribed and provided humidification even at low flow rates to prevent drying of the delicate respiratory mucous membranes. The nurses turned him slightly on his side by placing pillows behind his back every 2 hours. This change in position improved the V/Q matching and assisted in increasing his oxygenation. The nurses evaluated the effectiveness of these interventions by interpreting ABG values.

Although Mr. Smith was able to maintain a patent upper airway throughout his hospitalization, his lower airways were congested with the exudate resulting from his pneumonia. To ease this congestion, the nurses encouraged Mr. Smith to deep-breathe and cough 30 minutes after each albuterol treatment (which was given every 4 hours). Initially, in the ICU, he could not take a deep breath and his cough was weak, necessitating chest physiotherapy (CPT). After his albuterol treatments, the nurse and respiratory therapist performed CPT only to his right side. After CPT, his sputum production increased slightly and the nurse recorded the color, quantity, odor, and consistency of these secretions.

As Mr. Smith improved and his strength increased, the nurses and respiratory therapist shortened the rest periods, increased the frequency of deep breathing and coughing, and lowered the head of the bed during treatments.

To monitor his fluid volume status, the nurses were careful to monitor his weight on the same scale, at the same time each day, and in the same type of clothing.

When Mr. Smith was transferred to the medical nursing unit, Mrs. Smith expressed her concern to the nurse that when Mr. Smith got home, he would again feel that he couldn't breathe. She was reassured that he would be taught some ways to manage his COPD that would help him feel better and reduce his risk of another ARF episode. After conversations with both Mr. and Mrs. Smith, the nurse developed a teaching plan for managing his COPD more effectively.

After an evaluation of his room air ABG values, the nurse and doctor noted that Mr. Smith would require continuous home oxygen therapy after discharge. Mr. Smith decided on the liquid system, which would allow him mobility so he could continue to take Mrs. Smith shopping. The social worker arranged for a local supplier to deliver the liquid oxygen system to the Smiths' home.

Nursing management

The patient who survives an episode of ARF requires close supportive care during a difficult convalescence. Such care requires continual assessment and monitoring of the patient's respiratory function to evaluate therapy and verify that the patient's respiratory status has stabilized and is improving. Such monitoring is also important to watch for the development of new respiratory problems and to provide any necessary additional therapy promptly.

Inspection and monitoring

Frequent assessment of the patient's breathing is critical when the patient has *ineffective breathing pattern* or *impaired gas exchange.* Just watching the patient's chest expansion and respiratory muscle movements tells you quickly about the work of breathing and the condition of the lungs. The presence or absence of intercostal or sternal retractions tells you about airflow resistance, airway diameter, and lung compliance. Chest enlargement and upper abdomen retraction (especially in the area immediately below the ribs and sternum) indicate respiratory muscle dyscoordination, a sign of respiratory muscle fatigue. After an initial inspection, you can continue to monitor the patient's respiratory status with brief observations during subsequent patient contacts, adjusting to baseline changes as needed.

Watch breathing patterns. Monitor the respiratory rate and depth of each breath, the quality of breath sounds, and the level of consciousness for evidence of *ineffective breathing pattern.* Watch carefully for changes in rate or depth of respirations related to increased work of breathing and respiratory muscle fatigue. These signs may signal imminent respiratory arrest and require immediate intervention. Monitor breath sounds to evaluate air entry. Listen for wheezing. If it's worsening or not improving, current therapy is ineffective.

Watch for changes in level of consciousness. Because the brain is so sensitive to changes in O_2 level, a diminishing level of consciousness means the patient has *impaired gas exchange* and needs additional O_2 or a change in therapy to improve oxygenation. It also means that ventilation may rapidly deteriorate and that mechanical ventilation will be necessary. However, be aware that the absence of changes in level of consciousness does not necessarily indicate normal oxygenation; some patients can tolerate low levels of O_2 saturation.

The electronic apnea monitor helps you track breathing patterns in patients with shallow or irregular breathing. The monitor detects changes in chest size and tracks the patient's respiratory rate. It sounds an alarm when it detects apnea or a predetermined high or low respiratory rate; however, it may not detect very shallow or abdominal breathing. When using an electronic monitor, be sure also to assess respirations by observation at least once every hour to identify any change in their character.

Frequently assess the patient's respiratory status. If the patient is in severe distress with labored breathing, check his chest movement and respiratory rate at least every 5 minutes until you establish a baseline. Then check him every 15 minutes until the baseline stabilizes. After the patient has been breathing at the new rate for some time, you can space your assessments accordingly. As a rule, you should assess a patient in moderate respiratory distress (with increased work of breathing or shallow breaths) at least every 15 minutes until the rate is established as a baseline and then every 1 to 2 hours.

Assess the patient before and after administering respiratory therapy. Schedule your assessment according to the expected effect of the therapy. For example, expect to detect a decreased respiratory rate 15 to 30 minutes after starting O_2 therapy; and reassess breath sounds 20 to 30 minutes after treatment with an aerosol bronchodilator. To reduce the total number of assessments, combine pre- and post-therapy assessments with your routinely scheduled ones.

Measure pulmonary function and oxygenation. Though qualitative monitoring is often adequate for patient assessment, quantitative monitoring is sometimes needed as well. For example, when respiratory muscle weakness contributes to ARF, as in neuromuscular disease, specific measures of pulmonary function—such as VC, Vt, and NIF—are commonly used. These parameters help identify the point at which the risk of *ineffective breathing pattern* and ventilatory failure exceeds the potential risks of mechanical ventilation.

The pulse oximeter allows easy monitoring of the patient's SaO_2. This device measures oxygen saturation through a sensor placed on a finger or another well-perfused area, such as the bridge of the nose or an earlobe. When the monitored SaO_2 value is equivocal, obtain an ABG level to guide further therapy.

Check heart rate and rhythm. Cardiac monitoring can help detect changes in the heart rate and dysrhythmias that cause *decreased cardiac output* and reflect corresponding changes in oxygenation patterns. The heart rate increases with low oxygenation and increased work of breathing, and decreases to normal levels with improved oxygenation and decreased work of breathing. Patients with chronically low levels of oxygenation, such as those with COPD, commonly have dysrhythmias associated with acidemia—which may worsen in ARF. Reduced myocardial oxygenation and ischemia may cause new dysrhythmias to develop. Cardiac monitoring helps identify these dysrhythmias to allow prompt treatment.

Watch for sputum changes. Changes in the amount and color of sputum associated with fever and a rising WBC count signal *potential for infection.* Increased sputum production may also signal resolution of an infection. In early pneumonia, secretions consolidate in the lung and little sputum is produced. But as this consolidation breaks up and the involved tissue aerates, sputum production rises. In the latter situation, increased production of sputum is associated with a decreasing temperature and WBC count.

Evaluate therapy. The interpretation of assessment findings depends on whether ARF results from poor oxygenation or inadequate ventilation. For example, effective therapy for oxygenation failure should *decrease* the respiratory rate and depth; effective therapy for ventilatory failure should *increase* them. A general rule for evaluating ARF therapy is that it is effective when the patient's respiratory rate and depth return to normal with a decreasing work of breathing. When your physical assessment indicates effective therapy, obtain ABG levels for confirmation.

Managing complications
The major complication of ARF is unresponsiveness to therapy. Even mechanical ventilation will not provide adequate support if the respiratory system fails to oxygenate the blood. Therefore, the signs and symptoms of severe ARF complications depend on the tissue response to O_2 deprivation. Cerebral hypoxia causes

altered levels of consciousness, seizures, and coma. Myocardial hypoxia causes loss of contractility and dysrhythmias, which further reduce O_2 delivery to the tissues. Persistent hypoxia then leads to metabolic acidosis, which, superimposed on respiratory acidosis, can cause profound acidosis (with pH at or below 7.15). Such profound acidosis responds poorly to treatment.

Secondary respiratory infections also commonly complicate ARF. They often result from the use of artificial airways, mechanical ventilators, and O_2 delivery devices, which may harbor pathogens. Reducing the risk of such infection requires strict attention to infection control by all persons in contact with the patient. Other potential complications are those resulting from prolonged bed rest or from malnutrition.

Nursing interventions

Several nursing interventions are especially helpful for getting the ARF patient successfully through convalescence. They include positioning, teaching deep-breathing and coughing techniques, using tracheal suctioning, modifying diet, and maintaining fluid intake.

Maintain correct positioning. For the patient with *ineffective breathing pattern*, correct positioning should promote easier chest expansion to minimize the patient's work of breathing. Raising the head of the bed and bending the patient at the hips often work best, but these maneuvers may have to be modified according to the patient's condition. For example, an obtunded patient who can't maintain a patent airway should lie on his side rather than supine. A patient whose abdomen is large or distended should lie in a position that won't displace the abdominal contents upward. A quadriplegic patient should assume semi-Fowler's position in the highest elevation tolerable.

Encourage deep-breathing exercises. For the patient with *impaired gas exchange,* correctly performed deep breathing increases ventilation to collapsed and underventilated alveoli, thus improving V/Q matching, ABG levels, and airflow behind consolidated secretions. It is especially beneficial in patients with ARF who have atelectasis or retained secretions.

Instruct the patient to begin deep breathing with a slow, steady inspiration, and continue until he can't inhale any more air. At this point of maximal inspiration, ask the patient to try to continue inhaling for 3 to 5 seconds and then exhale without effort through pursed lips. This allows the patient to exhale a greater volume of air, increasing total ventilation and decreasing the total work of breathing. Patients with severe dyspnea may be unable to learn this technique but should be encouraged to do so once the dyspnea subsides. To avoid muscle weakness, the patient should perform deep breathing frequently for only a few breaths. He should limit the number of deep breaths to one or two but repeat the exercises every 10 to 15 minutes. The patient with severely limited energy should have a longer rest period between exercises.

Encourage coughing. For the patient with *ineffective airway clearance,* effective coughing improves sputum production, reduces rhonchi, and is the primary method for clearing retained secretions. If the patient's cough is weak and ineffective, identifying the cause will help select a technique to help the patient cough effectively. (See *Selecting an effective coughing technique,* page 212.) The patient's cough can be weak because of an inability to take a deep breath before the cough, because respiratory muscles are too fatigued to generate enough force to produce a cough, because fear of pain hinders the patient from coughing forcefully, or because of a decreased level of consciousness.

In patients with respiratory muscle weakness, the cough-friendly or quad-cough technique can help move accumulated secretions. Preliminary use of CPT can loosen secretions that have collected in smaller, more peripheral airways. CPT involves body positioning that uses gravity to help drain secretions from selected areas of the lungs, with percussion and vibration of the chest wall to loosen the secretions for drainage. However, in patients with ARF, the underlying disease may restrict the body positions that can be used for postural drainage. For example, a patient with a neurologic disease should not have his head positioned lower than his body. He can be turned onto one side without lowering the backrest elevation. Use cough techniques cautiously to avoid inducing bronchospasm and increasing the work of breathing.

Consider that deep-breathing and coughing exercises may tax the patient's energy unduly. So try to schedule them with other therapies to produce maximum benefit for the least energy

Selecting an effective coughing technique

When the patient is not coughing effectively, one of the techniques described below can make the cough effective. After each cough produced by one of the following methods, the patient should be allowed to rest briefly before repeating the cough. Encourage any spontaneous coughing that occurs during the deep-breathing phase of exercise.

Cascade cough
1. The patient takes three to four deep breaths and exhales slowly through the mouth.
2. During expiration after the fourth breath, the patient performs a series of three to four coughs until expiration is complete.

This cough is used if the patient has adequate strength to cough, no bronchospasm, and patent airways but is not coughing effectively.

Huff cough
1. The patient takes two to three slow, deep breaths and exhales slowly through the mouth.
2. The patient then takes one or two slow, deep breaths and ex-

hales in three short bursts of fast exhalation, or "huffs."
3. The patient takes a deep breath and exhales in faster, more forceful bursts with the glottis open, producing three to four strong huffs until expiration is complete.

The huff cough is useful for the patient who has bronchospasm, whose airways collapse easily, or who is afraid to perform the cascade cough—for example, because of postoperative pain.

Cough-friendly technique
1. The patient assumes a sitting position with his feet on the floor or on a stool.
2. The patient places a pillow or blanket over the abdomen and supports it with his forearms.
3. The patient bends forward, pressing his forearms against the abdomen while exhaling, then returns to the sitting position while inhaling deeply through the nose.
4. The patient repeats bending forward during exhalation and deep breathing for two or three breaths.

5. After the last deep breath, the patient presses firmly on the abdomen while bending forward and producing two or three staged coughs.

The cough-friendly method is used when the patient does not have enough strength in the chest wall, diaphragm, or abdomen to produce a forceful cough.

Quad cough
1. The patient lies supine with the head of the bed elevated 45 degrees or less.
2. The patient takes two or three slow, deep breaths, exhaling slowly through the mouth.
3. While the patient takes a deep breath, place the palm of your hand on his abdomen, above the umbilicus and below the ribs.
4. As the patient begins to exhale and attempts to cough, press sharply inward and upward on the abdomen two or three times during exhalation.

The quad cough is useful when the patient can take a deep breath but cannot generate enough force for a cough.

---

expenditure. For example, give bronchodilator therapy just before interventions to clear the airway, and cluster deep-breathing and coughing exercises just after giving pain medication.

Perform tracheal suctioning. If rhonchi persist in the larger airways after cough therapy, the patient still has *ineffective airway clearance*, and tracheal suctioning may be required. This helps patients with both ARF and artificial airways. It can also be used to stimulate deep breathing and coughing in obtunded patients. Keep in mind, however, that suctioning may induce bronchospasm, excessive coughing, hypoxemia, and dysrhythmias. To avoid these risks, use tracheal suctioning only if coughing is ineffective.

Promote adequate nutrition. Severe dyspnea interferes with nutritional intake in several ways and results in *altered nutrition: less than body requirements.* The dyspneic patient hasn't enough energy to eat properly. Moreover, eating may itself increase dyspnea by impairing diaphragm movement and using the patient's limited energy for digestion. Giving frequent small meals can help minimize respiratory impairment while providing adequate nutrition. The patient who can't manage even small meals will benefit from liquid nutritional supplements.

Carefully monitor nutritional intake so that you'll know when enteral or parenteral nutrition is necessary. Insufficient nutrition can deplete carbohydrate stores, causing general muscle breakdown. Because respiratory muscles in patients with ARF are already compromised, further loss of muscle mass and strength could worsen respiratory failure or, at least, delay recovery.

Maintain fluid intake. Adequate hydration keeps secretions moist, loose, and easy to clear. To maintain adequate hydration, keep the patient's fluid intake at 2 to 3 liters/day unless contraindicated, as in congestive heart failure or cor pulmonale. Monitor intake and output and assess for physical signs of *altered fluid volume* and *potential fluid volume deficit.*

Patient and family teaching

Once you've identified the patient's and family's *knowledge deficit* concerning his underlying disease, your goals are to teach the patient and his family about ARF and its treatment, to reduce the patient's anxiety, and to prepare the patient for discharge. (See *Patient-teaching checklist: Acute respiratory failure.*) Before you begin, consider the patient's ability to receive information. The patient who is excessively anxious, hypoxemic, or significantly obtunded is unlikely to benefit from your teaching. If the patient has severe dyspnea, you may have to wait until his respiratory status has stabilized to teach an effective breathing pattern. Afterward, focus your teaching on interventions that promote recovery. Assess the patient's and family's knowledge. Do they know that ARF is usually treatable? Reassure them that

▶ **PATIENT-TEACHING CHECKLIST**

Acute respiratory failure

Teaching the patient about acute respiratory failure (ARF) should include the following information:
☐ Explanation of ARF and its expected course
☐ Teaching related to the underlying chronic disease
☐ Explanation of therapy: what it does, any related discomfort, and side effects
☐ Effective breathing pattern: pursed lip, slow and deep, or effective deep breath
☐ Effective coughing technique for patient: cascade, huff, cough-friendly method, or quad cough
☐ Need for oxygen therapy, including when not dyspneic
☐ Need to stop activity and rest when tired to avoid excessive fatigue
☐ Importance of maintaining adequate nutritional and fluid intake
☐ Medications and their administration, including the sequence in which they should be taken and the need to avoid all over-the-counter respiratory medications
☐ How to avoid another episode of ARF
☐ How to recognize changing respiratory status that may lead to ARF if untreated
☐ Sources of additional community support and information for the underlying problem (such as the American Lung Association)

recurrence is often preventable if they follow the plan of care you'll have worked out with them.

Teach the patient an appropriate deep-breathing and coughing technique, and include his family in your teaching to increase compliance. Explain the use and importance of O_2 therapy. Emphasize that O_2 therapy is used to increase the amount of O_2 in his blood and not to treat dyspnea. The patient should know that even when his breathing has improved, he may need to continue O_2 therapy to maintain optimal blood oxygenation. Emphasize that he should continue to use O_2 when he's out of bed and active until the doctor tells him it's no longer needed.

If ARF was a complication of an acute disease that is unlikely to recur, the patient needs only limited teaching about ARF. However, if another episode of ARF is likely, teach the patient how to recognize early signs and symptoms of respiratory failure (decreased activity levels, fatigue, dyspnea, and respiratory infection) so that he can take prompt action to minimize its effects. If he has chronically shallow respirations, instruct him to continue deep-breathing exercises several times each day to minimize atelectasis and promote clearance of secretions. If retained secretions are a chronic problem, review the patient's coughing technique, and encourage him to set aside two or three sessions per day to focus on coughing and airway clearance. Also teach him how to maintain adequate fluid intake (2 to 3 liters/day unless contraindicated). If the patient's sputum is tenacious or copious, instruct family members how and when to perform CPT.

Inform the patient of the potential for infection and the associated risk of ARF. Teach him how to avoid these infections. Review typical changes—in sputum production, activity levels, frequency of dyspnea, and the need for bronchodilators—that mean such infection is causing deterioration of pulmonary function. Explain that untreated infection can lead to ARF. To prevent infection, encourage the patient to have an annual flu shot and a Pneumovax vaccination to protect against most pneumonias.

Discharge planning

As you continue to work with the ARF patient, you have an opportunity to guide him and his family to accept life-style changes that will promote an uneventful recovery and prevent

DISCHARGE PLANNING CHECKLIST

Acute respiratory failure

Discharge planning for the patient with acute respiratory failure (ARF) must consider nursing criteria, patient and family teaching, and required documentation.

Nursing criteria
Patient's documentation confirms...
- ☐ Vital signs stable and within normal limits for this patient
- ☐ ABG values normal or within acceptable limits
- ☐ Respiratory status (rate, depth, dyspnea, cough, and sputum) at pre-ARF baseline
- ☐ Adequate food and fluid intake
- ☐ Adequate self-care and family support or home care

Patient and family teaching criteria
Patient and family understand...
- ☐ ARF development and how to avoid it in the future

- ☐ Relationship of a chronic disease to ARF
- ☐ How to manage the chronic disease and have received appropriate literature about the disease
- ☐ Medications, including actions, dosage schedule and sequence, and side effects
- ☐ Patient's need to rest when tired to avoid becoming excessively fatigued
- ☐ Importance of maintaining adequate nutritional and fluid intake
- ☐ If home oxygen therapy is needed, when it should be used and safety practices to follow
- ☐ To obtain pneumonia vaccine and an annual flu shot
- ☐ Need to monitor patient for changes in sputum, activity level, and dyspnea level

- ☐ When to seek medical attention for identified respiratory changes in patient

Required documentation
Be sure to record...
- ☐ Respiratory status at discharge, including rate and character of respirations, cough, sputum, oxygen use, and dyspnea
- ☐ Level of activity, including any technique being used to limit dyspnea
- ☐ Plan to increase activity level after discharge
- ☐ Understanding that another episode of ARF is possible and when medical attention will be sought to avoid it
- ☐ Understanding of medications
- ☐ Patient and family teaching and discharge planning

a recurrence of ARF. Your nursing diagnoses will guide you toward this goal.

As the patient approaches discharge and becomes more active, instruct him to restrict his activity level to avoid stressing his respiratory system. If he is discharged with a tracheostomy tube in place, he will require extra instruction. At discharge, you may need to coordinate your teaching efforts with a medical equipment supplier and a home caregiver. For example, the patient may need a walker, a commode chair, a hospital bed, an oxygen delivery system, or other respiratory equipment. These require special teaching as well as arranging for home use. Your discharge planning should help the patient return to a nearly normal life with his family. (See *Discharge planning checklist: Acute respiratory failure.*)

Case study: Part 5

After Mr. Smith's ABG findings returned to their pre-ARF baseline level, he was considered for discharge. With a social worker, his doctor and nurse reviewed the discharge plan, including the availability of home oxygen, the completion of the patient teaching plan, and Mr. Smith's emotional readiness to return home. Before his discharge, Mr. Smith said he realized that a respiratory infection secondary to his COPD had led to ARF. Although much improved since admission, he recognized that he was not returning home to his baseline level of wellness. His short-term prognosis at discharge was good, but he would need a few days to regain the strength and energy expended during the episode of ARF. He was expected to regain his preadmission baseline level of wellness and eventually surpass it. Mr. Smith's COPD was now being optimally managed, and he was helping to manage it. With continuous supplemental O_2, he would be able to increase the amount of O_2 he had available for activity and also slow down development of cor pulmonale.

Mr. Smith's long-term prognosis, however, was poor. Over time, his lung function would continue to deteriorate because of the destructive changes inherent in COPD. He would continue to be at great risk for another episode of ARF that would threaten his survival.

CHAPTER 6
Adult respiratory distress syndrome

First recognized and described in 1967, adult respiratory distress syndrome (ARDS) strikes more than 150,000 people every year, a statistic that has remained constant for more than a decade. Thanks to abundant research, we now have a better understanding of the pathogenesis of ARDS and can intervene earlier and more appropriately. However, ARDS still proves fatal in half the cases; when accompanied by sepsis, it's fatal in 85%.

Because it may have a disarmingly subtle onset but can rapidly lead to profound respiratory failure, ARDS will challenge your nursing skills. Recognizing its subtle and nonspecific early signs requires special alertness because the typical ARDS patient is young and otherwise healthy, with no previous lung disease. Through close monitoring, however, you may uncover specific changes that herald ARDS or signal its progression; in many cases, these changes prove just as important as diagnostic tests in establishing the diagnosis and assessing the effects of therapy.

Once ARDS has been confirmed, you'll be expected to monitor and support respiration, ensure pulmonary hygiene, administer antibiotics and other drugs, monitor hemodynamic parameters, and monitor for complications. Your technical skills alone won't be enough, though. The patient and family's need for psychological support will challenge the art of nursing.

Case study: Part 1

Bob Lewis, a 62-year-old retired attorney, had lived a full life. Since retiring, he played golf twice a week and took frequent trips to Europe. Mr. Lewis had a significant medical history and saw his family doctor regularly. His essential hypertension and elevated serum cholesterol level had been discovered in his early forties; he had a history of duodenal ulcers.

Case study: Part 1 *(continued)*

At age 58, Mr. Lewis suffered a left cerebrovascular accident; fortunately, he'd been spared any residual effects. However, within the next few years, other health problems necessitated a cholecystectomy and a carotid endarterectomy. The latter procedure was complicated by airway obstruction from excessive bleeding, which necessitated a temporary tracheostomy. Mr. Lewis recovered fully, though, and was able to resume his normal activities.

About 4 months before his current admission to the hospital, he began to experience short periods of burning substernal pain that radiated to his neck and jaw; the episodes occurred when he played golf. An electrocardiogram (ECG) detected no myocardial damage, and nitroglycerin was prescribed for the pain.

Three months later, though, Mr. Lewis began to experience shortness of breath. A treadmill exercise test provoked chest pain and ECG changes reflecting myocardial ischemia. At his doctor's recommendation, Mr. Lewis agreed to undergo cardiac catheterization. His family, however, strongly opposed another hospitalization.

The cardiac catheterization proceeded without complications but revealed severe triple-vessel atherosclerotic coronary disease with well-preserved left ventricular function. The cardiologist recommended coronary artery bypass graft (CABG) surgery. Mr. Lewis consented and underwent the procedure 3 days after catheterization.

Unfortunately, problems arose in the operating room and continued afterward. During surgery, Mr. Lewis developed left ventricular failure, necessitating emergency insertion of an intra-aortic balloon pump. Then, on the first postoperative day, he had to return to the operating room so that surgeons could correct excessive bleeding and relieve cardiac tamponade.

Throughout the next 5 days, Mr. Lewis needed intensive nursing and medical care. For cardiovascular support, he received multiple vasoactive I.V. medications, including inotropic agents, antiarrhythmics, and vasopressors. He needed an endotracheal tube and mechanical ventilation to maintain airway and breathing. Because his hematocrit and platelet levels frequently fell below acceptable postoperative values, he also required multiple transfusions of blood products. The pulmonary artery (PA) and systemic artery catheters inserted before surgery remained in place to monitor Mr. Lewis' hemodynamic response to surgery and subsequent treatment.

Causes and characteristics

A form of noncardiogenic pulmonary edema, ARDS begins with a systemic or pulmonary illness or injury that directly or indirectly affects the lungs; it can quickly progress to acute respiratory failure. Always a secondary disorder, ARDS typically follows cer-

Clinical situations associated with ARDS

- Aspiration of gastric contents
- Cardiopulmonary bypass
- Disseminated intravascular coagulation
- Drug overdose
- Emboli
- Inhalation of noxious gases or smoke
- Massive blood transfusions
- Near-drowning
- Oxygen toxicity
- Pancreatitis
- *Pneumocystis* pneumonia
- Sepsis
- Shock
- Trauma

Sepsis: A special threat
Even when it originates outside the respiratory system, sepsis is the most common and important forerunner of adult respiratory distress syndrome (ARDS). A platelet count below 100,000/mm³ increases the risk of ARDS.

Sepsis is particularly likely to follow infection in patients with preexisting azotemia, congestive heart failure, diabetes mellitus, nosocomial infection, pulmonary hypertension, or immunosuppression. Although typically associated with gram-negative bacterial infection, sepsis may stem from infection by a viral, fungal, mycoplasmal, or gram-positive bacterial organism.

Because early detection and aggressive intervention are crucial to the treatment of sepsis, stay alert for such suggestive signs and symptoms as fever or hypothermia, skin lesions, altered mental status, hypotension, and thrombocyto-penia. In an elderly patient, altered mental status may be the first sign of sepsis.

In a patient with confirmed sepsis, hypotension and thrombocytopenia may herald the development of ARDS.

***Pneumocystis* pneumonia**
In this infection (common among patients with acquired immunodeficiency syndrome and other immunosuppressive conditions), *P. carinii* organisms attach to the alveolar wall and reproduce. Alveolar spaces then fill with a foamy, pink-staining exudate containing *P. carinii* organisms. The abnormalities that characterize ARDS—hypoxemia, intrapulmonary shunting, and decreased lung compliance—follow.

tain predisposing conditions (see *Clinical situations associated with ARDS*).

As ARDS evolves, the following respiratory abnormalities develop: hypoxemia (decreased arterial oxygenation), hypoxia (decreased tissue oxygenation), diminished lung compliance, reduced lung volume, and intrapulmonary shunting.

Pathophysiology
The precipitating lung injury compromises pulmonary perfusion and causes hypoxemia. Subsequent metabolic disturbances trigger the release of such chemical mediators as kinins, amines, and serotonin. These mediators damage Type I pneumonocytes, causing their junctures to widen and become uneven. The widened junctures then prevent the sodium-potassium pump from maintaining a normal ratio of extracellular-to-intracellular water; as a result, fluid, red blood cells, and other large molecules (such as plasma proteins) leave the pulmonary capillary and enter the interstitium. Excessive interstitial fluid raises interstitial osmotic

pressure, which leads to pulmonary edema. Changes at the alveolar epithelium then allow interstitial fluid to enter the alveoli (see *Alveolar fluid movement in ARDS*). Because diffusing gases must now move across a greater distance, through barriers posed by edema and particulate matter, gas exchange diminishes.

Meanwhile, in response to pulmonary hypoperfusion and hypoxemia, platelets and leukocytes aggregate within pulmonary capillaries, leading to peripheral and pulmonary vascular thrombosis. Embolization and occlusion of the pulmonary microcirculation result.

Microemboli, capillary compression (caused by edema), and hypoperfusion impair cellular nutrition. This, in turn, alters Type II pneumonocytes—the alveolar epithelial cells that produce surfactant to keep alveoli expanded. These cells' production of surfactant diminishes. Moreover, other factors—poor tidal volume, reduced ventilation, inadequate intermittent hyperventilation, and alveolar and interstitial edema and hemorrhage—also decrease surfactant production. Without adequate surfactant, alveoli collapse, gas exchange suffers, and atelectasis occurs. The lungs stiffen, reflecting reduced compliance, and breathing becomes labored.

Collapsed alveoli are airless and can't participate in gas exchange even if perfusion is adequate. Such unventilated alveolar regions create a ventilation-perfusion (V/Q) mismatch (intrapulmonary shunt) that allows unoxygenated blood to enter the arterial circulation, causing severe hypoxemia. (See *Pathogenesis of ARDS,* page 222.)

To compensate for these changes, the patient hyperventilates in an attempt to draw in more oxygen. However, oxygen can't cross the alveolocapillary membrane in sufficient amounts; carbon dioxide, which crosses more easily, is lost with each exhalation. Consequently, partial pressure of oxygen in arterial blood (PaO_2) and partial pressure of carbon dioxide in arterial blood ($PaCO_2$) fall.

As the $PaCO_2$ drops, arterial pH typically rises, causing respiratory alkalosis; if pH fails to rise, however, metabolic acidosis is present (from the lactic acidosis that accompanies shock and hypoxemia). If these abnormalities go unchecked, pulmonary edema worsens and pulmonary fibrosis sets in, further compromising gas exchange and reducing lung compliance.

Alveolar fluid movement in ARDS

The alveolocapillary unit has the following components.
• The *alveolus,* a tiny saclike dilatation of a terminal bronchiole, contains oxygen-rich air.
• The *alveolar epithelial membrane* consists of several cell types (including Types I and II pneumonocytes). Tight junctures between Type I pneumonocytes bar fluid from entering the alveolus but permit gases to diffuse readily across the membrane.
• The *capillary,* perfused with abundant blood flow, has an intact basement membrane and

endothelial layer that allow only minimal fluid to escape.
• The *alveolocapillary space* contains scant amounts of fluid (carried away by the lymphatic system) and no particulate matter to hinder gas diffusion.

Abnormal permeability
As ARDS develops, the capillary membrane becomes abnormally permeable, permitting fluid, plasma proteins, and other particles to enter the alveolocapillary space; eventually, the alveolus fills with fluid and particles.

FLUID MOVEMENT IN NORMAL LUNGS

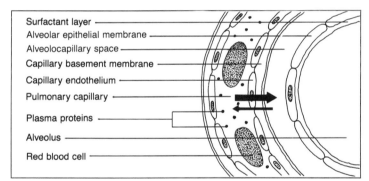

Surfactant layer
Alveolar epithelial membrane
Alveolocapillary space
Capillary basement membrane
Capillary endothelium
Pulmonary capillary
Plasma proteins
Alveolus
Red blood cell

FLUID MOVEMENT IN A.R.D.S.

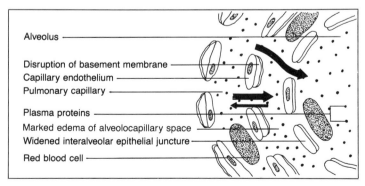

Alveolus
Disruption of basement membrane
Capillary endothelium
Pulmonary capillary
Plasma proteins
Marked edema of alveolocapillary space
Widened interalveolar epithelial juncture
Red blood cell

Pathogenesis of ARDS

ARDS begins with a systemic or pulmonary injury that affects the lungs and causes hypoxemia. Subsequent disturbances trigger a chain of pathologic events that can quickly lead to respiratory failure.

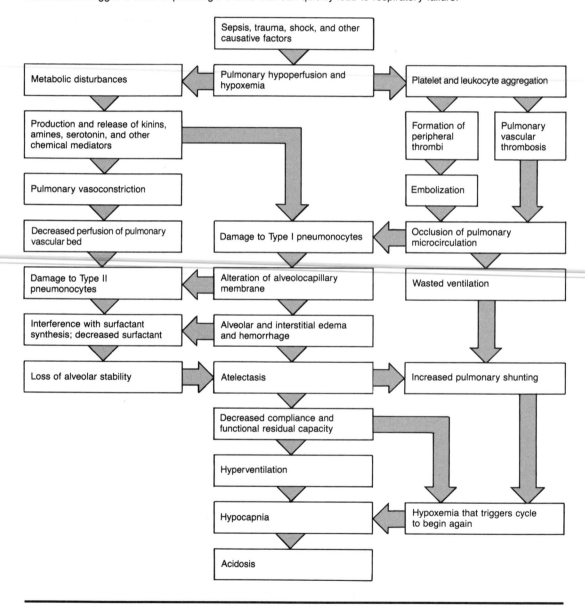

Case study: Part 2

Serious complications continued to mar Mr. Lewis' postoperative course. On the second day after surgery, he became agitated, frightened, and disoriented. Fearing that he'd harm himself, his intensive care unit (ICU) nurse monitored him continuously.

Suspecting that his agitation stemmed from sleep deprivation and pain, she began to give more frequent doses of the I.V. morphine that the doctor had ordered, administering one dose at least every 2 hours.

By the end of the second postoperative day, Mr. Lewis' cardiovascular condition had stabilized: Tissue perfusion improved, cardiac output measured 5 to 6 liters/minute, and pulmonary capillary wedge pressure (PCWP) measured 12 to 15 mm Hg. Gradually, he was weaned from the intra-aortic balloon pump.

The next day, however, Mr. Lewis' core temperature (as recorded by the tip of the PA catheter) reached 102.4° F (39.1° C). When the nurse reported this to the cardiothoracic surgeon who'd performed CABG surgery, the surgeon ordered emergency diagnostic tests, including a stat complete blood count (CBC), arterial blood gas (ABG) and venous blood gas (VBG) measurements, and a portable chest X-ray. He also requested blood, sputum, and urine cultures.

Laboratory results showed that Mr. Lewis' white blood cell (WBC) count had reached 19,400/mm³ (19.4 × 10⁹/liter) and his hemoglobin concentration measured 12.6 g/dl (126 g/liters).

The laboratory reported the following blood gas measurements:
• ABG values—pH, 7.42; $PaCO_2$, 39 mm Hg; PaO_2, 74 mm Hg; bicarbonate (HCO_3^-), 22 mEq/liter (22 mmol/liter); arterial oxygen saturation (SaO_2), 0.96 (96%)
• VBG values—partial pressure of venous oxygen (PvO_2), 29 mm Hg; venous oxygen saturation (SvO_2), 0.71 (71%).

As the nurse reviewed these values, she kept in mind that Mr. Lewis was on a mechanical ventilator with a fraction of inspired oxygen (FIO_2) of 0.4, a positive end-expiratory pressure (PEEP) of 5 cm H_2O, a tidal volume of 600 ml, and a ventilatory mode of intermittent mandatory ventilation (IMV) at a rate of 8 breaths/minute.

Cardiac output evaluation was as follows: cardiac output, 5 liters/minute; arterial oxygen content (CaO_2), 16.7 ml/dl; mixed venous oxygen content (CvO_2), 12.3 ml/dl; arterial–mixed venous oxygen gradient ($C[a-v]O_2$), 4.4 ml/dl; oxygen delivery (DO_2), 835 ml/dl; and oxygen consumption (VO_2), 220 ml/minute.

In response to these values, Mr. Lewis' PEEP was increased to 8 cm H_2O. ABG measurements taken 20 minutes after this change showed improved tissue oxygenation. The portable X-ray revealed a few patchy, irregular, interstitial infiltrates.

Case study: Part 2 *(continued)*

The cardiac monitor showed sinus tachycardia with no ectopic beats; graded peripheral pulses were palpable at 3 on a scale of 1 to 4. The arterial pressure monitor indicated a blood pressure of 116/74 mm Hg, with a corresponding cuff pressure of 112/70 mm Hg.

Mr. Lewis' breathing was rapid, with a ventilator respiratory rate consistently above 20 breaths/minute. Lung auscultation revealed fine, diffuse crackles at the lung bases, and endotracheal tube suctioning produced thick, purulent secretions.

On the fourth day after surgery, his respiratory rate was above 40 breaths/minute and he was restless again. His respirations were shallow and he'd begun to use accessory breathing muscles. Lung auscultation revealed harsh bronchial breath sounds throughout all fields.

ABG analysis revealed the following results: pH, 7.49; $PaCO_2$, 32 mm Hg; PaO_2, 58 mm Hg, $HCO_3{}^-$, 25 mEq/liter (25 mmol/liter), and SaO_2, 0.90 (90%). The morning chest X-ray disclosed diffuse, bilateral interstitial infiltrates—an indication of interstitial and intra-alveolar edema.

The patient was diagnosed as having noncardiogenic pulmonary edema secondary to shock and sepsis, with a superimposed pneumonia, as indicated by the gram-negative rods found in his sputum.

All the evidence pointed to one distressing conclusion—Bob Lewis was probably in the early stages of ARDS. His clinical course had included several conditions that can precipitate ARDS—a prolonged surgical procedure with pulmonary bypass, a postoperative hypoperfusion state (from bleeding and cardiac tamponade), multiple blood transfusions, and sepsis with an increased WBC count and a reduced platelet count.

Mr. Lewis' family was extremely upset, especially because they had tried to dissuade him from having the surgery. The nurse met with the family to help them deal with their anxiety and concern, and their anger with Mr. Lewis for not following their advice.

After she returned to the ICU, the nurse developed a plan of care by identifying the following nursing diagnoses:
• Impaired gas exchange related to decreased alveolar ventilation secondary to alveolar atelectasis and fluid accumulation
• Ineffective breathing pattern related to hyperventilation secondary to anxiety, decreased functional residual capacity (FRC), and decreasing lung compliance
• Ineffective airway clearance related to the presence of viscous secretions secondary to pulmonary infection
• Altered family processes related to inability of family members to communicate openly and constructively secondary to the critical illness of husband and father
• Potential for altered tissue perfusion: peripheral, cardiopulmonary, renal, cerebral, related to impaired circulation secondary to decreased myocardial contractility

• Potential for injury related to alterations in mentation secondary to inadequate cerebral tissue perfusion, sleep deprivation, or sensory overload.

Assessment and diagnosis

Generally accepted criteria for the diagnosis of ARDS include:
• hypoxemia that doesn't respond to oxygen administration
• history of a clinical condition that predisposes the patient to pulmonary injury
• clinical signs of respiratory distress, such as tachypnea, dyspnea, and labored breathing
• diffuse pulmonary infiltrates, as shown on X-ray
• pulmonary edema with no evidence of left ventricular failure (PCWP remains below 12 mm Hg).

During your initial assessment of a patient at risk for ARDS, review his history for any predisposing factors; early recognition and intervention may prevent a susceptible patient from progressing to ARDS or may halt ARDS at an early stage. The history usually reveals no previous health problems preceding the recent clinical condition associated with ARDS. Because ARDS can develop over several hours to days, initial signs and symptoms may not be definitive; however, stay alert for sudden respiratory distress several days into what seems like a normal recovery from the condition that necessitated hospitalization.

Stages of ARDS

For assessment purposes, ARDS can be divided into four phases.

Phase 1. After the initial injury, tissue perfusion decreases and breath sounds diminish. The lungs appear clear or slightly congested on chest X-ray. The patient hyperventilates and has dyspnea on exertion. He remains alert, with respiratory and heart rates at the high end of normal. ABG analysis reveals a normal or slightly reduced $PaCO_2$ (averaging 30 to 40 mm Hg).

Phase 2. The patient shows signs of subclinical respiratory distress—use of accessory breathing muscles; a dry cough with thick, frothy sputum; and bloody, viscous secretions. He seems anxious and diaphoretic. You may detect tachypnea, tachycardia, and elevated blood pressure. Auscultation may reveal basilar crackles.

The chest X-ray may still appear normal during this phase; however, the patient continues to hyperventilate. ABG measurements indicate persistent hypocapnia and hypoxemia despite administration of oxygen at high concentrations. The $PaCO_2$ typically ranges from 25 to 30 mm Hg. A V/Q mismatch (indicated by a respiratory quotient below 0.8) may develop, reflecting intrapulmonary shunting.

Phase 3. The patient appears gravely ill and may suffer severe dyspnea, tachypnea (with a respiratory rate above 30 breaths/minute), and tachycardia with dysrhythmias. He visibly struggles for air. Also expect pale or cyanotic skin, a productive cough, labile blood pressure, and decreased mentation. Auscultation may reveal crackles and rhonchi. As hyperventilation continues, the $PaCO_2$ drops to 20 to 35 mm Hg and the PaO_2 falls to 50 to 60 mm Hg. Intrapulmonary shunting may involve 20% to 30% of the cardiac output. Chest X-rays show pulmonary edema.

Phase 4. Now in acute respiratory failure, the patient has severe hypoxemia. Lacking spontaneous respiration, he lapses into a coma. Because he can't continue to compensate by hyperventilating, his $PaCO_2$ rises, reflecting a marked reduction in the number of functioning alveolocapillary units. About 50% to 60% of the cardiac output is now shunted. Other signs include bradycardia with dysrhythmias; hypotension; and pale, cyanotic skin. Chest X-rays now show a complete white-out (infiltrates in both lung fields), and pulmonary function tests reveal a dramatic FRC decrease. At this point, the patient is at grave risk for developing pulmonary fibrosis and possibly fatal pulmonary damage.

Secondary pulmonary infection, systemic sepsis, and cardiac dysfunction also develop late in ARDS. Manifestations of these problems include a high fever, purulent sputum, an elevated WBC count, severe hypotension, reduced tissue perfusion, bradycardia, and asystole. Sepsis initially causes high cardiac output with continued hyperthermia or hypothermia and warm, flushed skin; the patient may progress to septic shock. The combination of septic shock and cardiac dysfunction may be evidenced by falling cardiac output; cold, clammy skin; decreasing urine output; and increased lactic acid production, resulting in metabolic acidosis.

Diagnostic tests

For a patient with suspected ARDS, the goal of initial testing is to rule out cardiogenic pulmonary edema. This can be done by measuring PCWP via a PA catheter. With cardiogenic pulmonary edema, PCWP usually measures above 12 mm Hg, indicating poor ventricular function as the cause of pulmonary edema. With ARDS, PCWP typically measures 12 mm Hg or less.

Through the PA catheter, you may also collect pulmonary artery and mixed venous blood samples (to assess oxygen saturation) and measure pulmonary artery pressure (PAP) and cardiac output (by thermodilution techniques).

Assessment of bronchial fluid protein concentration also helps ARDS diagnosis by establishing the source of pulmonary edema. In noncardiogenic pulmonary edema (as in ARDS), the concentration of serum proteins in bronchial fluid typically exceeds 0.7; in cardiogenic pulmonary edema, the concentration usually remains below 0.5. Presumably, the higher concentration reflects ARDS-related damage to the alveolocapillary membrane, which allows large proteins to penetrate the alveoli.

Once noncardiogenic pulmonary edema is confirmed, differential diagnosis must exclude pulmonary vasculitis, diffuse pulmonary hemorrhage, drug ingestion (as shown by toxicology screening), pancreatitis (as shown by serum amylase measurement), and infection (as shown by culture and sensitivity tests on specimens collected from any suspected infection sites). Subsequent diagnostic tests include ABG analysis, chest X-rays, and various other tests that help evaluate pulmonary function. (See *Diagnostic profile: Findings in ARDS,* page 228.)

ABG analysis. Crucial to establishing the diagnosis of ARDS and monitoring therapeutic effectiveness, ABG analysis determines the patient's oxygenation, ventilation, and acid-base status. An increased $PaCO_2$ (or a $PaCO_2$ that fails to decrease when acidosis or hypoxemia exists) indicates poor alveolar ventilation. SaO_2, which reflects the percentage of hemoglobin saturated with oxygen, may be assessed from analysis of blood taken from an intra-arterial line; alternatively, SaO_2 may be monitored noninvasively with a pulse oximeter (see *Pulse oximetry: Noninvasive hypoxemia monitoring,* page 230).

Serial ABG studies for an ARDS patient initially show slightly decreased PaO_2 and $PaCO_2$, reflecting mild respiratory alkalosis.

▼ **DIAGNOSTIC PROFILE**

Findings in ARDS

Test	Normal findings	Expected findings
Radiography		
Chest X-ray	Clear	Clear in early stages; rapid development of bilateral infiltrates and complete white-out in later stages
Arterial blood gas analysis		
pH	7.35 to 7.45	Increased as $Paco_2$ value falls (respiratory alkalosis); decreased with lactic acid production (metabolic acidosis); decreased as $Paco_2$ rises (respiratory acidosis)
Pao_2	80 to 100 mm Hg	Decreased despite increase in FIO_2
$Paco_2$	35 to 45 mm Hg	Decreased in acute alveolar hyperventilation (respiratory alkalosis); increased in acute ventilatory failure
Sao_2	0.95 (95%) to 0.97 (97%)	Decreased
Hemodynamic parameters		
CVP	2.7 to 12 cm H_2O (2 to 6 mm Hg)	Normal unless patient is overhydrated
PCWP	6 to 12 mm Hg	Normal
Mean PAP	< 20 mm Hg	Normal
Pvo_2	35 to 40 mm Hg	Decreased
Cvo_2	15 ml/dl (15 vol%)	Decreased
Cao_2	20 ml/dl (20 vol%)	Decreased
$C(a-v)o_2$	5 ml/dl (5 vol%)	Decreased initially, then increased as cardiovascular system fails
Shunt studies		
Shunt fraction	< 6%	Increased
A-a gradient	< 15 mm Hg	Increased (may reach 500 mm Hg)
a-A ratio	0.8	Decreased
Pulmonary function studies		
FRC	Variable	Decreased from baseline value
PIP	Variable	Increased from baseline value

As gas exchange diminishes, the PaO_2 continues to drop and fails to rise despite increased concentrations of administered oxygen. Eventually, both respiratory and metabolic acidosis develop as minute ventilation decreases and the $PaCO_2$ rises. Anaerobic metabolism leads to lactic acid production; the resulting hypoperfusion and hypoxia contribute to metabolic acidosis.

Chest X-rays. Serial X-rays may show rapid progression from normal lungs in early-stage ARDS to the classic white-out pattern in later stages. Irregular, patchy bilateral infiltrates appear—interstitially at first, then in the intra-alveolar region. Gradually, the infiltrates spread, making the lungs look completely white.

Other parameters. Shunt studies, static compliance values, and peak inspiratory pressure (PIP) monitoring also aid ARDS diagnosis and help monitor therapeutic effectiveness.

The degree of intrapulmonary shunting can be calculated from various equations, using values obtained from ABG, VBG, and hemoglobin measurements. In a normal, healthy lung, only 3% to 5% of the cardiac output is shunted (passed from the heart's right to left side without participating in gas exchange). Shunting that exceeds 25% despite respiratory support strongly suggests ARDS.

You may determine your patient's shunt by calculating the alveolar-arterial (A-a) gradient. Usually, the A-a gradient is 5 to 15 mm Hg in a patient who's receiving an FIO_2 of 0.2; the gradient may reach 50 mm Hg when FIO_2 exceeds 0.4. In the typical ARDS patient, however, the gradient exceeds 450 mm Hg after administration of 100% oxygen for 15 minutes.

Compliance, which reflects lung distensibility, is measured as the volume change in the lung that results from applied pressure under static conditions. Compliance relates inversely to the work of breathing (as compliance diminishes, breathing becomes more labored) but relates directly to FRC (with reduced compliance, less air remains in the lungs after expiration). Compliance decreases in ARDS as interstitial and intra-alveolar fluid causes the lungs to stiffen.

In a mechanically ventilated patient, you may assess compliance by monitoring PIP (indicated on the ventilator) and static compliance (determined by a formula). Increased PIP for an

Pulse oximetry: Noninvasive hypoxemia monitoring

This relatively new method monitors ventilatory status noninvasively. Pulse oximetry uses light to continuously measure arterial oxygen saturation (SaO_2); it also measures pulse rate and amplitude.

The SaO_2 values obtained by pulse oximetry correlate closely with those determined from arterial blood gas analysis. Besides offering reliability, pulse oximetry eliminates the need for painful arterial punctures and avoids blood loss and other risks associated with indwelling arterial lines. Results are available instantaneously, allowing immediate action to correct any abnormal findings.

As an adjunct to physical examination, pulse oximetry can aid detection of hypoxia and can detect immediate changes after endotracheal intubation, suctioning, postural drainage, and adjustments of oxygen concentration and positive end-expiratory pressure. However, because the pulse oximeter measures only SaO_2, it can't be used when assessment of pH, bicarbonate values, and partial pressures of oxygen and carbon dioxide in arterial blood is needed to thoroughly evaluate the patient's respiratory status.

Keep in mind that pulse oximetry may yield false-low results in patients with poor tissue perfusion, such as those with reduced cardiac output, hypotension, hypovolemia, shock, or jaundice. False-high results may occur in patients who've undergone cardiac procedures involving the use of dyes.

How pulse oximetry works

Light-emitting diodes in the transducer (sensor) attached to the patient's body send red and infrared light beams through tissue. A light-sensitive photodetector opposite the transducer measures the transmitted light as it passes through the vascular bed, records the relative amount of color absorbed by arterial blood, and transmits the data to a monitor, which displays the information with each heartbeat. If the SaO_2 level or pulse rate exceeds or drops below preset limits, it activates visual and audible alarms.

EAR TRANSDUCER

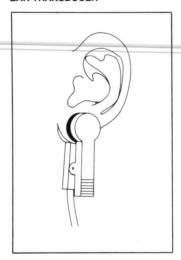

Both ear and finger transducers are available; for an ARDS patient, the ear transducer is preferred because of the hypo-perfusion state that usually accompanies the disease.

The transducer site requires no special preparation. However, if you choose an ear transducer, you may want to wipe the earlobe with an alcohol sponge for 15 to 30 seconds before applying the transducer to increase blood volume and thus obtain a stronger signal. Attach the transducer to the fleshy part of the earlobe, not the cartilage.

FINGER TRANSDUCER

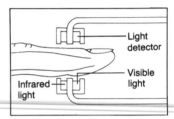

Light detector

Visible light

Infrared light

If you use a finger transducer, attach it to the patient's index finger at the heart level. Don't attach the transducer to an extremity that has a blood pressure cuff or an arterial catheter in place; occluded blood flow will hinder transducer performance.

Guard the transducer from exposure to bright sunlight and other strong light. Check the site frequently for transducer damage or displacement, and examine the patient's skin for abrasion and circulatory impairment. Rotate placement of the transducer every 4 hours and as needed to prevent skin breakdown.

established tidal volume (the amount of air inhaled or exhaled with each breath) may reflect decreasing lung compliance. However, always check for other causes of increased PIP, such as increased airway resistance (which may stem from accumulated secretions, air flow blockage caused by kinked tubing, or fighting the ventilator).

Static compliance, which reflects lung stiffness, decreases as FRC drops and returns to normal when FRC increases or tidal volume is optimized. Normally, static compliance measures 100 cm H_2O; in the patient with ARDS, it may drop below 50 cm H_2O. Once such mechanical factors as tubing obstruction are ruled out, decreased static compliance usually indicates a worsening shunt, which may warrant the addition of PEEP.

Case study: Part 3

To reverse Mr. Lewis' pulmonary deterioration, his doctors ordered mechanical ventilation to maintain airway and breathing; the intra-aortic balloon pump (inserted just after surgery) and initial postoperative medication (such as vasopressors and inotropic agents) maintained adequate circulation. Other medical interventions aimed to reverse hypoxemia, reduce oxygen consumption, improve tissue oxygenation, prevent complications, and maintain adequate nutrition.

Initially, the pulmonologist noted that Mr. Lewis' ABG values reflected both hypoxemia and hypocapnia, resulting in mild respiratory alkalosis. To treat hypoxemia, the following ventilator settings were selected: ventilatory mode, IMV; respiratory rate, 8 breaths/minute; FIO_2, 0.4; tidal volume, 600 ml; sigh volume, 900 ml; PEEP, 10 cm H_2O. The pulmonologist asked the respiratory therapist to increase PEEP by 3 cm H_2O, with repeat ABG measurements 20 minutes after each increase, until Mr. Lewis' PaO_2 rose above 70 mm Hg and his SaO_2 level exceeded 0.95 (95%).

Despite gradual PEEP increases to 20 cm H_2O, Mr. Lewis' PaO_2 remained between 50 and 60 mm Hg throughout the fourth postoperative day, indicating persistent hypoxemia. Also, as he continued to hyperventilate, his $PaCO_2$ initially fell, causing respiratory alkalosis to worsen.

Later that evening, as fatigue set in, Mr. Lewis' breathing became more labored and he could no longer maintain adequate minute ventilation. The laboratory reported the following ABG values: pH, 7.26; $PaCO_2$, 59 mm Hg; PaO_2, 55 mm Hg; HCO_3^-, 21 mEq/liter (21 mmol/liter); SaO_2, 0.89 (89%). To correct hypoxemia and hypocap-

Case study: Part 3 *(continued)*

nia to acceptable levels, the IMV rate was increased to 12 breaths/minute and PEEP was increased to 22 cm H_2O.

Hoping to ease his breathing and reduce his oxygen consumption, the pulmonologist removed Mr. Lewis from the volume-cycled ventilator and placed him on a servo-type pressure-support ventilator. She also increased his morphine dosage to 10 mg/hour, as needed, to reduce restlessness and agitation.

Mr. Lewis' fever, accompanied by chills and shivering, also increased oxygen consumption, so he was given acetaminophen and was placed on a cooling blanket.

Despite the increased morphine dosage and ventilator change, Mr. Lewis remained agitated throughout the fifth postoperative day. Because of concern that agitation would worsen his breathing patterns, pancuronium (Pavulon) was ordered; by paralyzing the chest muscles, the drug would eliminate the work of breathing, further reducing oxygen consumption. Sedation was continued.

Blood transfusions were given to maintain hemoglobin concentration above 12 g/dl (120 g/liter)—a level that would provide optimal oxygen-carrying capacity to meet the body's increased metabolic needs during illness—and the inotropic drugs dobutamine (Dobutrex) and amrinone (Inocor) at low dosages were given to improve myocardial contractility and maintain cardiac output above 5 liters/minute. Unfortunately, though, these drugs increased Mr. Lewis' heart rate and posed the threat of abnormal ventricular contractions—dysrhythmias that would increase myocardial oxygen consumption. For this reason, and because Mr. Lewis had developed dysrhythmias on the first postoperative day, an I.V. infusion of lidocaine at 2 mg/minute was started. Because high oxygen concentrations or excessive fluid administration could cause oxygen toxicity and lung injury, FIO_2 was kept at 0.4 and diuretics were used to maintain PCWP at approximately 10 mm Hg. The lower PCWP would help reduce fluid leakage from damaged capillaries while maintaining adequate circulating volume to minimize the adverse effects of PEEP therapy.

Culture and sensitivity tests were performed on blood, urine, and sputum specimens and appropriate antibiotics were started.

Enteral feeding was selected to maintain adequate nutrition because Mr. Lewis had a functioning GI tract. The nurses inserted the feeding tube and started feedings. Regular assessment for changes in bowel patterns and checks for residual food were important.

Mr. Lewis remained in the ICU for 14 postoperative days. When his PaO_2 and $PaCO_2$ began to stabilize on the sixth day, his pancuronium was discontinued; during days 7 through 10, his PEEP levels were reduced gradually. Chest X-rays showed progressive clearing of the pulmonary infection and pulmonary edema; by day 12, they showed marked improvement. On day 13, when he showed no signs of pulmonary infection or edema, Mr. Lewis was extubated; nurses monitored him closely that night for signs of respiratory distress. The next morning, his lungs sounded clear and his chest X-ray appeared normal; later that day, he was transferred to a surgical unit for further recovery and postoperative teaching.

Treatment options

Treatment for the patient with ARDS typically includes continuous positive airway pressure (CPAP) or mechanical ventilation with PEEP, fluid management, drug therapy, pulmonary hygiene, and nutritional support therapy. These interventions are aimed at correcting hypoxemia, reducing oxygen consumption, improving tissue oxygenation, preventing complications, and maintaining adequate nutrition. Treatment may also include administration of steroids.

Correcting hypoxemia

The immediate treatment goal in ARDS is to reduce or eliminate hypoxemia by increasing the PaO_2 above 60 mm Hg. Usually, a PaO_2 increase also reverses hypoxia (by maintaining adequate tissue perfusion) and restores the capillary membrane to its normal impermeable state.

Oxygen therapy, the key to reversing hypoxemia, improves gas exchange at the alveolocapillary membrane. ARDS patients must receive oxygen by a method that maintains positive airway pressure; most require mechanical ventilation with PEEP, but those who can breathe spontaneously without mechanical ventilation may receive oxygen via CPAP.

Three types of ventilators are used to treat ARDS patients. The *volume-cycled ventilator* ends inspiration after delivering a preset tidal volume; the *high-frequency jet ventilator* delivers small tidal volumes at a respiratory rate of 60 to 100 breaths/ minute; the *pressure-support ventilator*, a highly sophisticated microprocessor model, has multiple functions (see Chapter 8, Mechanical ventilation, for details on this ventilator).

PEEP therapy. The addition of PEEP to mechanical ventilation prevents airway pressure from falling to atmospheric levels during the expiratory cycle. Normally, alveoli expand during inspiration and remain expanded throughout the respiratory cycle. But in ARDS, alveoli collapse at the end of expiration and fail to reexpand on inspiration. PEEP maintains constant pressure across the alveoli throughout the respiratory cycle, preventing alveolar collapse and increasing the size and number of alveoli available for ventilation. Because alveoli remain expanded during expiration, FRC increases, resulting in a rise in the PaO_2 with the same or an even lower FIO_2.

PEEP also redistributes alveolar fluid by pushing it to the alveolar wall. Consequently, total lung volume increases and lung compliance improves. The shortened distance between capillaries and alveolar gas facilitates diffusion across the alveolocapillary membrane.

PEEP therapy usually begins at 3 to 5 cm H_2O and increases by small increments. The goal is to achieve a PaO_2 above 60 mm Hg with an FIO_2 of 0.4 or less—without causing deleterious cardiopulmonary effects. Once the optimal PaO_2 has been achieved, PEEP should be reduced and the patient monitored closely for signs and symptoms of reduced cardiac output and barotrauma.

Keep in mind that during mechanical ventilation, hypoxemia may persist or even worsen. If this happens, FIO_2 may be increased. However, if your patient's FIO_2 is 0.5 or higher for more than 24 hours, he may have an increased risk of oxygen toxicity and pulmonary fibrosis.

Also remember that abrupt discontinuation of mechanical ventilation with PEEP brings on immediate alveolar collapse with hypoxemia following as closely as 1 minute later. Once reinstated, PEEP increases the patient's PaO_2; however, PEEP takes 20 to 30 minutes to become fully established, so some collapsed alveoli may not reexpand.

CPAP therapy. In an ARDS patient who can breathe adequately on his own without mechanical ventilation, CPAP may be used to maintain an airway pressure above the atmospheric level throughout the respiratory cycle. Providing a constant positive airway pressure, CPAP increases FRC and improves lung compliance and arterial oxygenation.

CPAP may be delivered continuously via a tight-fitting mask or an endotracheal tube. Mask delivery may cause discomfort, skin excoriation, gastric distention, vomiting, and aspiration (the mask forces air into the stomach through the esophagus). A nasogastric tube should be inserted to prevent aspiration from vomiting if a mask is used. With either delivery method, CPAP may cause carbon dioxide retention from patient fatigue. If this happens, the doctor may switch to mechanical ventilation with PEEP.

Reducing oxygen consumption

In ARDS, the patient's oxygen needs may exceed his oxygen supply. To prevent or correct an oxygen imbalance, medical and nursing interventions will reduce oxygen requirements by decreasing the work of breathing and minimizing metabolic demands (such as from fever, shivering, agitation, and anxiety).

Labored breathing. Unfortunately, both CPAP and PEEP increase the work of breathing if the patient is breathing spontaneously. That's because even in healthy people, alveolar pressure must drop below atmospheric pressure to initiate inspiration; with CPAP or PEEP, alveolar pressure must drop even further.

To minimize breathing work, the ventilator should be set on the IMV mode; then, with the machine breathing at or below the respiratory rate, the patient can breathe spontaneously without added positive pressure between machine breaths. Alternatively, the assist-control mode may be used so that a slight negative pressure on inspiration triggers the ventilator to deliver a breath. A third option for reducing the work of breathing, pancuronium administration paralyzes the respiratory muscles, allowing the ventilator to assume the total work of breathing.

Metabolic demands. Controlling body temperature also helps equalize oxygen supply and demand by decreasing oxygen consumption associated with the work of breathing. Aggressive antipyretic therapy can control fever and thus avoid the muscular demands of shivering and chills, which may raise the metabolic rate as much as 50%.

Anxiety, which also increases oxygen demand, can be managed through the use of effective interpersonal skills, administration of anxiolytic or sedative drugs, and inclusion of supportive family and friends in the patient's treatment plan.

Improving tissue oxygenation

Measures used to improve oxygen delivery fall into two main groups—those that maintain adequate cardiac output and those that ensure sufficient blood oxygenation.

Maintaining adequate cardiac output. ARDS may reduce cardiac output directly; PEEP therapy may reduce it indirectly. To ensure normal circulating blood volume, strict fluid management may be necessary to avoid both fluid excess (which can worsen pulmonary edema by exacerbating interstitial fluid leakage) and fluid deficit (which can reduce cardiac output, leading to impaired tissue perfusion and circulatory shock).

In either case, I.V. fluids must be administered at the exact rates ordered and any changes in hemodynamic or clinical parameters reported immediately. Continue to monitor the patient closely throughout fluid replacement therapy, taking frequent PCWP readings and correlating the results with the patient's cardiac output, heart rate, urine output, and breath sounds.

The choice of fluid administered to an ARDS patient remains controversial. Some clinicians recommend colloids, which replace albumin and blood, contending that colloids restore oncotic and hydrostatic pressures in the vessels and interstitium, thereby reducing capillary leakage. Others favor crystalloids, contending that ARDS reflects discontinuity of the air-blood barrier, not oncotic pressure changes, and that colloid therapy only exacerbates fluid shift from vessels to interstitium.

Diuretics may also play a part in fluid management. For example, furosemide, a loop diuretic, may be ordered to reduce intravascular volume and restore the proper hydrostatic-oncotic pressure balance. However, the patient may not respond to diuretics and may require hemodialysis or ultrafiltration to relieve pulmonary edema. Hemodialysis removes toxins and fluids via a semipermeable membrane and dialyzer. Ultrafiltration, which involves use of a dialysis circuit without dialysate, reduces plasma volume by increasing venous resistance to blood flow. It also increases oncotic pressure and may help repair the alveolocapillary membrane.

Improving blood oxygen content. Because oxygen must combine with hemoglobin for delivery to the tissues, blood oxygen content depends on hemoglobin concentration. Administration of packed red blood cells helps ensure optimal oxygen-carrying capacity by maintaining hemoglobin concentration between 12 and 15 g/dl (120 to 150 g/liter).

Hemoglobin's ability to carry and release oxygen at a given PaO_2 hinges on its position on the oxyhemoglobin dissociation curve (see *Oxyhemoglobin dissociation curve,* page 238). Because abnormal blood pH, abnormal $PaCO_2$, fever, and hypothermia can alter oxygen release by hemoglobin, treatment may include measures to correct such abnormalities.

Preventing complications

Systemic or pulmonary infection may precede or accompany ARDS; impairment of the lungs' natural defense mechanism against bacteria is a characteristic feature. In patients with ARDS, increased production and retention of pulmonary secretions, intubation, and trapping of protein-rich fluid in the alveoli produce special vulnerability to gram-negative bacterial pneumonia. Consequently, expect to administer antibiotics; the agent selected depends on results of culture and sensitivity tests.

Some clinicians recommend prophylactic administration of broad-spectrum antibiotics from the onset of ARDS, reasoning that the extensive invasive procedures the patient will require heighten his infection risk and that alveolar fluid provides an excellent medium for bacterial growth. Others avoid prophylactic use of antibiotics because these drugs may promote development of drug-resistant bacterial organisms or secondary infection (especially by *Candida* organisms).

Whether or not the patient is receiving treatment with antibiotics, meticulous pulmonary hygiene helps prevent superimposed pulmonary infection—a leading cause of death in ARDS patients. Expect to suction the patient as necessary and perform chest physiotherapy to help mobilize secretions from small, inaccessible airways into larger bronchioles for removal.

Maintaining adequate nutrition

Intensive nutritional support bolsters the immune system in its fight against infection, promotes respiratory epithelial regeneration, and helps prevent progressive respiratory muscle weakness. Mechanically ventilated patients require 2,500 to 3,000 calories daily; sepsis increases the requirement to 10,000 calories and usually necessitates total parenteral nutrition. *Note:* Some ventilators calculate the patient's metabolic rate, which can help determine his nutritional requirements.

If appropriate for the patient, enteral feeding is preferable to avoid the risks associated with parenteral nutrition—poor

Oxyhemoglobin dissociation curve

To assess your patient's tissue oxygenation, you may monitor the oxygen pressures plotted on his oxyhemoglobin dissociation curve. As shown by the curve's S shape, arterial oxygen saturation (SaO_2) relates to oxygen pressure in a nonlinear fashion (in other words, a given increase or decrease in oxygen pressure doesn't always cause an equivalent rise or fall in oxyhemoglobin saturation).

Such factors as body temperature and acid-base status may shift the curve to the left or right. With a shift to the right, SaO_2 decreases for a given oxygen pressure, and hemoglobin more readily releases oxygen to the tissues. A shift to the left, in contrast, causes SaO_2 to increase for a given oxygen pressure; however, the hemoglobin molecule attaches more tightly to oxygen, so less oxygen is released.

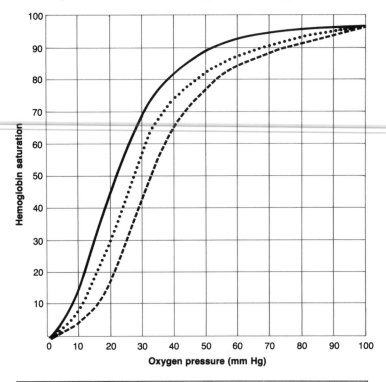

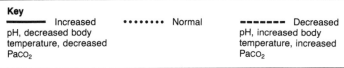

Key

——— Increased pH, decreased body temperature, decreased $PacO_2$

••••••• Normal

- - - - - - Decreased pH, increased body temperature, increased $PacO_2$

glucose control, fluid and electrolyte disturbances, and catheter-related problems (such as infection). Enteral feedings also carry a lower risk of stress ulcers and subsequent GI bleeding.

With either enteral or parenteral nutrition, carbohydrate content is an important consideration. A high carbohydrate load leads to increased carbon dioxide production. For the ARDS patient, eliminating the excessive carbon dioxide from the body may prove impossible or, at the very least, will further tax his compromised respiratory system.

To reduce the risk of pulmonary embolism, a potential complication of prolonged bed rest and pulmonary microemboli, the patient may receive low-dose heparin. To reduce the risk of stress ulceration from increased acid production or steroid use, the patient may receive concomitant antacids or histamine$_2$-receptor agonists.

Steroid therapy

The use of steroids in ARDS patients remains controversial. These agents may have a beneficial effect because they help stabilize cell membranes and prevent lysosomal enzyme release, thereby reducing inflammation, preventing WBC aggregation in the lungs, increasing surfactant production, and reducing pulmonary fluid leakage (by acting on endothelial cells to preserve vascular tone and thus correcting vascular permeability). However, steroids suppress the immune response, prevent complement activation, and may mask signs of infection.

Case study: Part 4

During Mr. Lewis' postoperative recovery, his ICU nurse developed a care plan based on appropriate nursing diagnoses. Keeping in mind the pulmonary deterioration that continued despite his cardiovascular stabilization, she used the following nursing diagnoses to devise nursing care strategies that would meet his and his family's changing needs: *impaired gas exchange, ineffective breathing pattern, ineffective airway clearance, altered family processes, potential for altered tissue perfusion,* and *potential for injury.*

Knowing that hypoxemia poses the gravest threat to the ARDS patient, the ICU nurses managed Mr. Lewis' deteriorating respiratory status by monitoring his ABG and VBG values closely to assess his arterial oxygen status. They also performed a physical examination every 1 to 2 hours and as needed to check for signs of hypoxemia, such as restlessness, confusion, agitation, tachypnea, dyspnea, and tachycardia.

Case study: Part 4 *(continued)*

Depending on his blood gas measurements, Mr. Lewis' ventilator settings were changed as specified.

To improve his gas exchange, Mr. Lewis sat in high Fowler's position, with the head of his bed elevated about 75 degrees. The ICU nurses turned him from side to side every 1 to 2 hours to promote gas exchange to all lung areas and to prevent skin breakdown.

Although positioning changes were aimed mainly at improving gas exchange, they also helped mobilize secretions. Respiratory assessment was performed every 1 to 2 hours. As ARDS progressed, Mr. Lewis' breath sounds changed from scattered crackles to loud gurgles throughout all lobes. Because of his severe respiratory distress and air hunger, Mr. Lewis couldn't comply when urged to slow his breathing and didn't respond to efforts to calm him through quiet conversation and therapeutic touch. Administration of pancuronium, to ensure adequate breathing, and his severe anxiety required high-dose morphine.

Mr. Lewis required frequent endotracheal suctioning, which produced thick, purulent secretions. When his secretions got thicker, sterile saline solution was instilled into the tube before suctioning to help liquefy them.

Because Mr. Lewis' chest X-rays showed that his right lung was more congested than his left, the nurse positioned him more frequently on his left side. This allowed gravity to increase circulation to the healthier lung and thus increase gas exchange.

Sputum specimens were sent to the laboratory for culture and sensitivity testing to identify any infectious organisms, and strict sterile technique was used when suctioning to prevent nosocomial infection.

Mr. Lewis' wife and children reacted to his illness with anxiety and anger. Hoping to reduce family strife, his nurse scheduled an appointment for the entire family to see a psychiatric clinical nurse specialist, who opened a discussion of the stress caused by a loved one's critical illness. After three conferences with the clinical nurse specialist, the children seemed less hostile and more accepting of their father's illness.

Mr. Lewis was evaluated often for signs of inadequate tissue perfusion, such as decreasing cardiac output; rising blood pressure; tachycardia; confusion; cool, clammy skin; and weak peripheral pulses. Monitoring his fluid intake and output determined that his hydration and renal perfusion were adequate. To maintain myocardial contractility, I.V. inotropic medications were given through the ninth postoperative day, when they were gradually tapered; on day 10, the drugs were discontinued.

Throughout the first 10 days after surgery, hemodynamic parameters were monitored to evaluate Mr. Lewis' right- and left-sided cardiac filling pressures and cardiac output. After the initial cardiovascular instability that followed CABG surgery, the nurses maintained Mr.

Lewis' hemodynamic values in the normal range by slightly modifying fluid administration rates and inotropic agent dosages, as ordered.

As Mr. Lewis became severely confused and agitated from hypoxemia, sleep deprivation, and the sensory overload of the ICU, the nurses grew concerned that he might harm himself. To help reduce Mr. Lewis' confusion, the nurses directed his attention to a clock and told him the date and day of the week every 4 hours. Even when he seemed unresponsive, they turned on his television so he could watch his favorite programs and baseball games.

When Mr. Lewis was ready for transfer to a step-down surgical floor, the nurses explained to him and his family the routine they could expect there.

Nursing management

The multiple serious threats posed by ARDS make nursing care of the ARDS patient intense, challenging, and sometimes frustrating. Be prepared to perform continuous, meticulous assessment and care to detect early signs of complications and disease exacerbation, to prevent iatrogenic complications, and to ensure optimal therapeutic effectiveness.

Continuous assessment

Be aware that many clinical changes in the ARDS patient are subtle; some may stem from the underlying condition. Because of your continuous presence at the bedside, you're the best judge of these changes and of the trends in your patient's condition. Always compare your assessment results with baseline findings and correlate them with the patient's clinical status. Reporting significant changes will ensure prompt treatment.

Monitor ABG values. Pulmonary edema, V/Q mismatch, and intrapulmonary shunting lead to *impaired gas exchange* and reduced arterial oxygenation. To identify and evaluate the degree of hypoxemia, monitor ABG values at least every hour during the acute disease stage, whenever the patient shows signs of respiratory distress, and 15 to 30 minutes after ventilator or PEEP adjustments. Avoid frequent and painful arterial punctures by drawing ABG samples from an indwelling arterial catheter.

In early-stage ARDS, expect normal ABG measurements as the patient compensates for his failing respiratory system. In later stages, watch for ABG values that reflect metabolic acidosis—an ominous sign of lactic acid build-up from prolonged hypoxemia. Report all ABG changes to the doctor.

Through serial A-a gradient calculations, you can assess the degree of oxygen diffusion across the alveolocapillary membrane and thus gauge the extent of intrapulmonary shunting (see *How to calculate an intrapulmonary shunt*). In most cases, a calculated shunt exceeding 30% is considered incompatible with prolonged spontaneous ventilation; notify the doctor immediately if your patient has a shunt of 30% or more and isn't on a mechanical ventilator.

Decreased CaO_2 and cardiac output impair oxygen delivery to the tissues. To determine tissue oxygenation, assess the patient for changes in skin color, mentation, and capillary refill.

Also monitor PvO_2 and CvO_2 by obtaining samples from the distal lumen of the PA catheter. Normally, PvO_2 is 40 mm Hg; CvO_2, 15 ml/dl (15 vol%); and CaO_2, 20 ml/dl (20 vol%). In ARDS, these values decrease.

The difference between CaO_2 and CvO_2 ($C[a\text{-}v]O_2$) reflects the amount of oxygen extracted by the blood as it passes through the tissues. Normally, this difference is 5 vol%. Stay alert for an increase in this value, which indicates decreasing cardiac output and inadequate tissue perfusion.

Monitoring PvO_2 as an assessment of cardiac output (decreasing cardiac output can lead to decreasing PvO_2) can aid in evaluating the consequences of PEEP therapy.

Monitor for hypoxemia. You may use pulse oximetry for noninvasive continuous hypoxemia monitoring. This method provides instant values, thus eliminating the need to await laboratory ABG results.

Monitor your patient's hemoglobin concentration and report any dramatic changes. Also note where hemoglobin falls on the oxyhemoglobin dissociation curve. Assess the patient for alkalosis, acidosis, hypothermia, hyperthermia, and altered $PaCO_2$ levels—conditions that hinder oxygen release by hemoglobin.

Promote tissue oxygenation. Change the patient's position every 30 to 60 minutes, and keep the head of the bed elevated 30 to 50 degrees whenever possible. Positioning changes help minimize gravity's effects on oxygen and fluid distribution throughout the body; elevating the head of the bed reduces the

How to calculate an intrapulmonary shunt

By using any of several equations, you can determine your patient's intrapulmonary shunt at the bedside.

Calculating a shunt from venous blood samples
This most accurate method requires samples of blood drawn simultaneously for measurement of arterial blood gas levels, hemoglobin (Hb) concentration, and mixed venous oxygen and carbon dioxide levels. (The mixed venous blood samples must be drawn from the distal lumen of the pulmonary artery catheter.)

To obtain data for the equations, first administer high concentrations of oxygen for 15 to 30 minutes before collecting the blood samples from which measurements are made. Usually, 50% oxygen is adequate; however, some doctors still specify 100% oxygen, the previously recommended level.

You can then calculate the shunt and the oxygen content of perfused and ventilated pulmonary capillary blood (CcO_2) by applying the collected data to the following equations:

$CcO_2 = (Hb \times 1.34) + (PaO_2 \times 0.003)$

$CaO_2 = \dfrac{(Hb \times 1.34 \times \% \text{ sat})}{100} + (PaO_2 \times 0.003)$

$CvO_2 = \dfrac{(Hb \times 1.34 \times \% \text{ saturation})}{100} + (PvO_2 \times 0.003)$

Shunted blood, expressed as a ratio of the total blood flow (Qs/Qt), can then be calculated as shown here:

$$Qs/Qt = \dfrac{(CcO_2 - CaO_2)}{(CcO_2 - CvO_2)}$$

Calculating a shunt from oxygen content
A simpler calculation uses partial pressures for oxygen content and requires fewer equations. It assumes that hemoglobin is fully saturated with oxygen.

$$Qs/Qt = \dfrac{([PAO_2 - PaO_2]\,0.003)}{(CaO_2 - CvO_2) + (PAO_2 - PaO_2)\,0.003}$$

Calculating a shunt from the A-a gradient
This method is less accurate than the others because it doesn't account for cardiac output changes. However, it's faster and easier to use for bedside monitoring. The equation compares estimated partial pressure of oxygen in aveolar blood (PAO_2) with measured partial pressure of oxygen in arterial blood (PaO_2). The result (difference) is known as the A-a gradient:

$$\text{A-a gradient} = PAO_2 - PaO_2$$

Then, to estimate the degree of shunting when the patient is breathing 100% oxygen, use this equation:

$$\% \text{ shunt} = \dfrac{(P[A-a]O_2)}{100} \times 5\%$$

Arterial-alveolar (a-A) ratio
You may prefer to assess your patient's shunt by calculating the a-A ratio because this value varies with the $PaCO_2$ level and the ventilation-perfusion ratio but not with FIO_2. Use this equation:

$$\text{a-A ratio} = \dfrac{PaO_2}{PAO_2}$$

---

risk of hypostatic pneumonia. Try to position the patient so that his less compromised lung is dependent; this maximizes blood flow to the healthier lung, helping to improve the V/Q ratio.

Other nursing interventions that reduce oxygen consumption and improve tissue oxygenation include maintaining normal body temperature; relieving pain by administering routine or around-the-clock analgesics, as ordered; and reducing restlessness and agitation by offering reassurance and encouragement, administering ordered sedatives or anxiolytics, and (in a mechanically ventilated patient) administering pancuronium, as ordered. (If your patient is receiving pancuronium, keep in mind that the ventilator must be set to the control mode because the patient can't breathe spontaneously. Also remember that pancuronium doesn't relieve pain or eliminate awareness, so the patient must also continue to receive sedatives and analgesics.)

Maintain ventilator efficiency. Frequently check the accuracy of ventilator settings to ensure specified delivery of oxygen, PEEP, and other parameters. Check PIP frequently to assess for airway resistance and to detect any mechanical problems (such as obstructed tubing).

Be aware that oxygen toxicity is a rare but serious threat to the ARDS patient, possibly leading to progressive lung consolidation and fibrosis. ARDS typically calls for an FIO_2 above 0.5 for several days; but the risk of oxygen toxicity increases when FIO_2 exceeds 0.5 for 2 to 3 days. Carefully observe for early signs of toxicity, including tracheobronchitis (beginning near the carina), cough, and inspiratory pain. Notify the doctor immediately if you detect any of these signs and symptoms.

Assess respiration. Decreased lung compliance and resulting fatigue may lead to *ineffective breathing patterns.* Perform frequent respiratory assessments to determine breathing adequacy and detect patient fatigue at its onset. Monitor the patient's vital signs at least every hour, especially noting respiratory rate, rhythm, and depth. Observe for tachypnea, accessory muscle use, and nasal flaring. Consider dyspnea a sign of deteriorating respiratory function.

Auscultate your patient's lungs for evidence of fremitus. Depending on the degree of atelectasis, expect decreased or diminishing breath sounds; basilar crackles signal increasing lung congestion. Palpation typically reveals decreased respiratory excursion as atelectasis spreads and lung compliance drops.

The patient may complain that he's out of breath. (If he's intubated, provide a communication board so that he can express such complaints.) As his breathing becomes increasingly ineffective, he may seem anxious and agitated; you may detect cool, diaphoretic skin. Notify the doctor of these and other indications of a change in respiratory status.

Mechanical ventilation may be necessary as the patient's fatigue worsens. If your patient is already on a ventilator, its settings or the PEEP level may need to be modified. Monitor PIP and static compliance values to assess lung compliance. A PIP level above 40 cm H_2O may indicate worsening lung compliance, accumulated airway secretions, airflow blockage from endotracheal or ventilator tube kinking, or incoordination of spontaneous and ventilator breaths (caused by patient agitation). If PIP doesn't decrease after suctioning or resolution of mechanical problems, notify the doctor.

Suction accumulating secretions. Decreased lung compliance and fatigue restrict deep breathing and effective coughing, resulting in *ineffective airway clearance.* Secretions may accumulate rapidly in the upper airways, preventing adequate ventilation. Suctioning helps remove secretions, thereby improving ventilation and helping to prevent secondary infection. When suctioning, use proper technique to avoid introducing new organisms into the respiratory system, inducing hypoxemia, and interrupting PEEP therapy. Just before placing the catheter into the endotracheal or tracheostomy tube, administer 100% oxygen. Never suction during catheter insertion—this decreases available oxygen. Also, avoid suctioning for more than 15 seconds at a time.

After you've finished suctioning, administer 100% oxygen for a few minutes. If copious secretions require additional suctioning, let the patient rest for a few minutes while you administer 100% oxygen, before resuming suctioning. Monitor vital signs and cardiac rate and rhythm during and after suctioning; auscultate breath sounds afterward and document any improvement. Also note the amount, color, and consistency of suctioned secretions.

As an alternative suctioning method for a mechanically ventilated patient, you may use the closed tracheal suctioning system (see *Closed tracheal suctioning,* page 246). This system has several advantages over conventional suctioning:
• The patient doesn't have to be disconnected from the ventilator during suctioning, so ventilatory support and PEEP therapy aren't interrupted.
• The system remains in place at all times, reducing the nursing time required for pulmonary hygiene.
• The closed system prevents dissemination of the patient's secretions into the air.

Closed tracheal suctioning

Unlike the conventional method, the closed tracheal suctioning system does not require interruption of mechanical ventilation and positive end-expiratory pressure therapy. It also offers the advantages of containing the patient's secretions and requiring less nursing time for the suctioning procedure.

The apparatus

The closed tracheal suctioning apparatus consists of a catheter in a sleeve that attaches to the ventilator circuitry as it joins the endotrachael or tracheostomy tube. Once attached, the catheter system can remain in place for 24 hours, reducing the risk of secondary infection during frequent suctioning. The catheter, which remains sterile, may have a bidirectional tip that allows you to suction both right and left mainstem bronchi; a side port

permits instillation of saline solution and catheter flushing after you've completed suctioning.

How to use it

To use the closed tracheal suctioning system, remove the tip protector and attach the control valve to the wall suction unit. The valve for activating suction pressure has a locked position to prevent accidental activation by the patient. Then turn on the wall suction, depress the thumb control valve, and set wall suction to the desired level. Next, attach the T-piece to the ventilator tubing and the endotracheal or tracheostomy tube. Keeping the T-piece parallel with the patient's chin, guide the bidirectional catheter into the left lung by rotating it to the right toward the 1 o'clock position and advancing it to the catheter (as shown). Use the blue line on the catheter as a guide. Then apply intermittent suction by depressing

the thumb control valve. Next, pull the catheter back slightly and turn it to the left by rotating it to the 11 o'clock position and advancing it into the patient's right lung. Again, apply intermittent suction by depressing the thumb control valve.

Keeping a grip on the T-piece, gently withdraw the catheter completely so that the extended length of the catheter is in the sleeve and the black mark on the catheter is visible at the back of the T-piece.

When you've completed suctioning, flush the catheter through the irrigation port by starting the suction, then slowly instill the flushing solution while maintaining suction. To prevent inadvertent suctioning, lift and turn the thumbpiece 180 degrees to the lock position on the suction control valve.

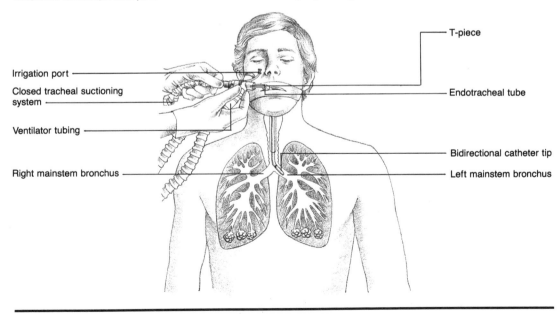

• The patient usually tolerates suctioning without prior hyperoxygenation.

• Gloving isn't necessary.

If your patient is extremely sensitive to small PaO_2 reductions, you may increase FIO_2 just before and during closed tracheal suctioning—but be sure to return it to the previous setting afterward. *Note:* Some ventilators can increase FIO_2 to 1.0 for short intervals, then automatically return it to the previous setting.

Perform chest physiotherapy. Frequent chest physiotherapy can help mobilize secretions from small, inaccessible airways into larger bronchioles for removal. You may want to perform chest physiotherapy over the entire lung field or just focus on the affected lobes (identified by auscultation and chest X-ray). Auscultate the lungs before and after chest physiotherapy, and document whether you noted any improvement in lung sounds.

Other nursing interventions aimed at improving airway clearance include providing adequate I.V. fluids to help liquefy and remove secretions, and changing the patient's position frequently to help mobilize secretions.

Monitor cardiac output. Mechanical ventilation and PEEP may cause *decreased cardiac output* because they increase intrathoracic pressure, which in turn reduces venous return. To detect early or subtle signs of reduced cardiac output, perform frequent physical examinations. Monitor vital signs, cardiac rhythm, central venous pressure (CVP), PAP, and PCWP at least every hour. Stay alert for such signs of decreased cardiac output as tachycardia; hypotension; cool, clammy skin; decreased peripheral pulses; reduced urine output; restlessness; and altered mentation.

Indices of preload, CVP, PAP, and PCWP also may reflect the patient's hydration status. Normally, CVP ranges from 2.7 to 12 cm H_2O (2 to 6 mm Hg), mean PAP is below 20 mm Hg, and PCWP measures 6 to 12 mm Hg. If your patient has below-normal CVP, PAP, or PCWP, suspect reduced venous return, possibly caused by fluid volume deficit or increased intrathoracic pressure that restricts venous return. Above-normal measurements may indicate fluid volume excess. Be sure to monitor all three parameters because any one could be erroneous or miscalculated.

The best time to take hemodynamic measurements remains controversial. When the patient is on a ventilator, measurements tend to increase, reflecting the ventilator's higher pressures. The important point is to maintain consistency by always taking measurements under the same conditions—with the patient on or off the ventilator—and documenting the ventilator status.

Optimal patient positioning during measurements is also debated. Nursing research indicates that the head of the bed can be elevated as much as 45 degrees without adversely affecting hemodynamic parameters, as long as the transducer's zero point is leveled at the right atrium position. Some authorities, however, believe the patient should be positioned flat during readings.

To maintain adequate cardiac output, administer ordered fluids and inotropic drugs, such as digoxin or dobutamine. As ordered, also give antiarrhythmics to control dysrhythmias.

Control fluid status. Precise fluid management can help correct or avoid *altered fluid volume.* Intensive fluid replacement aimed at increasing cardiac output may exacerbate interstitial fluid leakage. Assess the patient's hemodynamic parameters, vital signs, serum electrolyte levels, and urine output to determine any fluid imbalance. I.V. fluids must be administered at the exact rates ordered and any changes in fluid status reported immediately. Monitor the patient's response to diuretics—ventricular ectopy may signal hypokalemia.

If your patient must undergo hemodialysis or ultrafiltration to relieve pulmonary edema, monitor his vital signs frequently during and after the procedure to determine if removal of fluid has induced hypovolemia. Also observe for signs of abnormal bleeding, a potential adverse effect of the heparin given during either procedure. Weigh the patient afterward to help gauge whether the treatment was effective.

Stay alert for hematologic complications. ARDS may precipitate thrombocytopenia and disseminated intravascular coagulation, conditions that increase the risk of hemorrhage. Watch for petechiae; ecchymosis; increased bleeding time; bloody urine, stool, vomitus, or sputum; altered level of consciousness; cool, mottled extremities; and cyanosis. If any of these develops, alert the doctor right away—prompt treatment may prove lifesaving.

GI bleeding, a common and serious hemorrhagic complication of ARDS, may be brought on by stress ulcers. Notify the doctor immediately if your patient has bloody vomitus or stools, generalized abdominal pain, or vital sign changes.

Decreased cardiac output and *fluid volume deficit* can cause *altered tissue perfusion*, resulting in functional changes in the affected organ. Reduced renal perfusion, for example, can progress to renal failure. Assess your patient's urine output and urine specific gravity hourly to help determine the adequacy of renal perfusion and function.

Support adequate nutrition. *Altered nutrition: less than body requirements* may stem from respiratory distress, endotracheal intubation, mechanical ventilation, and generalized weakness—conditions that interfere with your patient's ability to eat. Also, the illness itself increases nutritional requirements. Consequently, expect to administer enteral or parenteral feedings to meet nutritional needs and prevent cachexia. With enteral feedings, assess tube placement, bowel sounds, and bowel function. To help prevent constipation and diarrhea, use a flow-control device and administer feedings at room temperature. Also assess for residual feeding in the patient's stomach. Keep in mind that a patient who has been heavily sedated for a prolonged period may develop paralytic ileus, so stay especially alert for constipation, abdominal distention, and decreased bowel sounds.

Elevate the head of the bed or turn the patient on his side when administering feedings to help prevent aspiration.

If your patient is receiving parenteral nutrition, watch for glucose abnormalities; infection originating from an I.V. line, a central catheter, or a catheter site; fluid overload; air embolism; and hemothorax or pneumothorax during catheter insertion. Monitor parenteral infusions closely, making sure to maintain the ordered flow rate. (The use of a flow-control device is highly recommended and, in most institutions, mandatory.) Check blood and urine glucose levels, urine specific gravity, and urine acetone levels at least once during each shift.

Remember that nutritional support therapy can increase carbon dioxide production from excessive caloric breakdown. This poses a special problem to the patient with compromised pulmonary function: By increasing breathing work, the excess carbon dioxide worsens tachypnea; if the lungs can't eliminate the excess, it leads to respiratory acidosis.

Prevent infection. Altered cell-mediated immunity, malnutrition, and the various invasive procedures necessary in treating ARDS increase the *potential for infection;* also, proteinaceous alveolar fluid serves as a perfect growth medium for bacteria. You'll need to assess the patient frequently for signs and symptoms of localized and systemic infection. Also, be sure to use sterile technique when suctioning, performing invasive procedures, and caring for indwelling line sites.

Other nursing diagnoses you may use for the ARDS patient include *anxiety, fear, impaired communication, ineffective individual or family coping,* and *pain.*

Patient teaching and discharge planning

As usual, you'll need to tailor your patient teaching to the patient's needs. Be prepared to reinforce your teaching frequently because the ARDS patient and his family may be too anxious to absorb information readily. In your teaching, include explanations of the disease process, treatments, hospital equipment, and the ICU activities surrounding the patient. Depending on the patient's condition, you may be able to teach him such helpful techniques as effective coughing.

Usually, the patient who recovers from ARDS regains satisfactory pulmonary function before discharge and thus requires minimal discharge planning (typically focusing on how to manage the clinical condition that precipitated ARDS). He probably won't need supportive care at home.

Case study: Part 5

Mr. Lewis' stay on the surgical step-down unit proceeded without complications. The nurses on that unit had ample time to assess the changing family dynamics and provide discharge teaching to the patient and his family. They encouraged him to take an active role in his care and let him help them plan his alternating periods of rest and activity. To encourage participation in his own care, they kept him fully aware of his condition. And by tailoring visiting hours to his family's needs, they ensured that he received plenty of emotional support to help him through this highly stressful experience.

Four weeks after CABG surgery, Mr. Lewis was discharged with instructions to see his cardiologist for routine follow-up visits. He expected to make a full recovery.

Chapter 7

Asthma

Asthma is a leading cause of death in North America and affects more than 8.5 million people in the United States alone. Every year, 1 million people visit emergency departments (EDs) with acute asthma attacks, and about 130,000 of them spend well over a million days in the hospital and lose about 5 million work days.

In the United States, asthma mortality is rising, with the greatest increase in children ages 10 to 14. Most asthma deaths occur in people over age 45 who have underlying heart and lung disease.

Despite recent advances in drug therapy, managing asthma continues to be difficult. However, more tests and treatments are being developed, including new bronchodilators that have more precise effects on the airways and fewer cardiac side effects, other drugs that can forestall allergic reactions that trigger asthma attacks, and more efficient drug delivery systems. But additional research is still needed before asthma is fully understood.

Case study: Part 1

Joanne Thompson, a 27-year-old asthmatic, came to the ED with breathing problems. She said that she'd had a sore throat for 3 days and had begun coughing up thick, yellow mucus, wheezing, and feeling short of breath. Although she'd used her nebulizer every 2 hours, it hadn't helped. Joanne's respiratory rate was 30 breaths/minute, and she had prolonged exhalation with an inspiratory-expiratory ratio of 1:6. Although her tongue, sublingual mucous membranes, and nail beds were pink, she was obviously in respiratory distress and was using the accessory muscles of her neck, shoulders, and abdomen to breathe. Chest auscultation revealed drastically diminished breath sounds with diffuse inspiratory and expiratory wheezes in all lobes.

Joanne's blood pressure was 140/86 mm Hg, with a paradoxical pulse of 12 mm Hg. Her heart rate was 120 beats/minute. Her radial and pedal pulses were full and bounding without deficits when compared to her apical heart rate. Her nail beds had a 1-second capillary refill time. Her skin was hot and dry, and her rectal temperature was 101° F (38.3° C).

Case Study: Part 1 *(continued)*

Arterial blood gases (ABGs) were drawn while Joanne breathed room air. The results were: pH, 7.41; partial pressure of oxygen in arterial blood (PaO_2), 62 mm Hg; partial pressure of carbon dioxide in arterial blood ($PaCO_2$), 42 mm Hg; arterial oxygen saturation (SaO_2), 0.92 (92%); and bicarbonate (HCO_3^-), 25 mEq/liter (25 mmol/liter). Based on these results, the doctor ordered 2 liters of oxygen per minute by nasal cannula.

Joanne's peak flow was 70, with a predicted peak flow of 378. So the doctor ordered albuterol (Proventil) by hand-held nebulizer. Peak flow after treatment was only 80, and breath sounds were unchanged, so the doctor ordered a theophylline level, a sputum Gram stain, a chest X-ray, and an electrocardiogram (ECG). The theophylline level was 3 mcg/ml; the sputum Gram stain revealed gram-positive rods in chains; the chest X-ray showed patchy atelectasis at both bases; and the ECG showed sinus tachycardia at a rate of 120 beats/minute with prominent P waves.

The doctor prescribed aminophylline (Aminophyllin), 200 mg by I.V. bolus followed by a maintenance dose of 500 mg in 500 ml dextrose 5% in water infused at a rate of 35 mg/hour; ampicillin, 1 g I.V. every 6 hours; and methylprednisolone sodium succinate (Solu-Medrol), 80 mg I.V.

Because Joanne didn't respond to initial treatments, she was admitted to the intensive care unit (ICU) for close observation and intensive therapy to prevent respiratory failure.

Causes and characteristics

The American Thoracic Society defines asthma as a clinical syndrome marked by increased responsiveness of the tracheobronchial tree to various stimuli. Its outstanding symptoms include paroxysmal dyspnea, wheezing, and coughing, which may range from mild and barely noticeable to intense, persistent, and life-threatening (status asthmaticus). (See *Status asthmaticus: Progression to respiratory failure.*) The primary physical symptom of asthma is variable airway obstruction that's usually at least partly reversible.

Asthma differs from other types of chronic obstructive airway disease in that it's not progressive and it rarely causes permanent pulmonary dysfunction. Status asthmaticus is an acute exacerbation of bronchial asthma that's marked by severe obstruction and that doesn't respond to standard treatments. In the past, asthma was divided into two categories: extrinsic, which is caused by an allergy or is immunoglobulin E (IgE)–mediated,

Status asthmaticus: Progression to respiratory failure

The patient with chronic asthma compensates by hyperventilating during an acute episode, so his $PaCO_2$ may remain subnormal. However, not every asthma patient always has a low $PaCO_2$; in some, a low level may signal the start of further respiratory deterioration, possibly leading to respiratory arrest.

As the attack becomes more severe, the patient tires and his breathing slows. Consequently, his pH and $PaCO_2$ reach normal or near normal levels. But as the attack continues, he becomes exhausted and hypoventilates. His $PaCO_2$ increases and his pH de-creases, causing respiratory acidosis. In many patients, respiratory acidosis precedes respiratory arrest.

To prevent the sudden onset of respiratory acidosis, pay particular attention to serial arterial blood gas values. An abnormal progression like the one charted below indicates a respiratory imbalance leaning toward respiratory arrest. The patient will probably require endotracheal intubation, mechanical ventilation, and increased sedation.

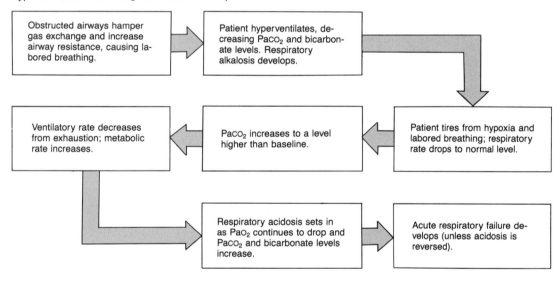

and intrinsic, which is not allergy-related and usually follows an upper respiratory tract infection. But these terms are no longer used as diagnostic classifications because the differences between extrinsic and intrinsic asthma aren't always clear and because most patients don't fit neatly into one category or the other.

Miscellaneous categories of asthma are drug-induced asthma and exercise-induced asthma. Such drugs as aspirin, indomethacin, and the additive tartrazine can induce a severe attack by discharging leukotrienes and prostaglandins from the mast cells. Exercise can cause asthma through the loss of heat and moisture in the upper airway. (See *Pathways of bronchial asthma development.*)

What separates asthmatics from other people? The sensitivity of their airways, which react with extreme bronchoconstriction to even mild stimuli. Increased airway sensitivity may predispose some people to asthma, but we still know little about how airway hyperreactivity develops. Three factors have been implicated: increased intrinsic reactivity of airway smooth muscle, an abnormality of autonomic nervous system control, and the collapse of airway defenses secondary to inflammation.

Most authorities estimate that up to 55% of asthma cases are allergy-related. An allergic reaction develops as follows: T lymphocytes identify an allergen, such as pollen, and give off IgE antibodies that apparently speed destruction of the allergen. Antigen-specific antibodies adhere to mast cells lining the skin, nose, throat, and digestive tract and to white blood cells (WBCs) and basophils in the bloodstream. When the IgE antibodies on the mast cell or basophil recognize the allergen, they alert the cells to release mediators, especially histamine, a powerful chemical that causes many common allergic symptoms. Then the mast cells and basophils produce still more mediators, including leukotrienes and muscle-constricting prostaglandins, which can cause asthmatic spasms.

Until about 10 years ago, allergists considered asthma a temporary crisis. They focused on a patient's immediate reaction to an allergen, such as cat dander or dust, and noted that three symptoms occur immediately and usually disappear within an hour: swelling, mucus secretion, and wheezing and dyspnea caused by bronchial airway constriction. What they didn't consider was that several hours later, patients have an extended period of inflammation, called the late-phase response. During this phase, the body produces a thick mucus composed of eosinophils and abnormal and deteriorating columnar respiratory cells. Also, some leukocytes probably travel to the lungs, where they discharge substances that cause tissue damage. For some reason, the late-phase response enhances lung sensitivity to asthma-producing stimuli, and this hypersensitivity can last for days or weeks, exposing the patient to new attacks. In fact, if a late-phase attack isn't treated, or isn't treated in time, bronchial

Pathways of bronchial asthma development

Extrinsic pathway	Intrinsic pathway

Extrinsic pathway

Inhaled allergen or antigen: pollen, dander

↓

Sensitization of bronchial mucosa by tissue-specific antibodies (immunoglobulins of the IgE, or type 1, class)

↓

Binding of IgE immunoglobulins to mast cells of tracheobronchial tree

↓

Reflex stimulation of parasympathetic nervous system receptors in bronchial mucosa

Release of histamine and other chemical mediators triggering bronchial smooth muscle contraction

↓

Increased vascular permeability causing leakage of proteins and fluid into tissue

↓

Tissue changes; increased IgE levels in serum

↓

Bronchial wall response
• Vasodilation with mucosal edema
• Smooth muscle contraction
• Increased mucus secretion

General response
• Dyspnea, cough, wheezing
• Prolonged expiration
• Eosinophilia

Intrinsic pathway

Viral infection, physical exertion, aspirin, smoke, fumes, psychological stress

↓

Lowered stimulus threshold of irritant receptors in tracheobronchial tree

↓

Mast cells activated by hyperreactivity to nonspecific stimuli

↓

Reflex stimulation of tracheobronchial receptors

↓

Vagal stimulation of bronchial smooth muscle contraction

Pathophysiology of bronchial asthma

Bronchial asthma is characterized by smooth muscle spasms that constrict airways. An inflammatory response further narrows airways by engorging blood vessels and swelling mucous glands and goblet cells. Eventually, epithelial denudation of the airway surface and thick-ening of the basement membrane result. Also, mucous secretions containing neutrophils, eosinophils, Charcot-Leyden crystals, Cursch-mann's spirals, clusters of epithelial cells, and bacteria or viruses plug the already narrowed airways.

NORMAL BRONCHIOLE

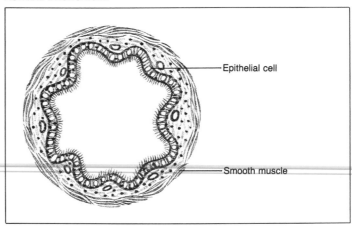

Epithelial cell

Smooth muscle

OBSTRUCTED BRONCHIOLE

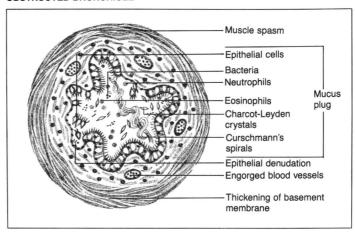

Muscle spasm

Epithelial cells
Bacteria
Neutrophils

Eosinophils
Charcot-Leyden crystals
Curschmann's spirals

Mucus plug

Epithelial denudation
Engorged blood vessels

Thickening of basement membrane

airways can become so obstructed with mucus and so inflamed that the patient suffocates. Because this late response involves airway inflammation, asthma is sometimes categorized as an inflammatory disease. (See *Pathophysiology of bronchial asthma.*)

Several factors exacerbate bronchoconstriction in asthma. They include allergens; exposure to irritants, such as air pollutants; bacterial or viral infection; drugs, such as beta blockers; psychological stress; cold air; and exercise. During an acute attack, airway resistance increases drastically as bronchial smooth muscles contract and mucosal edema and retained secretions narrow the lumen's airway. These abnormal changes prolong the forced expiratory time, diminish vital capacity, severely decrease forced expiratory volumes and flow rates, and cause overinflation of the lungs associated with changes in chest wall geometry and respiratory muscle activity.

Autopsies of asthma patients indicate that airway obstruction is related to increased and probably abnormal smooth muscle; to increased thickness of the airway wall from an exudative inflammatory reaction and enlarged mucous glands; and to mucus hypersecretion, causing plugged airways.

Case study: Part 2

While taking the history, the ICU nurse learned that Joanne had had asthma for 10 years and had been hospitalized several times. She was allergic to aspirin, cats, dogs, dust, and ragweed. As a teenager, she'd smoked a pack of cigarettes a day for 2 years. Both her sister and her aunt also had asthma. She'd been married for 4 years, had no children, and described her husband as "very supportive." She was worried about her mother, who lived alone and had recently had a heart attack. She'd been helping her with housework and felt that being exposed to dust, as well as feeling emotionally upset, exacerbated her asthma. She worked full-time as a computer programmer in an office where many of her co-workers smoked.

Joanne had also been dependent on steroids for a year, and whenever her doctor tried to lower the dosage, her symptoms immediately worsened. She was taking the following medications: prednisone (Deltasone), 10 mg by mouth every day; beclomethasone dipropionate (Vanceril), two puffs four times a day; theophylline (Slo-Phyllin), 250 mg four times a day; cromolyn sodium (Nasalcrom), one puff in each nostril three times a day; isoetharine hydrochloride (Bronkosol), 0.25 ml and 1 vial cromolyn sodium four times a day; and albuterol by inhaler as needed.

Case study: Part 2 *(continued)*

The effort of talking during the history taking was exhausting, and Joanne had to stop often to cough up thick, yellow secretions. During her physical examination, the nurse observed the following: Joanne had full range of motion and good strength in her arms and legs, but she used her sternocleidomastoid muscles to breathe, flared her nostrils, puckered her lips to exhale, and had prolonged expiration. She had tachypnea with a respiratory rate of 32 breaths/minute, inspiratory and expiratory wheezes, and decreased breath sounds in all lung fields. Chest percussion yielded dullness over both posterior lung bases, corresponding to the patchy atelectasis seen on her chest X-ray. Her lips and nail beds were still pink, the mucous membranes in her mouth were still very dry, and her skin was still warm and dry.

Joanne continued to receive supplemental oxygen. Repeat ABG values were as follows: pH, 7.42; PaO_2, 69 mm Hg; $PaCO_2$, 40 mm Hg; SaO_2, 0.93 (93%); and HCO_3^-, 25 mEq/liter (25 mmol/liter). Other laboratory results included an elevated WBC count of 16,000/mm³ (16 × 10⁹/liter), suggesting an infection, and an eosinophil count of 400/mm³, suggesting that an allergy had exacerbated the asthma attack. A repeat theophylline level was 14 mcg/ml, and serum electrolyte levels were normal. Because Joanne still had hypoxemia and her $PaCO_2$ was normal, the doctor increased her oxygen to 3 liters/minute by nasal cannula.

Joanne had suffered a potentially fatal attack of status asthmaticus. Warning signs included previous episodes of status asthmaticus, a peak expiratory flow rate (PEFR) below 100 liters/minute, pulsus paradoxus (a decrease in blood pressure of more than 10 mm Hg during inspirations), and an abnormal ECG. She remained in the ICU for further medical treatment and nursing care.

Assessment and diagnosis

Assessing and diagnosing asthma is a three-part process involving a detailed patient history, a physical examination, and diagnostic tests.

Patient history

Thorough history taking is the key to diagnosing and evaluating asthma. Its symptoms are typical and by careful questioning you can usually elicit a history of characteristic symptoms to support the diagnosis. Asking the right questions will also help you discover what agents cause your patient's asthma attacks so he can avoid them.

Most patients come to the hospital because of severe respiratory distress that isn't relieved by their usual medications. If the patient is too breathless to answer questions, question his spouse, parents, or whoever brought the patient to the hospital. Be sure to include the following categories and questions in your history.

Smoking. Do you smoke cigarettes, cigars, or a pipe? If so, how many years have you smoked and how much do you smoke every day? If you don't smoke now, did you ever? If so, how much and for how many years? A smoking history is critical because smoking can aggravate asthma symptoms and increase the risk of emphysema, lung cancer, and other smoking-related diseases.

Allergies. Do you sneeze often or have itchy, watery eyes? Are you allergic to any animals, foods, or medications, or to dust or pollen? Have you ever been tested or treated for allergies? Allergies can provoke asthma attacks.

Precipitating factors. Do certain things—such as cold air, exercise, medications (such as aspirin), colds, or respiratory tract infections—seem to trigger your asthma attacks? Singling out asthma "triggers" can help the patient recognize and possibly avoid them.

Home environment. Do you know of any allergens or irritants in your home? Cigarette smoke, feather pillows, and pets are some examples. Is your home near a factory? Have you taken any measures to reduce allergens and irritants in your home? Exposure to these substances can trigger an asthma attack.

Occupation. What is your present occupation? Your former occupations? Does your work expose you to chemicals, dust, or cigarette smoke? Exposure to these substances can trigger an asthma attack.

Hobbies. What are your hobbies? For example, do you paint or build models? Exposure to glues and other volatile substances used in these activities can provoke an asthma attack.

Coughing and sputum production. Do you cough frequently? If so, does it occur at certain times of the day? Do you cough up sputum? How much and what color and thickness is it? Does it have a foul odor? At what time of day do you produce the most sputum? Have you noticed a change in the color or amount of sputum recently? Most asthmatics cough up sputum, but changes—such as sputum turning from white to yellow—can signal a respiratory tract infection.

Dyspnea or wheezing. Do you ever wheeze or feel short of breath? Can you link these symptoms to certain activities, such as walking or climbing stairs? Do ordinary activities, such as washing, dressing, and cooking, leave you breathless or wheezing? Do you use an inhaler when these symptoms occur? If so, how many times a day do you use it? Patients with acute asthma may have to limit their physical activity to avoid wheezing and breathlessness; chronic asthmatics may have to perform activities of daily living at a slower pace.

Sleep pattern. Do you awaken during the night with coughing, wheezing, or other respiratory problems? If so, how often? Do you usually feel tired? Respiratory symptoms are often worse at night and in early morning, causing sleep disturbance. In acute asthma, fatigue accompanies decreased ventilation and rapid deterioration.

Family history. Do any family members have asthma or allergies? A family history of asthma is common. (See *Assessment profile: Acute asthma.*)

Physical examination
After taking a patient history, perform a thorough physical examination. Be sure to assess breathing and breathing patterns, coughing and sputum production, skin, mental status, nail beds, and blood pressure.

Breathing pattern. Watch for prolonged expiration or exhaling with pursed lips. The patient may use the accessory muscles (such as the sternocleidomastoid muscles) to breathe. He may also have dyspnea, one of the hallmarks of asthma. However, dyspnea isn't a good indication of the amount of respiratory distress because the amount of hyperventilation varies among patients. Also check the patient's respiratory rate for tachypnea. Auscultate the patient's breath sounds with a stethoscope, noting any adventitious sounds, such as wheezing; the quality of the breath sounds; and the amount of aeration. Patients with acute asthma usually wheeze during expiration, but some also wheeze during inspiration. However, the amount of wheezing may not correspond well to the severity of airway obstruction. Decreased

Acute asthma

Technique	Findings
Observation	Excessive use of accessory muscles of respiration Thoracic hyperinflation Tachypnea Dyspnea Nasal flaring Anxiety, restlessness Pursed-lip breathing ECG abnormalities Cyanosis (late sign)
Auscultation	Marked wheezing throughout lung fields Diminished or absent breath sounds Pulsus paradoxus > 10 mm Hg
Palpation	Tachycardia
Percussion	Dullness over lung bases (atelectasis)

breath sounds without wheezing may signal an obstruction so severe that air movement isn't sufficient to produce sound—so the absence of wheezing alone isn't necessarily a sign of improvement.

Coughing and sputum production. Observe the pattern of coughing and sputum production. During an acute asthma attack, a patient might not produce sputum for 24 to 48 hours. Coughing usually begins when he starts to improve, as inspissated mucus plugs that occluded the airways dislodge into the tracheobronchial tree and are expectorated.

Skin. Observe the patient's skin color. Are his lips, nail beds, or other highly vascular areas cyanotic? Cyanosis, which signifies extreme arterial oxygen desaturation, is an especially dangerous and late sign of severe asthma. Also check the skin and mucous membranes for dryness. Hyperventilation, diaphoresis, or inadequate fluid intake from general debility can cause dehydration. Last, check the skin for diaphoresis, which can signal fever, infection, or worsening asthma.

Mental status. Observe the patient for orientation to person, place, and time. Does he seem lucid or confused? Is he sleepy and difficult to arouse? Such mental status changes, which suggest hypoxemia and hypercapnia, can indicate that asthma is worsening and that the patient needs intubation for respiratory support.

Nail beds. Check the nail beds for clubbing—a painless, usually bilateral growth in soft tissue around the terminal phalanges of the fingers or toes. Clubbing causes the angle between nail and nail base to widen gradually until the nail base looks swollen and, later, convex. Clubbing is rare in uncomplicated asthma; its presence suggests concurrent problems, such as pulmonary neoplasm.

Blood pressure. Check for pulsus paradoxus, caused by marked shifts in intrathoracic pressure. The more obstructed the airway, the more serious the pulsus paradoxus.

Use this technique: With a sphygmomanometer or an intra-arterial monitoring device, inflate the blood pressure cuff 10 to 20 mm Hg above the patient's peak systolic pressure. Then deflate the cuff 2 mm Hg/second until you hear the first Korotkoff sound during expiration. Check systolic pressure. Watch the respiratory pattern while slowly deflating the cuff. The Korotkoff sounds will disappear during inspiration and reappear during expiration if the patient has pulsus paradoxus. Proceed with cuff deflation until you hear Korotkoff sounds during both inspiration and expiration. Check systolic pressure again. To calculate the degree of pulsus paradoxus, subtract the second reading from the first one—a difference of more than 10 mm Hg is abnormal.

Diagnostic tests

After the history and physical examination, the doctor usually orders several diagnostic tests to determine the severity of the patient's asthma. These tests include ABG levels, pulmonary function tests, oximetry, chest X-ray, ECG, blood studies, and sputum cultures. Skin tests and, possibly, the methacholine inhalation challenge test can help identify specific allergens and document airway hyperreactivity. (See *Diagnostic profile: Acute asthma.*)

ABG levels. ABG studies assess gas exchange in the lungs by measuring the PaO_2, $PaCO_2$, and pH of an arterial blood sample. The PaO_2 measures the amount of oxygen the lungs

▶ **DIAGNOSTIC PROFILE**

Acute asthma

Test	Normal findings	Possible findings
Forced expiratory volume in 1 second (FEV_1)	About 2 liters	< 0.5 liter
Peak expiratory flow rate	300 liters/minute	≤80 liters/minute
Total lung capacity	5,900 ml	Increased
Residual volume	1,200 ml	Increased
PaO_2	80 to 100 mm Hg	Decreased
$PaCO_2$	35 to 45 mm Hg	Increased (when FEV_1 is decreased by 20%)
pH	7.35 to 7.42	Decreased
HCO_3^-	22 to 26 mEq/liter (22 to 26 mmol/liter)	Decreased
Sputum	Normal	Increased viscosity and plug formation
Chest X-ray	Normal	Pneumomediastinum

transport to the blood, the $PaCO_2$ measures how effectively the lungs discharge carbon dioxide, and the pH expresses the acid-base level or hydrogen ion (H^+) concentration of the blood. Blood samples for ABG analysis are obtained through percutaneous arterial puncture or an arterial line.

Except in very mild asthma, when ABG levels may remain normal, these studies are fundamental in assessing decompensated asthma. In mild cases, $PaCO_2$ is slightly decreased, and pH may be slightly alkalotic because the patient is hyperventilating. In moderate cases, PaO_2 decreases and respiratory alkalosis is still present. In moderately severe cases, $PaCO_2$ begins to show an increase, but it may return to normal even though breathing is very labored (a confusing picture, since $PaCO_2$ and pH will both be normal). In severe asthma, patients have hypoxemia with acidosis caused by extreme airway obstruction and fatigue.

Pulmonary function tests

The most common bedside pulmonary function tests are spirometric measurements of volume (amount of exhaled air) and flow rates (speed of exhalation).
• Forced vital capacity (FVC) is the total amount of air that can be exhaled after maximum inhalation.
• Forced expiratory volume in 1 second (FEV_1) is the amount of air the patient can exhale at the beginning of an exhalation.
• The FEV_1-FVC ratio, the most common gross measurement of obstructive disease, represents the total exhaled volume the patient exhaled in the first second—in other words, how fast the patient exhales.
• Peak expiratory flow rate measures peak flow as the patient exhales as hard as possible into a peak flow meter. Peak flow is shown by an indicator on the unit. This test allows patients to evaluate their response to bronchodilator therapy and can help them to objectively evaluate the severity or progression of an asthma attack.

Pulmonary function tests. The two most common pulmonary function tests are spirometric measurements of volume (amount of exhaled air) and flow rates (speed of exhalation). (See *Pulmonary function tests.*)

In patients with asthma, these tests typically reveal the following abnormalities:
• decreased forced expiratory volume in 1 second (FEV_1), decreased PEFR, and decreased ratio between FEV_1 and forced vital capacity (FVC)
• a 15% or greater increase in the FEV_1 response to a bronchodilator
• diminished lung vital capacity
• increased lung functional residual capacity
• increased total lung capacity
• increased residual lung volume.

A simple technique called peak flow measurement is used to measure the severity of airway obstruction. Sometimes used in the ED, a peak flow meter gauges the patient's highest flow rate during exhalation; then these measurements are compared to those taken throughout the patient's hospitalization to chart his progress and treatment response.

During severe asthma attacks, even a bronchodilator may not clear airway obstruction and improve the patient's FEV_1. Why? Some experts believe that extensive viscous mucus plugs blocking the bronchi may bar the entry of inhaled drugs and that hyperventilation may diminish drug delivery to peripheral airways even more. Also, severe bronchial wall edema and spasms and hypertrophy in smooth muscles can block drug diffusion from the luminal surface to the site of action.

Oximetry. Electronic pulse oximeters are used to continuously measure SaO_2 and to detect decreasing saturation in patients with acute asthma. This procedure is valuable because it's noninvasive and can detect hypoxemia quickly.

Chest X-ray. All patients with acute asthma should have a chest X-ray to rule out pneumothorax, pneumomediastinum, pneumonia, atelectasis, and other complications. A chest X-ray may reveal hyperinflated lungs and patches of atelectasis, which may affect areas of varying size (from a small lung segment to an entire lobe) and may change in location from one hour to the next. These changes reflect relief of bronchospasm and mucus plugging with bronchodilators.

ECG. Because acute airway obstruction can affect cardiac function, asthma patients with tachycardia or other dysrhythmias should be placed on a cardiac monitor. Other reversible ECG abnormalities associated with asthma include sinus tachycardia, premature ventricular contractions, cor pulmonale, right axis deviation, right bundle branch block, clockwise rotation, right ventricular strain patterns, and nonspecific ST-T changes. As a rule, patients with the most severe obstructions and the most abnormal electrolyte and ABG levels are the most likely to have one or more ECG abnormalities.

Several factors can cause tachycardia and increased pulse rate, including a noticeable increase in breathing difficulty, hypoxemia or hypercarbia, acidosis, and the use of beta-agonists or theophylline. Although asthma therapy can halt many of these changes within a few hours, the ECG may not return to normal for 9 days.

Blood studies. Allergic reactions raise serum IgE and eosinophil counts, so knowing these results can help determine the origin of an asthma attack. The radioallergosorbent test is commonly used to measure allergen-specific IgE antibody serum levels. Electrolyte and serum hematocrit levels to determine fluid status are also useful because dehydration is common in patients with acute asthma.

Sputum cultures. Sputum cultures and Gram stains should be done to rule out bacterial infection as the cause of an asthma attack. These tests may reveal eosinophils in the sputum.

Skin tests. Skin testing can detect specific IgE antibodies to common allergens and can rule out allergy as the cause of an asthma attack. These tests are performed by applying a small amount of allergen to the skin. If the patient has specific IgE antibodies to that allergen, he'll have a positive wheal-and-flare reaction within 15 minutes. Skin tests aren't performed on patients during an acute asthma attack because they exacerbate allergic symptoms.

Methacholine inhalation challenge. This test helps diagnose asthma by establishing airway hyperreactivity. Because asthmatics are 100 to 1,000 times more sensitive to methacholine than people without asthma, inhaling increasing amounts of the drug can identify asthma by inducing bronchospasm and causing a decrease in FEV_1 (a 20% drop confirms asthma). The patient is then given a bronchodilator to reverse the spasm. This test isn't performed while patients are having an asthma attack because it may dangerously intensify their symptoms.

Case study: Part 3

Medical intervention to manage Joanne's status asthmaticus included bronchodilating drugs, oxygen, breathing exercises and chest physiotherapy (CPT), and antibiotics to prevent and treat infection. Joanne continued to receive 35 mg of aminophylline every hour. She also took metaproterenol sulfate (Alupent), a beta-adrenergic blocking agent; the cromolyn sodium spray she'd used at home; and I.V. methylprednisolone, a corticosteroid with anti-inflammatory, antiallergenic, and anti-immunologic properties.

After a full day of treatment, Joanne's peak flow had increased to 250, and her respiratory rate was 20 breaths/minute. On auscultation, her breath sounds showed increased aeration and decreased wheezing. She continued to receive oxygen therapy. Repeat ABG analysis showed that her hypoxemia had greatly improved since she was first assessed in the ED to: pH, 7.42; PaO_2, 78 mm Hg; $PaCO_2$, 38 mm Hg; SaO_2, 0.95 (95%); and HCO_3^-, 24 mEq/liter (24 mmol/liter).

To help clear her lung secretions, Joanne received breathing exercises and CPT. She also learned deep breathing with pursed-lip exhalation: inhaling through the nose, forming her lips into an "O" shape as if she were whistling, and exhaling slowly through her pursed lips. This technique prolongs expiration and keeps airways open during an asthma attack.

Joanne's sputum culture was positive for *Streptococcus pneumoniae*, suggesting that her asthma attack was triggered by a bacterial infection. The doctor prescribed ampicillin, first I.V., then by mouth.

Joanne's respiratory status improved significantly, and 2 days after her admission, she was transferred to a medical unit. There, bedside pulmonary function tests produced these results: FVC, 2,900 ml (predicted value 3,628 ml) 80% predicted; FEV_1, 1,900 ml 65% predicted; peak flow, 280 liters/minute (predicted value 378 liters/minute) 74% predicted.

The doctor began reducing drug dosages as Joanne's breathing returned to normal. By day 4, her breath sounds were normal with good aeration and no wheezing. ABG values taken on room air were pH, 7.40; PaO_2, 80 mm Hg; $PaCO_2$, 36 mm Hg; SaO_2, 0.95 (95%); and HCO_3^-, 24 mEq/liter (24 mmol/liter), so oxygen was discontinued.

Joanne's condition was back to normal. But before discharging her, the doctor ordered another series of bedside pulmonary function tests. The results were FVC, 3,266 ml (predicted value 3,628 ml) 90% predicted; FEV_1, 2,788 ml and 85% predicted; peak flow, 320 liters/minute (predicted value 378 liters/minute) 85% predicted. A repeat chest X-ray was also normal.

Treatment options

How acute asthma is managed depends on the severity of airway obstruction and on the patient's initial response to treatment. At first, treatment aims to decrease bronchospasm and increase pulmonary ventilation by administering bronchodilators and oxygen. If the patient is young and otherwise healthy, the doctor may substitute subcutaneous epinephrine (Adrenalin) or terbutaline (Bricanyl) for inhaled beta-adrenergics. But because these drugs can have adverse cardiovascular effects, they're not recommended for older patients or others with cardiovascular problems. Such patients receive $beta_2$-specific drugs given by metered-dose inhaler or nebulizer instead.

Theophylline may also be ordered initially; if it's not, it should be added later if the patient has a severe obstruction and hasn't responded well to inhaled beta-adrenergics. Corticosteroids should be given immediately if the patient has taken them recently, or if he doesn't respond to adrenergics or theophylline. Finally, ipratroprium can be administered by nebulizer every 4 to 6 hours if the patient's condition doesn't improve.

Treatment of acute asthma requires administration of oxygen, bronchodilating drugs, methylxanthines, corticosteroids, and anticholinergic drugs, as well as such interventions to aid ventilation as CPT and breathing exercises. Treatment may also include antibiotics, sodium bicarbonate, and various prophylactic treatments.

Oxygen to prevent hypoxemia

Treating life-threatening hypoxemia is the first priority with patients suffering from acute asthma. Because hypoxemia can increase pulmonary hypertension and airway resistance, impair cerebral function and cardiac contractility, prevent adequate renal perfusion, and increase dysrhythmias, all patients with acute

Epinephrine: Special alert

Some forms of epinephrine contain sulfites, which can cause allergic reactions, such as acute asthma attacks and anaphylaxis. Although such sensitivity to sulfites is probably rare in the general population, it appears to be prevalent in persons who have asthma. This potential risk should not discourage the use of epinephrine for treatment of severe allergic reactions in other emergencies for which epinephrine is the most effective treatment. However, sulfite sensitivity should be considered when the use of epinephrine produces decreased bronchodilation or paradoxical worsening of respiratory function.

asthma need supplemental oxygen in amounts determined by arterial PaO_2 measurements. Oxygen is usually given through a nasal cannula, usually at a flow rate of 2 to 4 liters/minute, to raise the SaO_2 to 90% or higher.

Bronchodilators to enhance airflow

The most potent bronchodilators are beta-adrenergics, which enhance airflow better than any other single drug. These drugs increase the amount of cyclic $3'$, $5'$-adenosine monophosphate (cyclic AMP) in airway smooth muscle cells, causing smooth muscle relaxation and bronchodilation. They include albuterol (Ventolin, Proventil), bitolterol (Tornalate), pirbuterol (Maxair), ephedrine, metaproterenol (Alupent, Metaprel), isoetharine (Bronkosol), terbutaline (Bricanyl), epinephrine, and isoproterenol (Isuprel). (See *Epinephrine: Special alert.*)

Mechanism of action. The effects of beta-adrenergic drugs can be divided into two classes: B_1 and B_2. B_1 effects are cardiotonic, including increased heart rate, increased contractility, and coronary vasodilation. B_2 effects are bronchodilatory, including bronchial and venous enlargement and smooth muscle relaxation. Although the perfect bronchodilator would have B_2 effects only, most drugs also have B_1 effects—but some drugs are more B_2-specific than others.

Besides bronchodilation, beta-adrenergic drugs also have other benefits for asthma patients. They increase ciliary movements, decrease chemical mediators of anaphylaxis, enhance bronchodilation by parenteral steroids, reduce capillary permeability, and decrease bronchoconstriction caused by exposure to allergens, exercise, or hyperventilation.

Routes of administration. Beta-adrenergic drugs can be given orally, intravenously, or subcutaneously, but inhalation via metered-dose inhaler or jet nebulizer is the preferred method. Inhalation is preferred for two reasons: First, it applies the drug directly to the respiratory tract, so small amounts are effective while resulting in a lower blood level and fewer adverse effects. Second, inhalation provides an onset of action that is just as fast as I.V. administration (5 minutes) and much shorter than oral administration (60 minutes).

Which inhalation method is best? In comparison tests, metered-dose inhalers and jet nebulizers had the same therapeutic effects. However, using a metered-dose inhaler requires correct inhalation technique, which some patients find difficult. A spacing device may help such patients use an inhaler effectively. The advantage of jet nebulizers is that they can be used without patient cooperation.

Patients with severe asthma who haven't responded well to inhaled drugs can receive beta-adrenergic drugs subcutaneously (epinephrine or terbutaline), or by slow I.V. injection or infusion (isoproterenol, albuterol, or terbutaline). Parenteral administration is probably more effective than inhalation in severe asthma because the drug travels through the systemic circulation to reach parts of the airway that may not be accessible by an aerosol. However, parenteral administration causes more side effects, especially in the cardiovascular system, so this route should be used cautiously in patients over age 40 or in those with cardiovascular disease.

Adverse reactions. Whatever the administration route, beta-adrenergic drugs can cause some adverse reactions because they stimulate both beta$_1$ and beta$_2$ receptors. The most common ones are palpitations, tachycardia and skin flushing (at high doses), and slight, dose-related increases in blood pressure. Tachycardia is the dose-limiting adverse effect of nonselective beta agonists; tremor is the dose-limiting adverse effect of selective beta$_2$ agonists. Side effects with higher dosages may include headache, dizziness, nausea, weakness, sweating, inhibition of uterine contractions, renin release, vasodilation of pulmonary arteries, slight worsening of the ventilation-perfusion (V/Q) ratio caused by a PaO$_2$ drop of a few mm Hg, and increased blood glucose levels (with I.V. administration).

Methylxanthines to relieve bronchospasm

The methylxanthines (theophylline preparations) are spasmolytics that relax and dilate the smooth muscles of the bronchial airways and pulmonary blood vessels. They can be administered orally, intravenously, or rectally, but rectal absorption is slow and erratic. This class of drugs includes theophylline, aminophylline, oxtriphylline, and theophylline sodium glycinate. Theophylline is the active ingredient in all these drugs, but the amount varies. Some theophylline salts increase solubility; some release theophylline in vivo. (See *Theophylline equivalents,* page 270.)

Theophylline equivalents

The table below compares the varying theophylline content of several common bronchodilators.

Theophylline salt	Percentage of theophylline	Equivalent theophylline dose
Theophylline (anhydrous)	100	100 mg
Theophylline monohydrate	91	110 mg
Aminophylline (anhydrous)	86	116 mg
Aminophylline dihydrate	79	127 mg
Oxtriphylline	64	156 mg
Theophylline sodium glycinate	46	217 mg

A sustained-release form of theophylline helps maintain therapeutic blood levels and promote patient compliance. Some forms, such as Theo-24, are administered only once a day. However, these products may be absorbed incompletely or erratically in some patients, so they must be used cautiously.

Mechanism of action. The following three processes have been suggested to explain the methylxanthines' mechanism of action in asthma.

• *Adenosine antagonism*—Adenosine and theophylline are similar in composition, and adenosine is known to cause bronchospasm in asthmatics. Theophylline antagonizes adenosine's effects.

• *Phosphodiesterase inhibition*—Cyclic 3', 5'-adenosine monophosphate, the intercellular mediator substance, is broken down by the enzyme phosphodiesterase, and theophylline inhibits this enzyme in vitro. However, this mechanism is questionable because the concentration of theophylline needed to inhibit the enzyme can't be achieved in vivo.

• *Calcium flux modulation*—Experiments have shown that theophylline helps release calcium from intracellular storage sites.

Effect on symptoms. How does theophylline alleviate asthma symptoms? First, it relaxes bronchial smooth muscle, stimulating the central nervous system (CNS) and enhancing the ventilatory response to hypoxemia. Then it increases skeletal muscle contractility in the diaphragm and decreases mast cell disturbance with accompanying release of mediator chemicals.

Adverse reactions. Theophylline can cause extreme CNS stimulation, including headache, restlessness, and seizures, as well as tachycardia, hypotension, nausea, and precordial pain.

Dosage. The theophylline dosage for acute bronchospasm varies, depending on the patient's current use of theophylline derivatives, smoking history, age, and cardiac and hepatic function. Before giving a loading dose to a patient who is already taking the drug or its derivatives, the nurse should determine the patient's serum theophylline level (although some clinicians give a small loading dose regardless). The recommended loading dose for patients already taking theophylline is 0.5 mg/kg, which causes a 1-mcg/ml increase in the serum theophylline level. Patients who aren't already taking the drug should receive a loading dose of 4.7 mg/kg.

To establish a steady-state therapeutic blood level of theophylline, a loading dose of I.V. aminophylline should be infused over 30 minutes at a rate not exceeding 25 mg/minute. A serum theophylline level should be drawn 30 minutes after the infusion to allow the drug to be distributed equally between blood and peripheral tissues, and to help estimate the constant infusion rate of aminophylline so the target serum concentration can be maintained. Although a therapeutic theophylline level is usually between 10 and 20 mcg/ml, some patients do well on lower levels. (See *Factors that alter theophylline clearance,* page 272.)

Corticosteroids to combat inflammation

In asthma patients, corticosteroids decrease airway inflammation, prevent the release of chemical mediators from mast cells, enhance the action of catecholamines, and produce an anti-allergenic and anti-immunologic effect. Commonly used corticosteroids include methylprednisolone, prednisone, beclomethasone, flunisolide, hydrocortisone, and triamcinolone acetonide. These drugs may be administered intravenously, orally,

Factors that alter theophylline clearance

Theophylline is eliminated from the body primarily by metabolism in the liver. Many factors alter theophylline clearance and, consequently, its dosage. For example, patients with liver disease need lower dosages because they have decreased theophylline clearance, and cigarette smokers need higher dosages because nicotine increases drug clearance. Some other factors that influence theophylline clearance include the following.

Factors that increase clearance	Factors that decrease clearance
• Age (2 to 18) • Chronic smoking of marijuana or tobacco • Low-carbohydrate or high-protein diet • Phenobarbital or phenytoin • Cystic fibrosis • Oral contraceptives • Withdrawal from caffeine • Ingestion of large amounts of charbroiled meat	• Age (neonates, elderly patients) • Acute and chronic liver dysfunction • Cardiac decompensation, including cor pulmonale • Macrolide antibiotics (erythromycin, troleandomycin), allopurinol • Histamine$_2$ antagonists

by metered-dose inhaler, and by nasal spray. Inhaled steroids have been improved—the oral inhalant form of flunisolide (Aerobid) needs to be given only twice a day; an oral inhalant form of triamcinolone (Azmacort) comes with its own spacer device.

Dosage. To treat status asthmaticus, most doctors recommend at least 100 mg of hydrocortisone (Cortef) or an equivalent every 4 hours, with 300 mg in 24 hours as an average dose; however, there is little agreement among doctors about the most effective dose. Some prescribe as much as 3,000 mg during the first 24 hours, and recent studies suggest that high initial doses give quicker results. The administration route (continuous or intermittent I.V. infusion) apparently doesn't influence these drugs' effectiveness.

Duration of therapy. The duration of treatment with an I.V. steroid depends on the patient's response and ability to tolerate the oral form of the drug. When a patient shows clear signs of improvement, the doctor may taper the I.V. steroid dose quickly, then prescribe a single daily dose of an oral steroid; then he may taper the oral dose further. Although metered-dose inhalers aren't used to administer these drugs during acute episodes, they are used during weaning from oral steroids.

Toxic effects. Corticosteroids can have toxic effects arising from withdrawal and from long-term high doses. Sudden withdrawal after prolonged use can provoke acute adrenal insufficiency, whose classic symptoms are fever, myalgia, arthralgia, and malaise. Prolonged therapy can suppress pituitary-adrenal function so it's slow in returning to normal. Other common complications of prolonged steroid use include fluid and electrolyte imbalances; hyperglycemia and glycosuria; heightened susceptibility to infections, including tuberculosis; peptic ulcers, which may bleed or perforate; osteoporosis; myopathy; behavioral changes; posterior subcapsular cataracts; arrested growth; and cushingoid syndrome (moon face, buffalo hump, supraclavicular fat pad enlargement, central obesity, striae, ecchymoses, acne, and hirsutism).

Administration by metered-dose inhaler causes fewer adverse effects than oral or I.V. administration. However, inhaled steroids can cause localized fungal infections (*Candida albicans* or *Aspergillus niger* in the mouth, pharynx, and larynx; hoarseness; dry throat and mouth; and irritated throat.

Anticholinergic drugs to relax bronchial smooth muscle

Anticholinergic drugs are generally used to supplement other drugs in treating bronchospasm, not to treat acute asthma attacks. One exception is atropine, which is sometimes used to treat acute asthma that doesn't respond to beta-adrenergics, theophylline, or corticosteroids. However, atropine causes CNS side effects that limit its usefulness. An atropine derivative, ipratropium bromide, is being used to treat asthma because it's not absorbed as much as atropine and it doesn't enter the CNS.

Anticholinergics are usually given as aerosol inhalants to provide local action and minimize adverse effects. Atropine is usually given via nebulizer, often combined with a beta-adrenergic drug. Ipratropium can be given either by nebulizer or metered-dose inhaler. The response to anticholinergic therapy varies.

Diaphragmatic breathing

Diaphragmatic breathing can help the patient slow down and deepen his respirations during episodes of respiratory discomfort. This breathing pattern uses less energy and oxygen than breathing with the accessory muscles.

Place the patient in semi-Fowler's position with his head slightly elevated, back well supported, and arms and neck relaxed. This position keeps the abdominal muscles relaxed, and allows the diaphragm to move freely and gravity to assist in lowering the diaphragm muscle.

Tell the patient to place one hand at the top of his abdomen just below the ribs. As he inhales gently, he should feel his abdomen rise; as he exhales, he should feel it sink back down.

If the patient has difficulty contracting his diaphragm, have him quickly sniff through the nose. He should feel a quick rise in his abdomen. Explain that he should try to achieve this rise slowly.

Once the patient has mastered this technique, he should try it in other positions (lying supine, with a pillow under his head, in Fowler's position, standing, and walking).

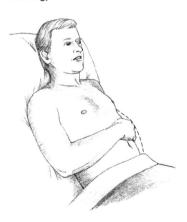

Adverse effects. Common effects of atropine include tachycardia, dry oral mucosa, blurred vision, urine retention, and constipation. Ipratropium frequently causes dry mouth. Limited absorption of this drug prevents many systemic adverse effects.

Interventions to aid ventilation

Depending on the severity of respiratory distress, patients with acute asthma may require CPT, bronchoscopy and lavage, intubation, or, rarely, mechanical ventilation.

CPT and breathing exercises. CPT may or may not be useful to treat severe asthma. Patients with status asthmaticus don't respond well to this treatment; moreover, they may not be able to tolerate tilting and other positions used for postural drainage. However, in less seriously ill patients, moderate chest percussion and forced expiration do help clear secretions, and deep breathing and pursed-lip exhalation help lengthen expiration and maintain small airway patency. Diaphragmatic breathing can also help. (See *Diaphragmatic breathing.*)

Bronchoscopy and lavage. One serious complication of asthma is mucus impaction with occasional gross atelectasis. If the main airways are obstructed by thick mucus, bronchoscopy or lavage may be performed to relieve it.

Tracheal intubation. When asthmatic patients need intubation, a large-bore endotracheal tube is usually used. Oral intubation is the preferred method because oral insertion is easier and avoids nasal polyps. Tracheotomy usually isn't necessary because most patients are extubated in a few days.

Mechanical ventilation. Patients with acute asthma need intubation and mechanical ventilation when their breathing fails to maintain sufficient gas exchange because of respiratory arrest, progressive hypercapnia with respiratory acidosis, or progressive mental status deterioration. Because these patients' airway resistance is high and usually changeable, a volume-cycled ventilator able to generate a high peak inspiratory pressure of more than 50 cm H_2O should be used. Hypercapnic patients or those who resist ventilation may need sedation with diazepam (Valium) or, rarely, temporary paralysis with pancuronium bromide (Pavulon). Ventilator inspiratory flow rates should be adjusted to provide enough exhalation time, and ABG levels should be measured frequently. In most patients with asthma, most of the obstruction should clear up within 48 hours; then patients can be extubated. Asthmatic patients are usually weaned quickly.

Antibiotics and sodium bicarbonate

Many doctors prescribe antibiotics for all patients with severe asthma. But recent studies reveal that bacterial infections are rare in these patients, so routine antibiotic use is being discouraged. Antibiotics should be reserved for patients with pneumonia, fever, leukocytosis ($>15,000/mm^3$ [15×10^9]), or bacteria on Gram stain.

Sodium bicarbonate may be used to restore normal pH in patients with severe acidosis. However, it should be used cautiously because patients may continue to have serious metabolic alkalosis even after bronchospasm is relieved and gas exchange improves. Improving gas exchange is the preferred method for treating acidosis.

Prophylactic medical treatments

Several treatments are being used to prevent further asthma attacks once the acute episode is over. These treatments include cromolyn sodium, immunotherapy, and several investigational drugs.

Cromolyn sodium. Cromolyn prevents allergic reactions by blocking mast cell degranulation and discharge of histamine and other mediators, which follow inhalation of certain antigens. Although this substance can help prevent allergy-induced bronchial asthma, it can't treat an acute asthma attack because it has no innate bronchodilator, antihistamine, or anti-inflammatory properties. However, it can be used before exercise to prevent bronchospasm.

Cromolyn is available as a metered-dose inhaler, a nebulizer solution, a capsule (inhaled with a Spinhaler device), a nasal spray, and an ophthalmic solution. The metered-dose inhaler and nebulizer forms—new treatments—cause less airway irritation and coughing than the powdered or capsule forms.

Common adverse reactions to inhaled cromolyn include dry, irritated throat; coughing; wheezing; and nausea. Reactions to other forms of cromolyn include bronchospasm, coughing, laryngeal edema (rare), nasal congestion, pharyngeal irritation, and wheezing.

Immunotherapy. Also called desensitization or hyposensitization, immunotherapy can help forestall allergic disorders through injections of small, concentrated, gradually increasing amounts of allergen. Because these injections create blocking antibodies that may decrease the late IgE-mediated allergic response, this treatment isn't effective during an acute asthma attack. Immunotherapy is also somewhat controversial because of poor standardization of allergen extracts and dose, ill-defined criteria for patient selection, and the lack of objective documentation of its benefits.

Investigational treatments. The Food and Drug Administration is currently testing several other drugs for possible use in asthma treatment. Two prophylactic drugs, ketotifen and nedocromil sodium, inhibit mediator release. Nedocromil sodium given by metered-dose inhaler has both anti-allergenic and anti-inflammatory properties. When used with bronchodilators and inhaled corticosteroids, it allows a 20% to 70% decrease in bronchodilator dosage and a moderate sparing effect in patients on steroids.

Case study: Part 4

After assessing Joanne, the nurses on all three units formulated nursing diagnoses. They all agreed that correcting Joanne's *impaired gas exchange* was their first priority. They also formulated the following other diagnoses and planned Joanne's nursing care around them: *ineffective breathing pattern, fluid volume deficit, ineffective airway clearance, potential for infection, anxiety, knowledge deficit,* and *ineffective individual and family coping.* They considered the following other possible diagnoses: *activity intolerance, self-care deficit: bathing and hygiene,* and *sleep pattern disturbance.*

During the first 24 hours, the nurses auscultated Joanne's lungs every 2 hours. Throughout Joanne's hospitalization, they checked her ABG levels to ensure adequate oxygenation, humidified the oxygen to keep her mucous membranes from drying out, and assessed her breathing patterns and her ability to clear airway secretions. They helped the respiratory therapist perform chest percussion, then recorded the color, odor, consistency, and amount of secretions and Joanne's treatment response.

The nurses positioned Joanne in high Fowler's position, and encouraged her to breathe slowly and deeply and to use pursed-lip breathing. They taught her an effective coughing technique: taking a few deep breaths, coughing three or four times until all inhaled air was expelled, and repeating this until her cough was productive. When they noticed that Joanne was having trouble using her metered-dose inhaler, they obtained a spacer device, which solved the problem.

To treat Joanne's dehydration, the nurses increased her fluid intake to at least 2,000 ml/day. They recorded intake and output every hour and also assessed her mucous membranes and skin turgor every shift to ensure adequate rehydration.

Because Joanne felt that stress exacerbated her asthma symptoms, the nurses taught her relaxation techniques and referred her to a stress management program. The hospital social worker set up a meeting with Joanne, her husband, and her mother to identify community services that could help Joanne's mother with cleaning, meals, and transportation.

Nursing management

Nursing care for the patient with acute asthma has three major aspects: assessment and interventions, patient teaching, and discharge planning.

Assessment and interventions

Patients with acute asthma need conscientious and continuous assessment to detect baseline changes, monitor response to treatment, and prevent complications.

Detect baseline changes. Evaluate the patient's respiratory status carefully. Auscultate the lungs for adventitious breath sounds and wheezing and for the quality of air movement, and check respiratory rate and depth. Developing or worsening tachypnea can mean worsening asthma. Review ABG levels, serum theophylline levels, and other laboratory test results. Monitor PaO_2, watching for sudden decreases below normal or below baseline. If PaO_2 does drop, observe for signs of hypoxemia: restlessness, confusion, and tachycardia. If $PaCO_2$ increases suddenly, watch for symptoms of hypercapnia: headache, somnolence, or mental status changes. Notify the doctor if you notice any of these symptoms. Also review the patient's chest X-ray and peak flow studies to learn more about his respiratory status.

To help the patient with *impaired gas exchange* and *ineffective breathing pattern* feel more comfortable, administer

Using a peak flow meter

A peak flow meter accurately measures peak expiratory flow, a valuable indicator of lung function. To use the peak flow meter, have the patient place the mouthpiece in his mouth, forming a tight seal with his lips. He should hold the meter in the vertical position so that the red indicator is at the bottom of the scale. Be sure his fingers don't block the opening.

Tell the patient to exhale as hard and fast as possible to move the red indicator up the scale. The final position of the indicator is the peak flow measurement. Record this value along with the date and time, then compare values to the average values provided with the instrument. Report results to the doctor, as ordered.

After use, slide the red indicator to the bottom of the scale, and remove the mouthpiece and rinse it.

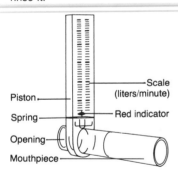

oxygen, use a hand-held nebulizer with a bronchodilator, and administer other prescribed respiratory treatments. Ease breathing by placing the patient in high Fowler's position, and support his arms on the overbed table to increase lung expansion. Teach pursed-lip breathing to ease breathlessness. Reducing the patient's hypoxia and breathlessness should help relieve anxiety.

Pulmonary function tests can determine the severity of gas exchange impairment and can point out any improvement or deterioration in the patient's condition. Explain to the patient that the doctor will also order peak flow measurements to help measure severity of airflow obstruction and response to treatment. (See *Using a peak flow meter.*)

Observe the patient carefully for wheezing, dyspnea, or abrupt decreases in peak flow, which can signal increased airflow obstruction. Document peak flow measurements, their closeness in time to bronchodilator treatments, and the patient's description of his symptoms.

Using oximetry to measure SaO_2 can also help evaluate the effectiveness of treatment. Be sure to explain the procedure to the patient before starting it. Oximetry can be performed by ear or by pulse. In ear oximetry, the earlobe is massaged with an alcohol sponge for 10 to 30 seconds, then a probe is attached. In pulse oximetry, the probe is attached to the patient's index finger. To prevent interference with the test, be sure the patient doesn't have long or false fingernails, and remove any nail polish.

For adults, set the default alarms at these settings: high saturation, 100%; low saturation, 85%; high pulse rate, 140 beats/minute; low pulse rate, 55 beats/minute. (Or individualize these guidelines according to the patient's pulse rate.) Remember: For patient safety, never turn the alarm off. Monitor SaO_2 readings, and document them in the patient's record. Watch for sudden drops in SaO_2, which can signal hypoxemia. If this occurs, the doctor will probably order additional ABG tests and increase the administration of oxygen. For adults, normal SaO_2 levels range between 95% and 100%, but they may be lower in elderly patients or those with chronic obstructive pulmonary disease. Once baseline readings are obtained, the doctor will order medications to halt the asthma attack and to correct the patient's *ineffective breathing pattern* and *impaired gas exchange.*

Monitor response to treatment. Check the patient frequently to see how well he's tolerating various drugs and how effective they are. Watch serum theophylline levels closely to be sure they're in the therapeutic range. Observe for signs of theophylline toxicity—nausea, vomiting, diarrhea, and headache—and for signs of subtherapeutic dosage—respiratory distress and increased wheezing. If the patient shows signs of overdose or underdose of this drug, notify the doctor so he can adjust the dosage.

Remember not to infuse I.V. aminophylline any faster than 25 mg/minute; otherwise, the patient may experience dizziness, faintness, light-headedness, palpitations, syncope, precordial pain, flushing, profound bradycardia, premature ventricular contractions, severe hypotension, or even cardiac arrest. When changing from I.V. aminophylline to oral theophylline, check the type of oral preparation being given to be sure the patient will continue receiving a therapeutic level. Wait 4 to 6 hours between discontinuing I.V. aminophylline and starting immediate-release oral theophylline, but give the first dose of slow-release theophylline immediately after stopping the I.V. drug.

Remember that certain drugs should be avoided in asthma patients. Sedatives and tranquilizers can be dangerous in asthma patients because they cause respiratory depression and disguise worsening airway obstruction. And, of course, don't give aspirin or aspirin compounds if the patient is hypersensitive to this drug.

Prevent complications. If the patient is taking systemic corticosteroids, observe for complications, such as psychosis and Cushing's syndrome. If the patient is taking steroids by metered-dose inhaler, watch for infections in the mouth and pharynx. Remember that steroids can mask infections, so be alert for signs of respiratory tract infection, such as a change in sputum color. Also check serum glucose levels and monitor urine for glucose and acetone, which can indicate hyperglycemia. When tapering steroid dosage for discontinuation, watch for signs and symptoms of acute adrenal insufficiency, such as fever, myalgia, arthralgia, and malaise. And remember not to give steroids on an empty stomach because they can irritate the GI tract.

To make the patient more comfortable, remove allergens and irritants from his room. Common irritants include strong-smelling cleaning fluids, flowers, fresh paint, cigarette smoke, and talcum powder. Also remove any known food allergens from his diet. These measures should help decrease bronchospasm and improve gas exchange.

Keep in mind that some patients develop a pneumothorax, which can further impair gas exchange. Signs and symptoms include sudden chest pain, restlessness, heightened respirations and pulse, decreased breath sounds, and hyperresonance when the affected side of the chest is percussed. A chest X-ray will confirm this diagnosis. If the pneumothorax is severe, the patient may need insertion of a needle or chest tube.

Before assessing the patient for other complications, check his vital signs, then compare them to his baseline. Monitor heart rate for tachycardia and other abnormalities that may signal worsening disease or medication toxicity. Also monitor blood pressure for pulsus paradoxus, indicating severe asthma, or hypertension, which may signal asthma-related hypoxia or complications such as pneumothorax.

Remember that during an acute asthma attack, patients may be too dyspneic to tolerate oral temperature taking, so you'll probably have to take the temperature rectally to establish a baseline. Temperature elevations suggest infection or dehydration and warrant further investigation for signs of *fluid volume deficit* and *potential for infection.*

Prevent dehydration. Patients with acute asthma are often too breathless, diaphoretic, and debilitated to drink much, so many develop a *fluid volume deficit.* Keeping these patients well hydrated can help them expectorate thick secretions and prevent mucus impaction, which can be fatal. Give the patient water if he can swallow without gasping, then insert an I.V. line for supplemental fluids and as an access for medication administration. Assess the patient often to determine his fluid needs, and replace fluids cautiously. Also monitor central venous pressure in elderly patients or those with cardiac problems.

Check the patient's oral mucosa and skin turgor for signs of dehydration, and monitor intake and output carefully, noting volume, specific gravity, color, and clarity of urine. *Fluid volume deficit* can affect heart rate and blood pressure, so take vital signs often. Dehydration also can lead to mental status changes, such as confusion and lethargy.

To treat *ineffective airway clearance,* observe for thick mucus or coughing up of mucus plugs, then auscultate the lungs, noting any adventitious or absent sounds. Watch how much and how severely the patient coughs, and note whether the cough is productive. If it isn't and rhonchi are present, teach effective coughing techniques. Also perform postural drainage and chest percussion to clear secretions if the patient can tolerate this. Intubated patients may need suctioning. Be sure to record the character of the sputum.

Keep the patient's room temperature comfortable and use an air conditioner in hot, humid weather. A humidifier will also help moisten secretions and clear the airway. If the airway obstruction doesn't improve with conservative treatment, the doctor may perform a bronchoscopy or bronchial lavage if the area of collapse is a lobe or larger.

Also, monitor the patient's *anxiety* level. Encourage him to express his fears and frustrations, offer reassurance, and offer relaxation techniques, such as massage; deep, pursed-lip breathing; and soothing music. Keep the patient's environment as quiet as possible, and provide privacy. Explain all procedures and medications, and encourage him to ask questions.

Patient teaching and discharge planning

To help reduce the number and severity of the patient's asthma attacks, focus on the patient's *knowledge deficit,* explaining the pathophysiology of asthma, factors that trigger attacks, drug treatment, correct use of metered-dose inhalers, prevention of future attacks, and guidelines for exercise. Include family members in your teaching sessions if possible. Knowing more about the disease may help patients feel less powerless and more in control.

Pathophysiology. Explain what asthma is and what occurs physiologically during an attack.

Asthma triggers. Discuss factors that commonly trigger attacks, such as allergens, exercise, cold air, and infection. Have the patient keep a diary to help him identify which factors trigger his asthma. (See *What triggers asthma?* page 282.)

Drug treatment. Describe prescribed drugs, including their names, dosages, actions, adverse effects, and special instructions. Warn the patient not to take any other prescription or over-the-counter drugs without first checking with the doctor. Emphasize that certain drugs can increase bronchospasm, sed-

---

What triggers asthma?

At home
• Foods such as nuts, chocolate, eggs, shellfish, and peanut butter
• Beverages such as orange juice, wine, beer, and milk
• Pollens from flowers, trees, grasses, hay, and ragweed; mold spores
• Animals such as rabbits, cats, dogs, hamsters, gerbils, and chickens
• Feather pillows, down comforters, and wool clothing
• Insect parts such as those from dead cockroaches
• Medicines such as aspirin and sulfite-containing perenteral adrenergic drugs used to treat status asthmaticus (ephedrine, epinephrine, isoetharine, isoproterenol)
• Vapors from cleaning solvents, paint, paint thinner, and chlorine bleach
• Sprays from furniture polish, starch, cleaners, and room deodorizers
• Spray deodorants, perfumes, hair sprays, talcum powder, and scented cosmetics
• Cloth-upholstered furniture, carpets, and draperies that gather dust
• Brooms and dusters that raise dust

• Dirty filters on hot air furnaces and air conditioners that put dust into the air

In the workplace
• Dusts, vapors, or fumes from wood products (western red cedar, some pine and birch woods, mahogany); flour, cereals, grains, coffee, tea, or papain; metals (platinum, chromium, nickel sulfate, soldering fumes); and cotton, flax, and hemp
• Mold from decaying hay

Outdoors
• Cold or hot air
• Excessive humidity or dryness
• Changes in seasons
• Smog
• Automobile exhaust

Any place
• Overexertion, which may cause wheezing
• Lying down, which allows mucus to collect in the airways
• Common cold, flu, and other viruses
• Fear, anger, frustration, laughing too hard, crying
• Smoke from cigarettes, cigars, and pipes whether inhaled directly or as second-hand smoke.

---

atives and tranquilizers can decrease respiration, and drugs containing epinephrine can cause cardiac adverse effects. (See *Patient teaching: Guidelines for using oral asthma medications.*)

Metered-dose inhalers. As many as 30% to 70% of asthma patients (most of them children and elderly patients) use these inhalers incorrectly, usually because of difficulty coordinating canister activation and inhalation. Placebo inhalers are available through drug companies for demonstration purposes. (See *How to use a metered-dose inhaler,* page 284.)

Guidelines for using oral asthma medications

For using theophylline
• To keep your blood concentration of theophylline at therapeutic levels, take theophylline on time and without missing doses.
• Know the signs of theophylline overdose and report them to your nurse or doctor immediately.
• Avoid excessive use of caffeine because it's chemically similar to theophylline and may increase any adverse effects.
• Take the drug with food, milk, or antacids to avoid GI irritation.

For using long-term steroids
• Wear a Medic Alert bracelet or necklace and carry a wallet card that identifies you as using steroid medications.
• Never stop taking steroids suddenly if you've been taking them a long time—taper them off gradually, exactly as your doctor recommended. Know the warning signs of acute adrenal crisis and report them immediately.

• Notify the doctor if you're under unusual physical stress (for example, if you're having oral surgery). He may decide to increase your dosage temporarily.
• Watch for potential adverse effects, including facial hair and puffiness.
• Be prepared to have mood swings while your dosage is being decreased. The well being and high energy you feel while on high doses may change to depression and listlessness.
• Take prednisone only once a day in the morning (unless your doctor directs otherwise) to reduce adverse effects and adrenal suppression. Some doctors prescribe steroids to be taken only every other day.
• Have regular eye examinations to detect cataracts or glaucoma, adverse effects of steroids. Inform your eye doctor that you're taking the drug.

Spacers or reservoir chambers attached to inhalers improve medication delivery to airways and make these devices easier to use for patients with poor hand-breath coordination. These devices help transport small droplets of medication to the airways and keep large droplets away from the oropharynx and major bronchi, where they are readily absorbed. Spacers also increase the effectiveness of steroid inhalers and decrease the incidence of oral candidiasis. Be sure to teach your patient how to clean his inhaler—it should be washed daily by removing the canister and washing the plastic case and cap with warm water. A new inhalation device called Ventolin Rotocaps provides a compact, breath-activated, propellant-free inhalation mode that facilitates bronchodilation therapy in patients who cannot use metered-dose inhalers effectively.

How to use a metered-dose inhaler

Before using the inhaler, insert the canister firmly and fully into the outer shell, and rotate it back and forth a few times. Shake the canister well, and then remove the mouthpiece cap.

Have the patient exhale fully until he can remove no more air from the lungs. Place the mouthpiece over his tongue and well into his mouth. Ask him to close his lips tightly around the mouthpiece, then press the top of the canister. For medication to completely penetrate the lungs (see illustration at left), the patient must inhale slowly and deeply, then hold his breath for 3 to 5 seconds. If he inhales quickly, for only 1 or 2 seconds, the medication may not reach the small airways (see illustration at right).

The patient can then release the pressure on the canister, remove the inhaler from his mouth, and exhale gently.

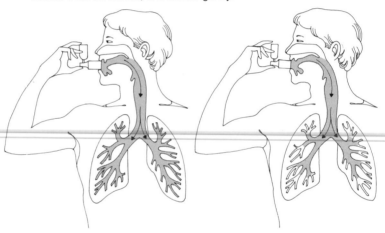

Complete penetration of the lungs   **Incomplete penetration of the lungs**

Patients using more than one inhaler need to know the correct order for use. Usually, beta-adrenergic bronchodilating agents are taken first to open airways and permit other medications to reach the lungs more effectively. Ipratropium bromide is usually taken second because it takes longer to act. Steroids and cromolyn sodium are taken last. Tell the patient to wait at least 5 minutes between inhalations. Also warn him against overusing beta-adrenergic inhalers, which can cause cardiac dysrhythmias and other adverse effects.

Prevention. To avert an acute asthma attack, give your patient this information:

• Know the signs of a respiratory tract infection, and notify the doctor immediately if one occurs so that antibiotic treatment can begin promptly.

• Ask the doctor about getting influenza and Pneumovax vaccines.

• Try to eliminate allergens and irritants from your environment. Avoid known allergens, such as animals, and use home furnishings made of allergen-free material or enclosed in allergen-proof covers, especially in your bedroom.

• Avoid exposure to irritants and volatile substances, such as chemicals, paint, perfume, and aerosols.

• Eliminate known allergens from your diet. Common allergens are peanuts; dyes in drugs and foods, such as tartrazine (Yellow Dye #5 and E102); monosodium glutamate; and preservative sulfites (sulfur dioxide, sodium or potassium bisulfate, and metabisulfite), which are often added to food in salad bars, to commercially prepared food, and to wine, beer, and seafood.

• Avoid exposure to cigarette smoke. Smoking or breathing second-hand smoke irritates airways and worsens respiratory symptoms besides increasing the risk of emphysema and lung cancer. If you smoke, a smoking cessation program, such as the one offered by the American Lung Association, can help you quit.

• Know how to use and clean any special equipment, such as a hand-held nebulizer or peak flow meter. A flow meter helps in measuring the amount of airway obstruction. Keep a record of peak flow readings and bring it to your medical appointments. Notify the doctor promptly if your peak flow drops suddenly—this can signal severe respiratory problems before other symptoms occur.

• Drink six to eight glasses of water daily to prevent dehydration, unless you must limit fluid intake because of cardiac disease or another medical problem requiring fluid restriction.

• Practice relaxation techniques, such as meditation, Jacobson's progressive relaxation techniques (alternately tensing and relaxing muscles), or listening to music or relaxation tapes. Or attend a stress management or relaxation program. Avoid unhealthy ways of coping with stress, such as smoking or drinking excessive alcohol. (See *Patient-teaching checklist: Asthma*.)

▶ **PATIENT-TEACHING CHECKLIST**

Asthma

Discuss the following points with your patient:

☐ How asthma causes bronchospasm, airway edema, and mucus production
☐ Complications such as status asthmaticus
☐ Asthma triggers
☐ Results of arterial blood gas analysis, pulmonary function tests, and other diagnostic studies
☐ Importance of allergy-free diet and adequate hydration
☐ Drugs and their administration
☐ How to use an inhaler and peak flow meter
☐ How to control an asthma attack
☐ When to call the doctor
☐ Warning signs and prevention of respiratory infection
☐ Medications to avoid, such as aspirin
☐ Eliminating allergens and irritants from environment
☐ Effective coughing techniques.
☐ Percussion and postural drainage
☐ Exercise guidelines
☐ Breathing exercises
☐ Energy conservation techniques
☐ Preferred relaxation and stress management techniques
☐ Availability of support groups, such as the American Lung Association

Activity and exercise guidelines. Asthma patients should be encouraged to exercise, but they need guidelines. The doctor or physical therapist will probably outline a home program of aerobic exercise, such as swimming, walking, or bicycling. Guidelines should include discussion of sexual activity because it may cause asthma symptoms. The doctor will discuss various ways to prevent bronchospasm during exercise or sexual activity—for example, by taking a beta-adrenergic or cromolyn sodium inhalant.

Asthma patients should also learn how to conserve energy. For example, they should sit while doing as many activities as possible because sitting expends less energy than standing.

Case study: Part 5

After 4 days in the hospital, Joanne's condition had noticeably improved. Her lungs were clear, she wasn't wheezing, and her pulmonary function tests and ABG levels were normal. She was also becoming much more knowledgeable about her disease, thanks to the nurses, who had emphasized prevention and prompt intervention in their teaching. Joanne also seemed much less anxious after the meeting with her husband and mother, and said that she didn't feel so burdened with her mother's care.

On her fifth day of hospitalization, the doctor discharged Joanne with prescriptions for the following medications: 300 mg of theophylline twice a day; 15 mg of prednisone every day, with orders to taper the dosage; two puffs of beclomethasone four times a day; 0.25 ml isoetharine hydrochloride and 1 ampule cromolyn sodium via hand-held nebulizer four times a day. She was to return in 1 week for a follow-up examination.

Joanne visited the medical unit several months later. She looked well and reported that she'd been following the suggestions made by her nurses during their teaching sessions. Although she'd had two colds since her discharge, she had avoided hospitalization. She'd also decreased the irritants and allergens in her environment by hiring a cleaning service for herself and her mother and by having her desk moved to a nonsmoking area at work. Joanne said that she now felt more in control of her asthma and her life.

CHAPTER 8

Mechanical ventilation

Once used exclusively in intensive care settings, mechanical ventilators are now common in other hospital settings as well. As hospital care focuses ever more sharply on acute illness, staff nurses are increasingly likely to include management of mechanically ventilated patients among their routine responsibilities.

Managing ventilator-dependent patients safely requires a thorough understanding of the physiologic mechanisms of respiration, the various functions of mechanical ventilators, their effects on other vital functions (especially on perfusion), and their potential for causing complications. It also requires the ability to recognize and deal with ventilator malfunction, to provide adequate ventilation while preserving the patient's ability to resume spontaneous breathing, and to provide the complex supportive care these patients need.

Mechanical ventilation supports respiration automatically by expanding the chest and delivering oxygenated gas to the lungs for patients who cannot maintain physiologic levels of oxygen and carbon dioxide by breathing spontaneously. Indications for mechanical ventilation include apnea, acute ventilatory failure, and impending acute ventilatory failure. The latter may result from interruption of the normal regulatory mechanism of respiration, paralysis of respiratory muscles, restriction of chest wall movement, or impaired gas exchange. (See *Understanding ventilation,* page 289.) In patients with such impairments, mechanical ventilation can supply adequate ventilation and oxygenation, reduce dyspnea, and promote rest and reconditioning of fatigued ventilatory muscles.

Negative-pressure ventilator

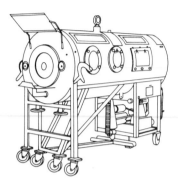

Pressure-cycled ventilator

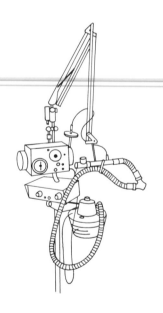

Types of ventilators

Various kinds of ventilators are available. They are classified according to their cycling mechanism: negative-pressure ventilators, pressure-cycled ventilators, and volume-cycled ventilators. A fourth type, the high-frequency ventilator, is investigational; it can be used as a high-frequency positive-pressure, high-frequency jet, or high-frequency oscillation ventilator.

Negative-pressure ventilators

Once commonly used for polio victims, negative-pressure ventilators generate alternating or intermittent negative pressure by removing air from inside a closed container. They can encompass the entire body (like the iron lung) or just the upper torso and anterior chest (like the cuirass). Negative-pressure ventilators mimic the normal changes in pressure gradients by causing thoracic expansion that creates negative pressure within the lungs. The positive atmospheric pressure then flows into the lungs. Negative-pressure ventilators do not require an artificial airway. (See *Negative-pressure ventilator.*)

Negative-pressure ventilators are noisy and restrictive and have other important disadvantages. By restricting access to the patient's body, they make nursing care difficult. They usually involve a risk of hypovolemic shock because negative pressure applied to the abdomen causes venous pooling in abdominal blood vessels; in turn, this decreases venous return and cardiac output. With the chest type of negative-pressure ventilator, a tight, effective seal is difficult to maintain.

Pressure-cycled ventilators

These commonly used ventilators terminate inspiration at a preset pressure of gas, which then allows passive expiration to take place; the preset pressure is reached independently of volume or time. Pressure-cycled ventilators include the Bennett PR-2 and the Bird Mark 7. (See *Pressure-cycled ventilator.*)

Pressure-cycled ventilators have the disadvantage of delivering varying amounts of tidal volume over varying time intervals because pressure within the lungs depends on lung compliance or airway resistance. Therefore, they deliver small tidal volumes to patients with stiff lungs, mucus plugs, or bronchospasm and

Understanding ventilation

Ventilation is the process that moves a mixture of gases into and out of the pulmonary system to allow gas exchange (respiration) within the respiratory units (the alveoli and their surrounding capillaries). Ventilation requires normal alveolar function and structure, adequate pulmonary perfusion, and a flow of gases. It occurs in two phases—inspiration and expiration—which are controlled by three mechanisms: chemical stimulation, changes in pressure gradients, and neurologic regulators.

Chemical stimulation

Central chemoreceptors located in the anterior medulla monitor ventilatory status by responding to changes in carbon dioxide (CO_2), oxygen (O_2), and pH. These chemoreceptors, which are particularly sensitive to changes in $Paco_2$ and acid-base balance, stimulate the respiratory centers to increase respiratory rate and depth when they detect a rise in hydrogen ion levels. When expiration of CO_2 lowers carbonic acid levels, diminished stimulation of chemoreceptors decreases respiratory rate and depth. If blood levels of CO_2 fall below normal, these chemoreceptors induce apnea until cellular metabolism produces sufficient CO_2 to stimulate the respiratory centers, which again trigger breathing.

Peripheral chemoreceptors, located in the aortic and carotid bodies, primarily monitor the blood O_2 level. Diminishing O_2 concentration in the blood also diminishes the O_2 content of interstitial fluid around the peripheral chemoreceptors; in response to decreasing O_2 levels, the peripheral receptors stimulate the respiratory centers to increase the rate or depth of respiration and thereby increase the amount of available O_2.

Changes in pressure gradients

In spontaneous breathing, gas flow follows changes in intra-alveolar pressure. Contraction of the inspiratory muscles—the diaphragm and intercostals—causes expansion of the chest cavity. This expansion generates a negative intrapulmonary pressure with respect to the atmosphere and causes gases to flow from the atmosphere into the lungs. Stretch receptors located in the bronchial and bronchiolar smooth muscle and in smooth muscle around the trachea react to rising pressure within the lungs by inhibiting further inspiration to prevent overdistention of the lungs. This reflex, known as the Hering-Breuer reflex, inhibits afferent impulses in the inspiratory center, interrupting respiratory muscle contraction. As the inspiratory muscles relax, normal elastic recoil returns the lung to its normal volume or size. This contraction of the chest cavity creates a positive intrapulmonary pressure and causes passive expiration of gases.

Inspiration usually takes up to a third of the respiratory cycle with a 1:2 ratio of inspiration to expiration.

Neurologic regulators

These regulators for the mechanical aspects of breathing are located in the medulla oblongata and the pons. In the medulla, neurons associated with inspiration and expiration apparently interact to regulate the respiratory rate and depth. They react to impulses from other areas, particularly the pons. In the pons, two neuron groups, or centers, regulate respiratory rhythm by interacting with the medullary respiratory center to smooth the transitions from inspiration to expiration and back. The apneustic center of the pons stimulates inspiratory neurons in the medulla to initiate inspiration. In turn, these inspiratory neurons stimulate the pneumotaxic center of the pons to initiate expiration. They do this in two ways: by inhibiting the apneustic center and by stimulating the expiratory neurons in the medulla. Thus, the pons, as pacemaker, regulates rhythm and the medulla regulates rate and depth.

Conscious control of breathing through nerve impulses from the motor areas of the cerebral cortex can override the involuntary respiratory centers. This permits voluntary breath control for such activities as speaking, singing, and swimming. This conscious control is limited, however, and the respiratory centers can override cortical impulses to meet ventilatory needs.

Volume-cycled ventilator

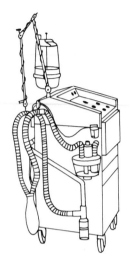

High-frequency ventilator

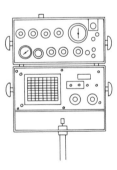

larger tidal volumes to patients with normal lungs, resulting in an increased risk of barotrauma. Pressure-cycled ventilators are used mainly for short-term support, such as during recovery from drug overdose.

Volume-cycled ventilators

Volume-cycled ventilators, which include the MA-1 and the Bear 2, terminate inspiration at a preset volume of gas and allow passive expiration to occur. They deliver the preset volume regardless of the pressure needed to deliver it. (See *Volume-cycled ventilator.*)

Volume-cycled ventilators are equipped with different settings, modes, and special adjuncts to mechanical ventilation therapy to meet the patient's needs. Such ventilators can set the tidal volume, respiratory rate, and inspiratory-expiratory (I:E) ratio, and can set a larger tidal volume (sigh) intermittently, usually one to three times per minute. Sigh is used to reexpand alveoli and prevent atelectasis. Sigh is usually not used when the patient is on positive end-expiratory pressure (PEEP), to avoid excessively high pressures. (See *Understanding airway pressures.*)

Volume-cycled ventilators offer the following adjustments:
• Inspiratory time can be adjusted by adjusting the flow rate of the delivered gas.
• Oxygen concentration, determined as the fraction of inspired oxygen (FIO_2), can be selected in concentrations from 21% (room air) to 100% to provide the amount of oxygen necessary to maintain an adequate partial pressure of oxygen in arterial blood (PaO_2).
• Modes available include continuous or controlled mandatory ventilation, assist-control ventilation, intermittent mandatory ventilation, and synchronized intermittent mandatory ventilation.
• Adjuncts include continuous positive airway pressure (CPAP) and PEEP.

Volume-cycled ventilators are now the most commonly used because they offer distinct advantages of safety and versatility. For example, they are equipped with several alarms, including a pressure limit alarm that is activated by high peak airway pressures, thus helping to prevent lung damage from high pressures. A pop-off safety valve relieves excessively high pressures. Volume-cycled ventilators can deliver adequate tidal volumes to most intubated patients when an increase in airway pressure or lung compliance increases airway resistance. This makes these ventilators useful for patients with acute chest disease or surgical intervention.

High-frequency ventilators

High-frequency ventilators (HFVs), using high ventilatory rates (usually four times greater than the patient's normal respiratory rate) and small tidal volumes (less than or equal to the patient's dead space volume), are used to ventilate the alveoli with less risk of barotrauma and cardiovascular changes. The three types of HFVs include high-frequency positive-pressure ventilator (HFPPV), high-frequency jet ventilator (HFJV), and high-frequency oscillation. (See *High-frequency ventilator.*)

HFPPV. This type of ventilator generates a breath when a volume of compressed gas is delivered via a pneumatic valve. An angled side arm directs most of the gas to the patient during active inspiration. Expiration is passive. The patient receives the same FIO_2 as the compressed gas. HFPPV is the oldest type of HFV and has largely been replaced by the technologically more advanced form, HFJV.

HFJV. This type of ventilator delivers the gas through an extra lumen of an endotracheal tube or a transtracheal cannula. The gas, compressed under 10 to 50 psi, travels through a fluidic-controlled ventilator with a flow interrupter and an electric timer. Small pulsed jets of gas enter the airway at high respiratory rates (100 to 1,000 breaths/minute) and at low tidal volumes (100 to 300 ml). As the jet stream is propelled into the tube, entrained gases are propelled down the trachea. Expiration is passive and the percentage of inspiratory time equals 30%. With HFJV, the patient may also be on a volume-cycled ventilator with CPAP. This ventilation pattern keeps airway pressures low and produces only minimal alveolar distention, thus increasing functional residual capacity (FRC), stabilizing alveolar ventilation, and improving arterial oxygen tension. Because the tidal volume

Understanding airway pressures

An understanding of airway pressures is important to understand ventilator settings.

Peak airway pressure is the maximum pressure in the airways required to deliver the tidal volume (Vt). Peak pressure is the highest pressure noted on the airway pressure gauge at the end of inspiration. Peak airway pressure represents the lungs' resistance to expansion in relation to the Vt or dynamic compliance.

Dynamic compliance is calculated by:

$$\frac{Vt}{peak\ airway\ pressure}$$

Static airway pressure measures the inspiratory pressure that persists after airflow has stopped but before the breath is exhaled or escapes. Measure static airway pressure or compliance at the end of the respiratory cycle by occluding the expiratory line or activating inflation hold. The airway pressure gauge will give peak airway pressure; read static pressure as the pressure falls and stabilizes (zero movement of air). An accurate reading requires the patient to be relaxed and not actively inspiring. It also requires an airtight system.

Static compliance is calculated by:

$$\frac{Vt}{static\ airway\ pressure}$$

Increased peak airway pressure occurs with stable static pressure in patients with mucus plugs or bronchospasm; and with increased static airway pressure in those with tension pneumothorax, atelectasis, pulmonary edema, or pneumonia.

combines entrained gases and jet flow, the exact tidal volume and FIO_2 are difficult to calculate. The cascade humidifier of the volume ventilator and an infusion of normal saline solution into a portion of the endotracheal tube humidifies the delivered gases.

High-frequency oscillation. This pattern provides a continuous to-and-fro movement of gas rather than intermittent delivered volume. The rate is delivered in cycles per minute ranging from 180 to 2,400 cycles/minute. This type of high-frequency ventilator is suitable mainly for patients with severe respiratory distress syndrome (RDS) because of the limited tidal volume it displaces.

Modes of ventilation

The mode of mechanical ventilation is the mechanism that ends expiration and signals the mechanical ventilator to initiate inspiration. Modes of ventilation used with the volume-cycled ventilator include continuous mandatory ventilation (CMV), assist-control ventilation (ACV), intermittent mandatory ventilation (IMV), synchronized intermittent mandatory ventilation (SIMV), and pressure support ventilation (PSV). Modes are selected according to their specific advantages and disadvantages with respect to the patient's respiratory need and underlying pathophysiology. (See *Modes and adjuncts of ventilation,* pages 294 and 295.)

Continuous mandatory ventilation

CMV delivers a preset tidal volume at a preset rate regardless of the patient's inspiratory effort. In this mode, the patient cannot take a spontaneous breath. CMV is commonly used in patients with apnea secondary to central nervous system or neuromuscular dysfunction (such as nerve damage or paralysis, severe brain trauma, Guillain-Barré syndrome, spinal cord injury, and poliomyelitis), drug overdose, or status asthmaticus. Because CMV does not allow the patient to breathe spontaneously, its use in semiconscious or alert patients may cause anxiety, agitation, and a tendency to "fight" the ventilator. Such patients may need sedation or neuromuscular blocking agents.

CMV offers the advantage of decreasing the patient's work of breathing, consuming less oxygen, and producing less carbon dioxide. It has two important disadvantages, however: It does not allow activation of normal ventilatory compensatory mechanisms in response to increasing carbon dioxide levels, and its passive use of the patient's respiratory muscles risks muscle atrophy and increases the need for muscle reconditioning during weaning. CMV also has undesirable cardiovascular effects: decreased venous return and reduced cardiac output related to alkalemia and increased intrathoracic pressure.

Assist-control ventilation

ACV augments spontaneous ventilation in patients with normal respiratory drive but weak respiratory musculature. In this mode, a decrease in pressure (usually -1 cm H_2O) triggers the ventilator to begin inspiration and to instill the preset tidal volume. If the patient becomes apneic, the ventilator takes over and controls ventilation at a preset rate. The ventilator can be set to varying levels of sensitivity; that is, it can respond to varying levels of negative pressure, allowing greater or lesser work of breathing. For example, at a highly sensitive setting, little patient effort is required to trigger a ventilator-assisted breath.

Because ACV allows the patient to initiate respirations, it doesn't risk the loss of respiratory muscle tone needed for successful weaning. ACV also allows the patient to increase his respiratory rate in compensatory response to rising carbon dioxide levels. Its cardiovascular effects are the same as those of CMV.

Intermittent mandatory ventilation

IMV provides a positive-pressure breath at a preset volume and rate independent of patient effort; concurrently, the patient can breathe spontaneously while the ventilator delivers humidified, oxygenated air from a separate circuit. With IMV, the patient does part of the work of breathing.

IMV requires a preset ventilatory rate, tidal volume, and time intervals. The tidal volume is between 10 to 15 ml/kg of the patient's ideal body weight. The rate is usually the lowest necessary to maintain normal arterial blood gas (ABG) values and pH while allowing the patient to perform part of the work

Modes and adjuncts of ventilation

The mode of mechanical ventilation is the mechanism that ends expiration and signals the mechanical ventilator to initiate inspiration. Modes of ventilation include continuous mandatory ventilation (CMV), assist-control ventilation (ACV), intermittent mandatory ventilation (IMV), synchronized intermittent mandatory ventilation (SIMV), and pressure support ventilation (PSV). Modes are selected according to their specific advantages and disadvantages with respect to the patient's respiratory needs and underlying pathophysiology.

Two adjuncts to assisted ventilation, positive end-expiratory pressure (PEEP) and continuous positive airway pressure (CPAP), are used to supplement mechanical ventilation, increasing functional residual capacity (FRC) and improving gas exchange.

Mode or adjunct	Advantages	Disadvantages
CMV Delivers tidal volume at a preset rate regardless of patient's inspiratory effort. Commonly used in patients with apnea secondary to central nervous system or neuromuscular dysfunction (nerve damage or paralysis, severe brain trauma, Guillain-Barré syndrome, spinal cord injury, and poliomyelitis), or drug overdose.	• Decreases patient's work of breathing, consumes less oxygen (O_2) and produces less carbon dioxide (CO_2)	• Prevents activation of normal ventilatory compensation mechanisms in response to increased CO_2 levels, risks respiratory muscle atrophy, and increases need for muscle reconditioning during weaning • Reduces venous return and reduces cardiac output related to alkalemia and increased intrathoracic pressure
ACV Augments spontaneous ventilation in patients with normal respiratory drive but weak respiratory musculature.	• No loss of respiratory muscle tone needed for successful weaning • Allows increased respiratory rate to compensate for rising CO_2 levels	• Cardiovascular effects same as those with CMV
IMV Provides positive-pressure breath at a preset volume and rate independent of patient effort; also allows patient to breathe spontaneously while ventilator delivers humidified, oxygenated air from separate circuit.	• Allows delivery of all inspired gases at same temperature, humidity, and O_2 concentration (ventilator or spontaneous breath) • Produces less negative effect on cardiac output secondary to lower mean airway pressures; when used with PEEP, produces lower incidence of barotrauma than CMV with PEEP • Causes less anxiety and agitation, requiring less use of sedatives, narcotics, and muscle relaxants • Allows increased respiratory rate to compensate for rising CO_2 levels	• Contraindicated in patients whose ventilatory drive suddenly changes or is impaired (as in apnea) • Contraindicated in patients whose work of breathing and O_2 consumption must be kept to a minimum
SIMV Type of IMV; synchronizes mandatory machine-delivered breath with patient's next spontaneous breath.	• Same advantages as IMV, but synchronized breathing more efficient	• Delayed cycling of ventilator-assisted breaths, which increases work of breathing
PSV Investigational; provides positive pressure only in response to a spontaneous breath so rate of delivery (times/minute) is determined by patient.	• Can be combined with SIMV, PEEP, or CPAP • Reduces work of breathing and maintains respiratory muscle function while reducing muscle fatigue • Provides more patient comfort, less anxiety, and decreased dyspnea	• Risks barotrauma, especially if used with PEEP or CPAP; resulting high intrathoracic pressures may have adverse hemodynamic effects

Modes and adjuncts of ventilation (continued)

Mode or adjunct	Advantages	Disadvantages
PEEP An expiratory maneuver that limits unimpeded expiratory flow at a preset level of system pressure. Useful in patients with acute diffuse restrictive lung disease and hypoxemic respiratory failure refractory to mechanically delivered O_2 alone. Occasionally used to increase intrapulmonary pressure in patients with intrathoracic bleeding.	• Decreases work of breathing needed to reexpand collapsed alveoli during inspiration (alveolar recruitment) • Maintains airway pressure in lungs that increases FRC, reexpands collapsed alveoli, and keeps them open • Improves arterial oxygenation and decreases intrapulmonary physiologic shunting • Can be used with IMV	• Risk of barotrauma greater when PEEP levels exceed 20 cm H_2O; less when PEEP is used with IMV rather than CMV or ACV • Contraindicated in patients with untreated hypovolemia secondary to hemorrhage, dehydration, or neurogenic causes (anaphylactoid or septic shock); in patients with drug-induced decrease of cardiac output; and in those with compromised circulation • Also contraindicated in patients with chronic obstructive pulmonary disease with hypoxemia, pulmonary hyperinflation, and elevated FRC with decreased or normal compliance • High-level PEEP contraindicated in patients with increased ICP
CPAP Increases oxygenation by increasing FRC and lung compliance. Essentially PEEP in a spontaneously breathing patient, except that it maintains positive airway pressure throughout respiratory cycle, not just on expiration. Useful for oxygenation failure or for weaning from ventilator. Often used with PEEP.	• Can be used in patients with pulmonary surfactant deficiency (such as those with adult respiratory distress syndrome, smoke inhalation, toxic lung damage, or neonatal respiratory distress syndrome) • Can be used cautiously with PSV	• Applied through endotracheal, nasotracheal, or tracheostomy tube, or through tight-fitting face mask, which interferes with mouth, upper airway, and skin care; tolerated for 12 to 36 hours • With intubation, increased risk of respiratory muscle fatigue and failure of weaning

of breathing. The IMV rate should be adjusted by changes in the pH. The IMV rate may also be increased when the spontaneous respiratory rate rises above 25 breaths/minute or if tidal volume falls to less than twice the patient's anatomic dead space or to 250 ml.

With IMV, peak inspiratory pressure limits should be set between 10 to 15 cm H_2O above the peak inspiratory pressure. A high-pressure relief valve eliminates the risk of stacked breaths (a ventilator breath superimposed on a spontaneous breath).

IMV offers several advantages. It allows delivery of all inspired gases at the same temperature, humidity, and oxygen concentration (ventilator or spontaneous breath). It also has less negative effect on cardiac output secondary to the lower mean airway pressures and, when used with PEEP, produces a lower incidence of barotrauma than CMV with PEEP. Moreover, because IMV allows the patient to control his own respirations, it causes less anxiety and agitation and therefore requires less use of sedatives, narcotics, and muscle relaxants. This system also allows the patient to increase his respiratory rate in compensatory response to rising carbon dioxide levels. The continued active use of his diaphragm and respiratory muscles helps prevent weakening or atrophy of these muscles.

IMV is contraindicated in patients whose ventilatory drive suddenly changes or is impaired (patients at risk for apneic episodes either during sleep or as a response to medication). It should also be avoided in patients whose work of breathing and oxygen consumption must be kept to a minimum.

Synchronized intermittent mandatory ventilation

A variation of IMV, SIMV synchronizes a mandatory machine-delivered breath with the patient's next spontaneous breath. A preset timing sequence is established to set the rate for the machine-delivered breath. The positive-pressure breaths are then triggered by the patient's inspiratory effort or the generation of a negative inspiratory pressure at preset intervals. If the spontaneous breath does not occur within the preset time, the ventilator automatically delivers a breath and then returns to the cycle of sensitivity to the patient-initiated breath.

SIMV offers the same advantages as IMV, but the synchronized breathing is more efficient. Its disadvantage is the delayed cycling of the ventilator-assisted breaths, which increases the work of breathing.

Pressure support ventilation

PSV is a new, investigational mode of mechanical ventilation that provides pressure in response to a spontaneous breath. With a spontaneous breath, the airway pressure rises to a preset level, holding at that level until the ventilator senses a drop occurring in the inspiratory flow rate. Only the newest ventilators can sense the minute changes in airway pressure that signal the need for pressure support.

Because PSV supplies pressure only when it senses inspiratory effort, the rate of delivery (times per minute) is determined entirely by the patient. It cannot be used if the patient is receiving ACV or CMV, which deliver a predetermined tidal volume with each breath. PSV supplies pressure support only when the patient takes a spontaneous breath and delivers no predetermined tidal volume. Of course, very high-pressure support (more than 10 cm H_2O) will affect the tidal volume.

To benefit from PSV, the patient cannot be apneic and must have an adequate respiratory drive. With this system, the patient's failure to take a spontaneous breath will result in apnea unless the ventilator has a built-in backup mode. For example, the Puritan-Bennett 7200 moves automatically into a "fail-to-cycle" alarm and provides ventilation if the patient fails to breathe. Other ventilators sound an alarm without providing mandatory ventilation.

PSV can be combined with SIMV or CPAP. SIMV is especially helpful if the patient cannot provide the required minute ventilation. When SIMV is combined with PSV, the required minute ventilation can be supplied, and any extra breaths that the patient takes can receive some limited flow support from the ventilator.

PSV reduces the work of breathing and maintains respiratory muscle function while reducing muscle fatigue. It usually provides more comfort, less anxiety, and decreased dyspnea.

A potential complication of PSV is barotrauma, especially if PSV is used with CPAP; if so, the preset pressure of PSV is added to that set for CPAP. Such high intrathoracic pressures may have adverse hemodynamic effects.

Adjuncts to assisted ventilation
Adjuncts to assisted ventilation include PEEP and CPAP.

Positive end-expiratory pressure
PEEP is an expiratory maneuver that limits unimpeded expiratory flow at a preset level of system pressure. It maintains an airway pressure within the lungs that increases FRC and reexpands collapsed alveoli and keeps them open, thus increasing

the number available for ventilation; it also improves arterial oxygenation and decreases intrapulmonary physiologic shunting. PEEP decreases the work of breathing needed to reexpand collapsed alveoli during inspiration (commonly called alveolar recruitment). PEEP levels should be increased or decreased in increments of 3 to 5 cm H_2O until the patient achieves a PaO_2 of 60 to 70 mm Hg and an FIO_2 of 0.5 or less without significant reduction of cardiac output. PEEP levels commonly range from 5 to 10 cm H_2O, but pressures as high as 40 cm H_2O can be used with the IMV ventilators. (See *Visualizing the alveolar effects of PEEP and CPAP.*)

Continuous positive airway pressure

CPAP increases oxygenation by increasing FRC and lung compliance. CPAP is essentially PEEP in a spontaneously breathing patient except that it maintains positive airway pressure throughout the entire respiratory cycle, not just during expiration. Because the patient is breathing spontaneously, he supplies the work of breathing at all times. CPAP decreases the negative effect of PEEP on venous return by generating negative pressure to trigger the inspiration of air in spontaneous ventilation (negative pressure is the stimulus for inspiration, the inflow of air into the pulmonary tree).

CPAP is useful for patients with oxygenation failure or as a means of weaning. It is indicated for the awake and alert patient who can maintain the work of breathing. Such a patient should have a current PEEP below 12 cm H_2O; a good tidal volume, vital capacity, and inspiratory force; a respiratory rate below 24 breaths/minute; a low to normal partial pressure of carbon dioxide in arterial blood ($PaCO_2$); and a normal pH.

CPAP is applied with a continuous flow system or a demand flow system through the ventilator circuitry with an endotracheal, nasotracheal, or tracheostomy tube or through a continuous flow, tight-fitting face mask. A nasogastric tube is usually inserted when a face mask is used to decrease the risk of gastric dilation, vomiting, and aspiration.

Patients usually tolerate CPAP for 12 to 36 hours; if it has been successful, they are then extubated. If it is unsuccessful,

Visualizing the alveolar effects of PEEP and CPAP

NORMAL ALVEOLUS
Functional residual capacity
(FRC) provides volume that
keeps the alveolus open for gas
exchange.

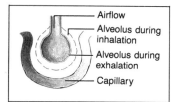

— Airflow
— Alveolus during
  inhalation
— Alveolus during
  exhalation
— Capillary

**ALVEOLUS WITH DECREASED
FUNCTIONAL RESIDUAL
CAPACITY**
Note that less area is available
for gas exchange, and the color
of blood in the capillary is
darker, indicating a lower PaO_2.

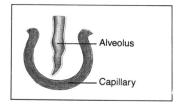

— Alveolus

— Capillary

**ALVEOLUS WITH RESTORED
FUNCTIONAL RESIDUAL
CAPACITY**
The problem of diminished FRC
has been resolved, using posi-
tive end-expiratory pressure
(PEEP) or continuous positive
airway pressure (CPAP).

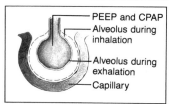

— PEEP and CPAP
— Alveolus during
  inhalation
— Alveolus during
  exhalation
— Capillary

they are intubated and returned to positive-pressure ventilation.
An important limitation of mask CPAP is the need for a mask,
which interferes with mouth, upper airway, and skin care. In
patients who are intubated on CPAP, the additional work of
breathing through a small airway may cause respiratory muscle
fatigue and failure of weaning.

   Indications for PEEP and CPAP. PEEP is helpful for patients
with acute diffuse restrictive lung disease or hypoxemic respiratory failure that is unresponsive to mechanically delivered oxygen alone. If the patient can ventilate adequately but has
ineffective oxygenation because of decreased FRC, CPAP is in-

Levels of PEEP

The following terms are used to describe the level of positive end-expiratory pressure (PEEP) to be used.
• Optimum PEEP is the level of PEEP achieving the lowest physiologic intrapulmonary shunting without a physiologically significant decrease in cardiac output.
• Optimal PEEP is the level that provides maximum oxygen delivery and the lowest ratio of dead space to tidal volume.
• Appropriate PEEP is the level that produces the least dead-space ventilation.

dicated. Refractory hypoxemia (adequate ventilation with normal $PaCO_2$ but low PaO_2) occurs in patients whose compromised FRC results from such problems as atelectasis (especially postoperatively), secretions that occlude the airway, and fluid that may fill alveoli and cause pulmonary edema. PEEP can also be used in patients with pulmonary surfactant deficiency (those with adult respiratory distress syndrome, smoke inhalation, toxic lung damage, and neonatal RDS). In patients with surfactant deficiency, PEEP and CPAP can prevent the collapse of alveoli until adequate levels of surfactant are produced. Occasionally, PEEP is used to increase intrapulmonary pressure in patients with intrathoracic bleeding. Increased pressure helps control bleeding by reducing venous return; however, this effect on venous return may require fluid therapy to prevent hypovolemic shock.

In some patients with pulmonary edema, PEEP and CPAP can help decrease the alveolar fluid–volume ratio. Expanding the size of alveoli while the amount of fluid remains the same increases the area available for gas exchange. Some clinicians believe that positive pressure in the alveoli helps push fluid back into alveolar capillaries. (See *Levels of PEEP*.)

Complications of PEEP. Decreased cardiac output results from decreased venous return effected by high intrathoracic pressures. Correcting it may require administration of fluids and, rarely, of inotropic or pressor agents. Insertion of a flow-directed balloon-tipped pulmonary artery catheter can facilitate monitoring of fluid status. Such monitoring is important to monitor for fluid overload and accumulation of fluid in the lungs.

Pulmonary barotrauma, the result of increased intrapulmonary pressure, may cause pneumothorax or subcutaneous emphysema. The risk of barotrauma increases when PEEP levels exceed 20 cm H_2O and decreases when PEEP is used with IMV rather than CMV or ACV. Barotrauma requires insertion of a chest tube.

Contraindications. PEEP is contraindicated in patients with untreated hypovolemia secondary to hemorrhage, dehydration, or neurogenic causes (such as anaphylactic or septic shock); those with a drug-induced decrease in cardiac output; and those with compromised circulation. High-level PEEP is contraindicated in patients with increased intracranial pressure (ICP) because it raises central venous pressures, thereby raising ICP. Using PEEP in such patients requires close monitoring of carbon dioxide and ICP levels.

PEEP is also contraindicated in chronic obstructive pulmonary disease patients with hypoxemia, pulmonary hyperinflation, and elevated FRC with decreased or normal compliance. The elevated FRC in overinflated areas leads to vascular compression and increased shunting, venous admixture, and hypoxemia. However, if diminished FRC occurs after intubation, low-level PEEP may be helpful.

Unilateral lung disease is a relative contraindication for PEEP, which would further alter distribution of the blood and ventilation. PEEP can be used cautiously in patients with bronchopulmonary fistula and recent lung surgery if a chest tube is inserted.

Complications of mechanical ventilation

Airway pressure therapy with mechanical ventilation has profound and widespread physiologic effects with great potential for complications and injury. Such complications may follow either correct or incorrect use of mechanical ventilators. They may include respiratory distress, airway malfunction, changes in acid-base balance, diminished venous return, cardiac dysrhythmias, barotrauma, atelectasis, gastrointestinal effects, oxygen toxicity, infection, asynchronous breathing, ventilation dependence, and adverse psychological effects. Understanding these complications and anticipating them can help prevent them or limit their potential for irreversible injury. (See *Ventilator alarms,* page 302.)

Respiratory distress

In mechanically ventilated patients, the usual source of reversible respiratory distress is ventilator malfunction. The most common causes of malfunction are:
• alarm failure, disconnection, or mechanical breakdown
• kinked ventilator tubing or accidental extubation, which follows inadequate stabilization of ventilator tubing

Ventilator alarms

Most ventilators are equipped with several alarms. These alarms must be set properly and must *always* be turned on. They may signal the following problems.

Low-pressure alarm
• Tube disconnected from the ventilator
• Displaced endotracheal tube above the vocal cords or extubated tracheostomy tube
• Low cuff pressure and leakage of tidal volume (insufficient cuff pressure, hole in cuff, leak in the one-way valve, or ruptured cuff)
• Ventilator malfunction
• Leakage in ventilator circuitry (loose tubing or connection, loss of temperature sensing device, hole in ventilator tubing, or cracked humidification jar)

High-pressure alarm
• Increased airway pressure
• Biting on oral endotracheal tube
• Secretions in airway
• Right mainstem bronchus intubation
• Patient coughing, gagging, or attempting to talk
• Increased airway pressure and decreased lung compliance
• Worsening of disease
• Atelectasis, pneumothorax, tension pneumothorax, or pulmonary edema
• Wheezing secondary to suctioning or bronchospasm
• Repositioning with resistance to chest wall expansion, abdominal pressure against the diaphragm, chest wall injury, external restrictions, and abdominal contractions during coughing
• Failure of fail-safe valve

Spirometer alarm
• Low cuff volume or cuff rupture
• Displaced artificial airway
• Ventilator malfunction (delivers less than desired tidal volume)

• electrical failure of the ventilator power source
• incorrect temperature setting, which may cause tracheobronchial burns if it's too high or inadequate humidification and possible bronchospasm if it's too low
• malfunction of the fail-safe valve, which prevents the patient from exhaling air.

In all the above circumstances, the patient experiences air hunger or inability to inhale an adequate amount of oxygenated air and displays obvious signs of respiratory distress. Respiratory distress in the arousable patient who is not paralyzed is evident in an increased heart rate and respiratory rate and "fighting" the ventilator or asynchronous ventilation.

In response to such signs of respiratory distress, treat the patient, not the ventilator. If alarms are activated or the patient is in obvious distress, remove the patient from the ventilator and ventilate him manually. Perform manual positive-pressure ventilation with a self-inflating bag in which appropriate levels of oxygenation and PEEP can be given. A PEEP attachment should be added to any resuscitation bag if the patient is to receive over 10 cm H_2O of PEEP.

Airway malfunction
The next most common complication, airway malfunction may result from obstruction (most commonly by mucus plugs) of the patient's airway or of the indwelling tube; from cuff malfunction; or from tube displacement (extubation or bronchial intubation) or disconnection from the ventilator.

Airway complications are classified according to the time of their occurrence during the initial intubation, during maintenance of the indwelling artificial airway, or during extubation. The longer an artificial airway is kept in place, the greater the risk of complications. Two-thirds of all patients who have artificial airways in place for longer than 30 days develop some form of airway complication. The risk of such complications is greater if the intubation is traumatic, if traction or rubbing of the tube occurs, or if cuff pressure is excessive. A greater risk of complications is also linked to metabolic impairment (which inhibits healing), edema, upper respiratory obstruction, dehydration, the presence of nasogastric or duodenal tubes, inadequate removal of secretions, neck surgery, or postintubation attempts to speak.

Several anatomic factors also predispose the mechanically ventilated patient to develop complications. For example, the thinner the epithelial layer of the trachea, the greater the risk of tracheal damage resulting from intubation. This layer tends to be thinner in women and infants. Similarly, the trachea and vocal cords vary in size; they are larger in men. Consequently, using the same size cuff for men and women is likely to exacerbate airway malfunction. Infants, elderly patients, and those who have anatomic abnormalities of the airways typically tolerate airway intubation poorly.

To prevent airway malfunction, good tube care and the use of appropriate cuff pressure (18 to 22 mm Hg) with minimal occlusive leaking is essential. (See *Correct inflation of the cuff.*)

Acid-base imbalance

Managing the airway to provide appropriate oxygenation is the key to safe and effective mechanical ventilation. Inadequate ventilation causes retention of carbon dioxide, which raises $PaCO_2$ (hypercapnia) and leads to respiratory acidosis. The acidotic patient experiences lethargy, cerebral vasodilation with increased cerebral blood flow, increased ICP, and possible coma. Treatment of respiratory acidosis requires increased ventilation by increasing the respiratory rate or tidal volume.

Hyperventilation increases diffusion of carbon dioxide from the venous blood to the alveoli, reducing $PaCO_2$ (hypocapnia) and raising pH (respiratory alkalosis). In turn, respiratory alkalosis leads to cerebral vasoconstriction with hypokalemia, increased risk of dysrhythmias, tetany, seizures, and coma. Alkalosis causes a shift to the left of the oxygen-hemoglobin curve with increased hemoglobin affinity for oxygen. The resulting hypoxemia and hypoxia cause restlessness, anxiety, apprehension, dysrhythmias, headache, angina, confusion, disorientation, impaired judgment, decreased blood pressure, increased heart rate, dyspnea, and tachypnea. Ultimately, alkalosis causes tissue hypoxia and failure to wean.

Correct inflation of the cuff

Underinflating a cuff on a tracheostomy or endotracheal tube allows air to leak around the cuff; overinflating it can cause cuff rupture or tracheal damage. To ensure correct inflation of the cuff, follow these steps:
1. Suction oropharynx and trachea.
2. Insert syringe into valve at end of pilot balloon. Deflate cuff.
3. Inflate cuff to minimally occlude trachea.
4. Place stethoscope over laryngeal area and inflate cuff until no movement of air is heard with ventilation above larynx.
5. Remove 0.10 to 0.5 cc of air until small air leak is heard at peak inspiratory pressure.
6. Maintain cuff pressures below 25 mm Hg. (Arterial supply to the tracheal wall occurs at a pressure of 25 to 30 mm Hg. A cuff pressure over 25 mm Hg could occlude arterial blood supply to the tracheal wall.) *Note:* For higher inspiratory pressures or increased levels of positive end-expiratory pressure, increased cuff pressure may be necessary to adequately ventilate the patient.
7. Measure cuff pressure every 8 hours, making sure patient is in same position each time.

Treatment of alkalosis requires reduction of the respiratory rate or tidal volume, if it is inappropriately high, or increasing the mechanical dead space (distance of ventilator circuit tubing).

Diminished venous return

Positive pressure of mechanically delivered gases increases the pressure in the alveoli and airways; this pressure is then transmitted to the surrounding pulmonary vasculature, where it impedes blood flow. As this pressure rises with higher levels of PEEP, it impedes venous return. The diminished blood flow to the chest cavity decreases preload. If PEEP is added, the additional pressure with decreased venous return ultimately decreases cardiac output. Reduced cardiac output is more evident in normovolemic patients with congestive heart failure, in patients in hypovolemic shock, and in patients who receive high levels of PEEP. Subsequently, reduced cardiac output raises the heart rate and reduces blood pressure and urine output. In such patients, maintaining fluid volume by administering fluids may increase right ventricular preload. If administration of fluids or blood fails to improve severely reduced cardiac output, inotropic agents, such as dopamine, are used to increase cardiac contractility.

Cardiac dysrhythmias

With physiologic stress in the cardiovascular system, the heart increases its work load, which increases myocardial oxygen consumption. The difference between the supply of oxygen and oxygen demand widens when decreased cardiac output decreases coronary blood flow. The resulting myocardial hypoxia and acidemia leads to dysrhythmias. Multifocal atrial tachycardias are commonly associated with acidosis, hypoxia, and hypokalemia. Ventricular dysrhythmias occur when coronary artery disease further impedes coronary blood flow.

Barotrauma

Such injury to lung tissue results from excessive pressures or volumes that cause the alveoli to leak gas into the extraparenchymal structures. Barotrauma is most common in patients with severe preexisting chronic lung disease, chest trauma or surgery, closed chest compression, subclavian vein needle puncture, or acute restrictive lung disease requiring PEEP at levels exceeding

10 cm H_2O. During mechanical ventilation, the risk of barotrauma increases as the peak inspiratory pressure (PIP) rises above 40 cm H_2O.

Alveolar leaks are usually caused by tears in the parietal pleura. Such tears may result from trauma, chest tube insertion, rib fracture, pulmonary tissue damage, rupture of blebs, or a ruptured bronchus.

The most common causes of barotrauma are pneumothorax, tension pneumothorax, and pneumomediastinum.

Pneumothorax. The presence of air in the pleural space collapses part of the lung. As the amount of air within the pleural space increases, the resulting compression of lung tissue decreases the alveoli available for gas exchange and leads to hypoxemia. Pneumothorax produces respiratory distress, elevated PIP, diminished breath sounds over the affected lobe, decreased chest movement on the affected side, subcutaneous emphysema, restlessness, changing vital signs, and cyanosis; chest X-rays show a shift in the trachea, mediastinum, and other structures and a loss of lung markings. Depending on the degree of severity, pneumothorax may require immediate removal of the air by needle aspiration and insertion of a chest tube.

Tension pneumothorax. This more severe form of pneumothorax involves the rapid intrusion of air into the pleural space. The greater-than-atmospheric pressure in the pleural space rapidly leads to collapse of the lung and compression of the mediastinum, great vessels, atria, and ventricles; it also causes total circulatory collapse and failure of ventilation. The patient with tension pneumothorax shows severe dyspnea and restlessness, cyanosis, weak and rapid pulse, falling blood pressure, a sudden increase in PIP with a decrease in tidal volume, decreased PaO_2 or increased alveolar-arterial oxygen difference ($A\text{-}aDO_2$), asymmetry of the thorax, tracheal deviation, hyperresonance to percussion, decreased or unilateral vocal fremitus, cardiac arrest, and shock. This condition is rapidly fatal unless thoracic decompression with a large-bore needle and insertion of a chest tube is performed immediately.

Pneumomediastinum. Air in the mediastinum is detected by auscultating a crunching or bubbling sound on inspiration in synchrony with the heartbeat. Depending on the amount of air trapped in the mediastinum, the resulting pressure could compress the heart muscle and significantly decrease cardiac output.

Atelectasis

The collapse of lung parenchyma or alveoli follows occlusion of the airway, usually by increased secretions, with eventual reabsorption of gas distal to the occlusion. Atelectasis may be lobar or segmental. Its causes include failure to ventilate the alveoli because of small tidal volumes or obstruction, inadequate humidification of inspired gases, insufficient pulmonary hygiene, inadequate tracheal aspiration, and infrequent position changes.

The clinical effects of atelectasis include low-grade fever, (usually less than 101° F [38.3° C]), decreased breath sounds, crackles on auscultation, worsening ABG values, increased alveolar-arterial (A-a) gradient, decreased compliance, and infiltrates on chest X-ray.

Atelectasis can be prevented by periodically increasing the tidal volume through sighing, incentive spirometry, delivery of humidified gas and appropriate suctioning, chest physiotherapy, and frequent repositioning. Meticulous pulmonary nursing care plays a major role in preventing atelectasis. However, in patients with mucus plugs and copious secretions, fiberoptic bronchoscopy may become necessary.

GI effects

Because physiologic stress increases gastric acid secretion, prolonged ventilatory support can induce stress ulcers and gastric bleeding. Other GI complications include air swallowing with gastric dilation and adynamic or paralytic ileus. GI complications are most common in patients with a preexisting GI ulcer or on long-term steroid or salicylate therapy.

To prevent GI complications, antacids and histamine$_2$-receptor antagonists are administered to maintain gastric pH above 3.5. Early and frequent nasogastric or duodenal feeding also decreases gastric irritation; patients receiving tube feeding should be carefully monitored for gastric distention. Bowel sounds should be assessed every 4 hours to monitor for paralytic ileus. Monitoring should include routine testing of stomach aspirate and all stools for occult bleeding.

Oxygen toxicity

The prolonged administration of oxygen concentrations of 40% or higher can lead to oxygen toxicity: impaired surfactant activity, progressive capillary congestion, fibrosis, edema, and thickening of the interstitial spaces.

Clinical effects of oxygen toxicity include retrosternal distress, paresthesias in the extremities, nausea and vomiting, anorexia, fatigue, lethargy, malaise, dyspnea, coughing, and restlessness. Late signs include progressive respiratory distress, cyanosis, severe dyspnea, and asphyxia. Pulmonary changes include decreased compliance and vital capacity with an elevated A-a gradient.

Monitoring for oxygen toxicity requires frequent ABG measurements to maintain a PaO_2 of 55 to 60 mm Hg and an arterial oxygen saturation (SaO_2) of 90% on the lowest FIO_2 level. The preferred FIO_2 is less than 0.4.

Infection

Within 48 hours of any respiratory therapy, the patient's upper respiratory tract is colonized by hospital-acquired flora. Such colonization can be contained as long as the tracheal wall is intact. The intact wall and the normal flora maintain good oxygenation of local tissue with nutrients supplied by good blood flow. However, during mechanical ventilation, many factors combine to encourage infection. Any injury to the tracheal mucosa, secondary to suctioning and tube placement, provides an opening for bacteria. Inflation of the artificial airway cuff impedes blood flow to the tracheal wall. The indwelling tube blocks protective reflexes from clearing the upper air passages by coughing. Use of respiratory equipment to administer aerosols can introduce microbes into the respiratory tract, as can unsterile or frequent suctioning. In a debilitated patient, decreased resistance and immunosuppression exaggerate the risk of infection. Insertion of centrally placed lines and tissue injury resulting from aspiration of gastric contents also provide sites of opportunity for infection.

Signs of respiratory tract infection include a temperature above 102° F (38.9° C) and increased purulent secretions. Such infection requires culture and sensitivity tests to identify the causative organism and appropriate antibiotic treatment. To prevent cross-contamination by respiratory caregivers, meticulous hand washing is mandatory.

Asynchronous breathing

The usual causes of asynchronous breathing are inappropriate ventilator settings that create air hunger, a partially obstructed airway, ventilator malfunction, or anxiety caused by loss of respiratory control. As a result, the patient tries to take a breath between and occasionally against the ventilator breaths. This stacked breathing can lead to excessive intrapulmonary pressure. To prevent such effects, promptly remove the patient who exhibits signs of air hunger from the ventilator and ventilate him manually while rapidly assessing for a patent airway and the ability to ventilate. Such assessment must include a check of vital signs, breath sounds, and hemodynamic parameters. Suctioning of the patient's airway ensures that the endotracheal tube or tracheostomy tube is patent. ABG levels should be measured and any adjustments in ventilatory support completed. If the airway is patent, ABG values are acceptable, and manipulation of the ventilator for increased inspiratory or peak flow does not ease the patient's air hunger, the patient may need sedation. Pharmacologic paralysis should be considered only if other methods cannot achieve ventilatory support. Throughout ventilator therapy, calmly reassuring the patient and family can help ease the patient's anxiety and thus help prevent asynchronous breathing.

Ventilator dependence

Eventual weaning from the ventilator should be a major consideration from the beginning of mechanical ventilation. The more respiratory muscle function maintained, the easier the weaning. Factors that contribute to unsuccessful weaning are discussed in the section on weaning.

Adverse psychological effects

The patient loses control of breathing and all other decisions while the ventilator is providing total or partial support for respiration. The unfamiliar surroundings, inability to communicate because of the endotracheal tube, mechanical equipment, and invasion by tubes and catheters magnify the patient's fear, sense of aloneness, and loss of control; the mounting sense of anxiety increases autonomic nervous system stimulation and induces stress.

The stress response increases the heart rate, raises blood pressure and respiratory rate, and causes dilated pupils, dry mouth, and peripheral vasoconstriction. Even if the patient accepts hospitalization calmly, frequent checks of the ventilator and of vital signs cause sleep deprivation and loss of rapid eye movement sleep, increasing the patient's level of stress and fear. Recurring interruption of sleep causes disorientation. To prevent severe disorientation, maintain the patient's orientation to time with a calendar and clock, maintain his contact with his family to keep up with significant events, and try to schedule care to allow 4-hour periods of uninterrupted sleep. Reassuring the patient that he is responding appropriately to treatment and establishing an effective method of communication help enhance the patient's comfort.

Nursing management

Nursing care of the mechanically ventilated patient requires meticulous assessment for adequate ventilation, careful checks of mechanical function, and continual monitoring for complications and other problems.

Assessment

A complete body system review is required to establish a baseline for recognizing significant changes in clinical status.

Neurologic function. Review the patient's level of consciousness and check for recent changes in mentation. Intact neurologic function supports adequate ventilation, airway protective reflexes, and the capacity to sense and respond to changes in $PaCO_2$ and pH. Normal mentation and the capacity for communication help the mechanically ventilated patient deal with fear and anxiety.

Cardiovascular function. The increased intrapulmonary and intrathoracic pressures associated with mechanical ventilation require careful monitoring of cardiovascular function. Check the patient's heart rate and rhythm, blood pressure, central pressures (right atrial pressure; pulmonary artery systolic, diastolic, and mean pressure; and pulmonary capillary wedge pressure). Direct or indirect measurement of cardiac output helps evaluate perfusion to the brain, heart, and kidneys.

Respiratory function. Throughout mechanical ventilation, check the patient's respiratory rate and rhythm, effort of breathing, use of respiratory muscles, thoracic shape and excursion, and synchrony of ventilatory effort with the ventilator. Check for and record the location of bronchial, bronchovesicular, and vesicular breath sounds and any adventitious sounds. Also check the artificial airway for appropriate type and size, the current cuff pressure, and the presence of an air leak; the amount, color, consistency, translucency, and odor of secretions; and the frequency of suctioning necessary to maintain airway patency. Also observe skin color, though this is an unreliable indicator of hypoxemia.

Chest X-ray and ABG values reflect changes in the patient's disease condition and in gas exchange; they should be monitored frequently to maintain adequate ventilation. Bedside measurements should include minute ventilation (MV), respiratory rate, tidal volume (Vt), vital capacity (VC), maximal inspiratory flow, PIP, plateau pressure, and static compliance; such measurements determine the effectiveness of ventilation or weaning. Derived measures, such as A-aDO$_2$, intrapulmonary shunt fraction (Qs/Qt), and ratio of dead space ventilation to total ventilation (VD/VT), also help evaluate ventilation.

Abdomen. Examining the abdomen for normal bowel sounds and gastric distention is essential. Confirming the patient's ability to maintain adequate nutrition and recognizing conditions that interfere with metabolism will influence nutritional status and, in turn, affect respiratory muscle strength and carbon dioxide levels, which if allowed to rise will tax an already compromised respiratory system. Checking gastric secretions for the pH, amount, and presence of blood and watching for melena help monitor the integrity of the GI mucosa. All GI aspirate and stools should be tested for occult blood. Remember that metabolic and electrolyte abnormalities profoundly affect respiratory functions.

Intake and output. Monitoring the patient's fluid intake and urine output helps evaluate renal and cardiac function. Daily weights can signal fluid retention and the patient's metabolic needs. Testing urine specific gravity, glucose, acetone, and electrolyte levels, and osmolality may indicate fluid volume status. Measuring serum osmolality and electrolyte levels helps detect metabolic and acid-base imbalances.

Nutrition. Carefully review the patient's nutritional status, which influences weaning and recovery. Check recent weight gain or loss, albumin levels, and skin condition, which indicate hydration and the need for calories. Closely monitor supplemental feedings because their metabolic breakdown commonly increases carbon dioxide production.

Emotional status. Support effective methods of communication with the ventilated patient; this is essential to prevent anxiety. Whenever possible, schedule care so that the patient can maintain a normal sleep-wake cycle to support orientation and emotional health.

Mechanical checks and special monitoring

Routinely do the following to detect ventilator malfunction:

• Check ventilator function every 1 to 2 hours and as needed.

• Check ventilator settings as listed in the doctor's written order, including ventilator mode (CMV, ACV, IMV, SIMV, HFV, PSV), adjuncts (PEEP, CPAP), Vt, respiratory rate, I:E ratio, FIO_2, sighs/minute, and temperature.

• Monitor and measure Vt expired, PIP, plateau pressure, and static compliance.

• Respond to alarms and solve any problems.

When ventilator therapy includes use of PEEP or CPAP, the patient should have special monitoring of cardiovascular function and of ventilatory and hemodynamic measurements.

Cardiovascular monitoring. Whenever PEEP or CPAP is increased or decreased, monitor vital signs every 5 minutes for 15 minutes, every 15 minutes until stabilization, and then every hour to check for reduced cardiac output. Watch for a systolic blood pressure decrease of 20 mm Hg, an increased heart rate, decreased urine output, or altered neurologic status; these signs may indicate hypovolemia. Assess breath sounds for early signs of pulmonary barotrauma (absence of breath sounds with decreased pulmonary excursion) at least once every 4 hours.

Ventilatory measurements. Such measurements should include Vt, respiratory frequency, MV, peak and plateau pressure, PEEP or CPAP level, static compliance, ABG and mixed venous gas (PaO_2, arterial oxygen content [CaO_2], pH, $PaCO_2$, and venous oxygen saturation [SvO_2]) levels, A-aDO_2 or shunt, and, if available, arterial minus the end-tidal carbon dioxide gradient.

Hemodynamic measurements. Such measurements should include blood pressure, heart rate, cardiac output, SvO_2, pulmonary artery pressure (PAP), and pulmonary capillary wedge pressure (PCWP). Arterial blood pressure should maintain a mean arterial pressure of 70 mm Hg, which supports adequate cerebral, coronary, and renal blood flow. Monitor heart rate for adequate ventricular filling time; it is adequate when the patient maintains a cardiac output of 4 to 8 liters/minute and a cardiac index of 2.5 to 3.5 liters/minute/m² without angina. ECG monitoring is necessary to recognize dysrhythmias that increase myocardial oxygen needs and decrease filling time and cardiac output. Central pressures should be maintained at a level to provide adequate cardiac output and a urine output of 0.5 ml/kg of body weight. Normal central pressures in healthy persons include right atrial pressure, 2 to 6 mm Hg; pulmonary artery systolic pressure, 20 to 30 mm Hg; pulmonary artery end-diastolic pressure, 8 to 12 mm Hg; mean PAP, below 20 mm Hg; and pulmonary artery wedge pressure, 4 to 12 mm Hg. Note that the patient with myocardial infarction requires higher pressures to maintain stroke volume.

An SvO_2 of 60% is considered within the normal range when the patient's hemoglobin, oxygen delivery, and cardiac output are adequate. The A-a gradient reflects oxygen uptake by the peripheral tissues. Levels between 300 and 350 are considered normal.

PCWP should be measured at the end of expiration. If the PEEP level is less than 15 cm H_2O, the patient should not be removed from the ventilator for such measurements. The increased alveolar pressure secondary to PEEP is probably offset by absorption of the increased pressure by the extraparenchymal structures. In patients with PEEP levels greater than 15 cm H_2O, the PCWP will be falsely elevated; consider such secondary elevations when treating elevated PCWP. Monitor the range of PCWP values and each increase in PEEP to determine the actual increase in central pressure relative to that increase. Usually, the patient cannot tolerate removal from the ventilator for measurement of actual values; however, if the patient can tolerate it, compare actual and monitored values once per shift. During monitoring by trending (following the pattern of PCWP), consider that PEEP at high levels raises PCWP. Much nursing controversy exists over whether removing the patient from the ventilator for PCWP readings aids treatment. The hemodynamic measurement obtained during mechanical ventilation with high PEEP levels reflects what is happening to the patient moment by moment. When recording central pressures, be sure to specify whether measurements were taken on or off the ventilator.

Nursing diagnoses

Consider the following patient problems that are common in mechanically ventilated patients.

To prevent *impaired gas exchange,* frequently check the mechanically ventilated patient's breath sounds and ventilator settings for changes in status. Make sure the tape or securing device has not loosened and allowed the endotracheal tube to slip out of position. The weight of the ventilator hoses may pull on the tube. Avoid routinely retaping an endotracheal tube, however; retaping it creates more trauma to the vocal cords. Retape only if the tape is soiled or loose enough to allow dislodgment of the tube or if local irritation of the skin is present.

Ineffective airway clearance commonly requires suctioning, but certain precautions are necessary to minimize the potential risks. For suctioning the patient on PEEP therapy, if the PEEP level is 10 cm H_2O or greater, consider continuing PEEP during suctioning with a resuscitation bag with a PEEP attachment. An in-line suction apparatus is available for easier suctioning. To prevent hypoxemia and to replace the oxygenated air removed by the suction catheters, you must hyperoxygenate and hyperventilate the patient before and after suctioning with FIO_2 at 100% and manually or mechanically ventilate at a tidal volume 1½ times the normal ventilated tidal volume. If hypoxemia is severe, hyperventilate the patient at a rate faster than the mechanical rate; if oxygenation is adequate, ventilate at the preset rate. The net goal is to prevent a large drop in PaO_2.

Impaired verbal communication results from intubation and mechanical ventilation. The endotracheal tube passes through the vocal cords and holds them open. Inability to speak causes the alert patient to feel anxiety and frustration. If the patient tries to speak so that someone may read his lips, the vocal cords will reflexively abduct around the tube, causing trauma and vocal cord edema. Therefore, mechanically ventilated patients must communicate using other tools, such as a magic slate, letter board, or pen and paper. Felt-tipped markers, which write with little pressure, are especially appropriate for use by debilitated patients.

Altered nutrition: less than body requirements is a potential problem in all ventilated patients and can delay weaning if it is severe enough to allow loss of muscle mass. To prevent such loss, high-calorie, per-ounce tube feedings are the preferred nutritional choice if the patient's GI tract is intact. If trauma or surgery has disrupted the patient's GI tract, total parenteral nutrition (TPN) with supplemental intralipid infusions may be used for more precise nutritional control. However, TPN increases the risk of infection.

Fluid volume deficit must be avoided to maintain intravascular volume, blood pressure, cardiac output, and the fluidity of bronchial secretions. *Fluid volume excess* must be avoided to prevent pulmonary edema and further impairment of gas exchange. Monitor intake and output and daily weight to assess fluid status.

Impaired physical mobility commonly decreases muscle strength and promotes joint stiffness. To prevent such effects, impose active and passive range-of-motion exercises as soon as possible. Teach family members to assist the patient with these exercises.

Impaired skin integrity can also cause impaired mobility by causing pain. By taxing the patient's immune system, pressure sores increase the risk of infection. To protect the patient's skin, turn him every 2 hours, keep sheets wrinkle-free, and provide special beds or mattresses that minimize pressure. Change wet or soiled sheets promptly, and keep the patient's skin clean and dry.

Sleep pattern disturbance is a special problem in patients who receive prolonged treatment in the intensive care unit; it contributes to physical weakness and psychosis. In turn, physical weakness can cause inability to wean. Schedule nursing care to provide adequate uninterrupted sleep.

Fear and *powerlessness* associated with mechanical ventilation understandably cause anxiety, which itself can interfere with effective ventilation. To prevent overpowering anxiety, frequently offer reassurance, try to anticipate the patient's physical needs, and respond to the patient's call bell as promptly as possible. If the patient expresses anxiety by becoming too demanding, offering reassurance and setting reasonable limits may help him feel more relaxed and cooperative.

Home care
Ventilator-dependent patients who are medically stable can be discharged and maintained on mechanical ventilation at home. Appropriate candidates for home ventilation include patients with neuromuscular disease or chronic lung disease who have no complications of other major systems. (See *Patient-teaching checklist: Teaching patient and family before discharge,* page 316.)

Weaning
Most patients can be weaned from mechanical ventilation as soon as the source of respiratory distress has been corrected. However, successful weaning requires preparation that should begin at intubation and continue throughout mechanical ventilation.

Managing mechanical ventilation to facilitate weaning requires special planning, including:
• selection of ventilator settings to maintain respiratory muscle function
• using IMV or ACV to maintain spontaneous breathing
• keeping the duration of mechanical ventilation to the minimum necessary
• maintaining respiratory muscle conditioning.

Criteria for weaning
Weaning is the gradual withdrawal of mechanical ventilatory support. Certain prognostic factors can indicate whether the patient will be able to breathe spontaneously after discontinuation of mechanical ventilation. The criteria for successful weaning are, in effect, the reverse of those for improving ventilatory support. First, the pathophysiologic changes that created the need for respiratory support must be corrected. Such resolution of the

Teaching patient and family before discharge

Teach the patient and a designated family member the following procedures.

Airway assessment
☐ Show the family caregiver how to assess the patient's respiratory rate and recognize variations in breathing patterns, including shortness of breath and apnea.
☐ Teach how to describe the quality and amount of secretions.

Bagging technique
☐ Identify appropriate equipment.
☐ Connect the hand-held resuscitation bag to oxygen.
☐ Connect the hand-held resuscitation bag to the tracheostomy tube.
☐ Use the hand-held resuscitation bag to give oxygenated ventilation at a comfortable rate.

Clean suctioning
☐ Explain the need for sterile technique while in hospital.
☐ Wash your hands.
☐ Select appropriate equipment (catheter, gloves, hand-held resuscitation bag, sterile packet of normal saline solution).
☐ Demonstrate clean suctioning technique.

Cleaning inner cannula of tracheostomy tube
☐ Review aseptic technique. Wash your hands.
☐ Gather the necessary supplies: gloves, mixture of half hydrogen peroxide and half normal saline solution or other

appropriate solution, brush, pipe cleaners, sponges, tracheostomy tapes, and 4″ x 4″ dressing. An extra tracheostomy set will already be at the bedside.
☐ Unwrap equipment and disconnect the ventilator from the patient. Then put on gloves.
☐ Remove the inner cannula.
☐ Submerge the inner cannula in a mixture of half hydrogen peroxide and half normal saline solution. *Caution:* Assess the patient's respiratory status continuously while cleaning the inner cannula.
☐ Clean the inner cannula with the brush.
☐ Feed the pipe cleaner through the inner cannula.
☐ Shake excess fluid off the inner cannula.
☐ Reinsert it and lock it in place.
☐ Connect the ventilator to the patient.
☐ Remove the 4″ x 4″ dressing around the tracheostomy.
☐ Clean peristomal skin with a mixture of half hydrogen peroxide and half normal saline solution, as ordered.
☐ Record the peristomal skin condition.
☐ Place the new 4″ x 4″ dressing around the tracheostomy.
☐ Change the tracheostomy tapes only if another person can help. This can be the patient if he's able.
☐ Explain the danger of the outer cannula coming out. Describe what to do: Immediately replace it with a sterile or clean tracheostomy tube and tie securely, notify the doctor, and assess respiratory status.

Troubleshooting ventilator problems
☐ While giving routine respiratory care, the caregiver will learn for how long the patient can tolerate being off the ventilator. Tell the caregiver that if he can't troubleshoot the ventilator, he should provide needed ventilatory support and call the respiratory therapist, doctor, or ambulance service immediately.
☐ If there's time to troubleshoot, he should identify possible causes of respiratory distress or triggers of the ventilator alarm. Explain how to deal with the following:
Obstructed tracheostomy tube
☐ Preoxygenate the patient using a hand-held resuscitation bag.
☐ Remove the inner cannula.
☐ Clean the inner cannula and replace it.
☐ Instill 3 to 5 ml of normal saline solution.
☐ Suction the patient.
☐ Connect the patient to the ventilator and assess his respiratory status.
☐ If the patient is still in distress, dial an emergency phone number to arrange transportation to the nearest hospital.
Water in tubing
☐ Disconnect the tubing from the ventilator.
☐ Empty water from the tubing.
Improper cuff pressure
☐ Inflate the cuff with an appropriate amount of pressure. (Explain the importance of proper cuff inflation.)
☐ During the patient's next medical visit, the caregiver should report problems and solutions.

underlying disease may occur quickly (as in drug-related respiratory depression) or may take months (as in neuromuscular disease). Thus, the criteria for weaning will vary with the underlying pathophysiology; however, certain guidelines help determine when weaning can begin. The patient must be able to maintain adequate ventilation with spontaneous respirations, must have a stable cardiovascular status, and must show resolution of large intrapulmonary shunts (to less than 20% of total pulmonary blood flow). Increased work of breathing increases oxygen demand by the respiratory muscles; if oxygen is not readily available, respiratory muscle fatigue occurs and prevents successful weaning. The patient's chest X-ray should be clear or clearing to indicate an improvement of the underlying lung disease or pulmonary edema. He should have a normal temperature (98.6° F [37° C], plus or minus 1 F degree), which indicates an eradication or control of infection and decreased metabolic needs.

Preserving the patient's respiratory muscle strength can be achieved by using ventilator settings that allow for the maximal work of breathing tolerated while providing adequate ventilation during the disease process. Maintaining adequate nutrition prevents the breakdown of muscle tissue and provides nutrients to meet energy needs. Metabolic studies to determine actual metabolic needs are helpful to prevent excessive feeding of carbohydrates. The metabolism of carbohydrates leads to an increase in carbon dioxide production and therefore an increase in work of breathing.

The patient should be able to maintain a PaO_2 of 60 mm Hg. However, if he has a chronic lung disease, knowing the previous oxygen levels is helpful. In patients with chronic lung disease, a PaO_2 of 55 mm Hg is usually acceptable.

Stable and acceptable hemodynamic parameters indicate the heart's ability to pump oxygenated blood. The patient's maintenance of adequate cardiac output and cardiac index is a key factor in confirming adequate oxygenation and supports a successful weaning process. Normal central pressures indicate adequate hydration and rule out fluid overload. Both instances decrease the heart's work load. A normal hemoglobin level is essential for oxygen-carrying capacity; in patients with polycythemia, a decrease in blood viscosity is essential to reduce af-

Criteria for weaning

The subjective and objective criteria listed below can indicate that the patient is a good candidate for weaning from mechanical ventilation. Not all patients who meet these criteria will be weaned successfully, and not all patients who are weaned successfully meet these criteria. Nevertheless, these criteria offer a place to begin evaluating the patient for weaning.

Subjective criteria
• The patient has recovered from the immediate effects of anesthesia or any other depressant drugs.
• The patient is alert.
• The patient has no neurologic deficits.
• The patient's airway protective reflexes are intact.

Objective criteria
• Spontaneous vital capacity is greater than 10 ml/kg.
• Spontaneous tidal volume is greater than 6 ml/kg.
• PaO_2 is greater than 60 mm Hg on FIO_2 of less than 0.4.
• $PaCO_2$ is within 35 to 45 mm Hg unless the patient has chronic lung disease; then at patient's baseline pH.
• Inspiratory force is greater than -20 cm H_2O.
• Forced expiratory volume in one second is greater than 10 ml/kg.
• Resting minute ventilation is less than 10 liters/minute.
• Maximal minute ventilation is greater than 20 liters/minute or twice the minute ventilation.
• Shunt is less than 15%.
• Alveolar-arterial gradient is 300 to 350 mm Hg.
• Compliance is greater than 35 cm H_2O.
• Circulation is stable.
• Respiratory rate is below 35 breaths/minute.

terload. A normal or slightly elevated potassium level will help prevent dysrhythmias and facilitate normal cardiac function.

Adequate oxygenation, adequate sleep, and stable hemodynamic parameters encourage an acceptable level of consciousness. Preferably, the patient should be awake, alert, and oriented. However, knowing the level of consciousness before intubation and ventilatory support helps in evaluating the patient's suitability for weaning. Depending on the course of the disease, a return to the patient's earlier functional level may not be possible. In that case, a decision on what is an acceptable level of consciousness must be made.

Throughout weaning, ABG values are acceptable when the PaO_2 is unchanged from baseline during partial ventilatory support and during T-piece or CPAP trials. The $PaCO_2$ value should remain the same (within 5 mm Hg) during partial support and nonsupported breathing periods. It may be allowed to climb to its pre-event level in patients with chronic lung disease. In such patients, weaning should be done over several days to weeks to allow time for compensatory production of bicarbonate (HCO_3^-) by the kidneys. The increased HCO_3^- will then buffer the additional hydrogen ions accompanying the elevation in carbon dioxide levels. This buffering maintains pH in the normal range of 7.35 to 7.45.

The weaning parameters used are VC, negative inspiratory force, forced expiratory volume in one second, MV, maximal minute ventilation, $PaCO_2$, PaO_2, Qs/Qt, A-a gradient, and VD/VT. The normalization of these parameters must accompany the other factors listed in *Criteria for weaning*.

Once physiologic factors are within an acceptable range, the patient must be psychologically prepared, emotionally ready, and cooperative. After prolonged mechanical support, these criteria may be the most difficult to meet.

Weaning techniques
Techniques for weaning vary, depending on whether oxygenation failure or ventilatory failure is the major underlying problem.

Oxygenation failure. When oxygenation failure is the underlying problem, weaning focuses on the ability to decrease PEEP and FIO_2. Thus, PEEP is decreased in increments of 3 to

5 cm H_2O to maintain a PaO_2 of at least 60 mm Hg on an FIO_2 of 0.5 or less. The ventilator rate, mode, and volume should be adjusted to keep the pH between 7.35 to 7.45. When PEEP is reduced to 5 cm H_2O or less, with an FIO_2 of 0.4, weaning can be completed. Extubation can then be considered after a successful trial of 2 to 6 hours of CPAP.

Ventilatory failure. When the underlying problem is ventilatory failure, the IMV technique, the ACV technique, or the T-piece technique may be used. The IMV or ACV technique is used for patients who are difficult to wean (elderly patients, debilitated patients, and patients with chronic pulmonary or neuromuscular diseases); these methods are used with the T-piece or CPAP mode.

IMV technique. This method decreases the number of ventilator breaths until the patient is self-supporting. It produces less hemodynamic impairment than T-piece weaning and avoids respiratory alkalosis. The lower mean airway pressure at a low IMV rate allows more uniform intrapulmonary gas distribution. Furthermore, the prevention of respiratory muscle atrophy is said to expedite weaning. Psychologically, this technique of gradually decreasing the assisted breaths is easier for a fearful patient.

Disadvantages of IMV weaning are the increased work of breathing with partial support associated with respiratory muscle fatigue, increased risk of hypercarbia, and cardiac decompensation in patients with underlying heart disease. Such weaning could become prolonged if the rate is changed infrequently. Prolonged weaning at IMV rates of 4 or less in a patient with a small airway could lead to increased work of breathing and promote respiratory muscle fatigue.

ACV technique. The ACV technique lowers the tidal volume at a rate of 50 to 100 ml/day until the patient's spontaneous tidal volume is achieved. At the same time, it increases the ventilatory rate to the patient's rate, which provides support for each breath. The ventilatory rate is then decreased to allow the patient added work of breathing; or the patient is placed on humidified, oxygenated air connected directly to the T-piece for short periods each hour. Each day during waking hours, the T-piece time is increased by 5 minutes until a full hour is reached; then it is increased by 15 minutes until 2 hours are reached; finally, it is increased by 30 minutes up to 4-hour intervals.

At this point, weaning continues by 4 hours off the ventilator followed by 1 hour on. Nighttime weaning is increased by an additional hour each night until it continues around the clock, 4 hours on and 1 hour off. At this point, CPAP or T-piece weaning is attempted. These intermittent periods of increasingly prolonged nonsupport with total support at night allow gradual strengthening of respiratory muscle function.

T-piece technique. The T-piece method is used for patients who have been intubated and ventilated for less than 2 days. Usually, such a patient has had cardiothoracic surgery, is emerging from coma, has status asthmaticus, or has had a brief exacerbation of a chronic lung disease. The patient is placed on the T-piece as soon as he is awake. ABG measurements within an acceptable range after 20 to 30 minutes, and repeated every 1 to 4 hours, indicate the readiness for extubation. For the patient who has a debilitating disease, has chronic lung disease, or has been on prolonged ventilation, use of the T-piece starts at 5 minutes/hour and increases to 4-hour periods. Encouraging adequate nighttime rest is essential for these patients to overcome the possibility of respiratory muscle fatigue. CPAP may be necessary to prevent airway closure and microatelectasis in spontaneously breathing patients.

Once the decision is made to wean, the patient and family should receive an explanation of the weaning plan. The patient should be placed in an upright position. If he is seated in a chair, weaning attempts should begin within 5 minutes after the change in position to prevent the effort of sitting up from interfering with weaning.

During weaning, baseline vital signs and ECG rhythm as well as frequent assessment of vital signs and ventilatory parameters are required. Ventilatory measurements should include the respiratory rate, Vt, MV, PIP, and VC. In T-piece weaning, the ventilator should be close by in case respiratory fatigue sets in before the preselected time has elapsed. In weaning by IMV, the caregiver must be available to reassure the patient and return him to the previous level of support when he completes his trial or return him to the ventilator for rest if the attempt is unsuccessful.

Weaning failure

Resuming ventilation is necessary when discontinuation causes the patient's blood pressure to rise or fall by 20 mm Hg systolic or 10 mm Hg diastolic; heart rate to rise by 20 beats/minute or to a rate greater than 120 beats/minute; respiratory rate to increase by 10 breaths/minute or to a rate greater than 35 breaths/minute; or when any of the following occur: cardiac dysrhythmias (frequent premature ventricular contractions), a decreased tidal volume, increased $PaCO_2$, or signs of increased work of breathing (use of accessory muscles, paradoxical breathing, intercostal retractions, flaring of the nostrils, apprehension, diaphoresis, fatigue, drowsiness, and decreased level of consciousness).

The causes of weaning failure include insufficient ventilatory drive caused by a high ventilatory requirement, hypoxemia, or respiratory muscle weakness. Respiratory muscle weakness can result from persistent lung disease and from decreased cardiac output. Low compliance and excessive work of breathing increase the work load and make weaning more difficult. Increased work of breathing is also related to excessive secretions, a weakened cough, impaired mucociliary clearance, or ineffective suctioning. Inadequately treated respiratory infections, inappropriate use of antibiotics, and absence of effective pulmonary physiotherapy further increase the secretion load. The resulting increase in airway resistance may exaggerate the ventilation-perfusion mismatch and cause deterioration of gas exchange.

Extubation

When weaning has been successful (with stable vital signs, an ability to maintain a patent airway, and acceptable ABG values and ventilatory parameters), the patient is extubated. The removal of an artificial airway (in a patient with orally or nasally inserted tubes) decreases the work of breathing by decreasing resistance in the upper airway.

For a patient with a tracheostomy tube, extubation may be delayed because reinsertion is a surgical procedure. For this patient, extubation begins with insertion of a fenestrated tube (a tube with holes through the outer lumen of the tracheostomy tube). If needed, the patient can be mechanically ventilated with the insertion of an inner cannula that serves to occlude these openings. If the fenestrated tube interferes with airflow, a stent may be placed to maintain the tracheostomy.

Before extubation, explain the procedure to the patient. Then position him with his head elevated and check vital signs. At the bedside, set up a high-humidity, oxygen-enriched gas source, a self-inflating resuscitation bag with mask, and 100% FIO_2. Also have intubation equipment readily available.

Before the doctor extubates the patient, the upper airway and the oropharynx are suctioned. The cuff is deflated with a 10-cc non-Luer-Lok syringe. The tube is removed at the peak of spontaneous or mechanical (self-inflating bag) ventilation. Encourage the patient to cough as the tube is removed. Appropriate levels of oxygen are given to prevent laryngospasm. Monitor the patient for signs and symptoms of laryngospasm, which include inspiratory stridor (a high-pitched sound) and dyspnea. Adding high humidity may decrease laryngospasm. The patient's vital signs should be checked and ABG levels measured 20 minutes after extubation.

Early postextubation complications include acute laryngeal edema, hoarseness, and aspiration. Late complications may include fibrotic stenosis of the trachea with dyspnea, stridor, or tracheoesophageal fistula and laryngeal stenosis requiring dilation, surgery, or a permanent tracheostomy.

Cardiopulmonary care plans

The following care plans present selected nursing diagnoses that are usually applicable to patients with acute cardiac or respiratory diseases. They include expected outcomes and specific interventions required to successfully manage such patients.

Nursing diagnosis	Expected outcomes	Nursing interventions
Altered tissue perfusion (cardiopulmonary, peripheral, cerebral, and renal) related to fluid volume deficit	• Systolic blood pressure > 90 mm Hg • Cardiac index 2.5 to 3.5 liters/m²/minute (cardiac output divided by body surface area = cardiac index) • Pulse pressure > 30 mm Hg (systolic − diastolic blood pressure = pulse pressure) • Strong, palpable peripheral pulses (2 on a scale of 4) • Urine output > 0.5 ml/kg/hour • Capillary blanch test < 2 seconds on feet or hands • Normal state of consciousness. • Warm, dry skin • Pink sublingual mucous membranes and tongue	• Assess for signs of decreased tissue perfusion, such as delayed capillary blanch test on extremities; hypotension; decreased or absent peripheral pulses; cold and moist skin; dusky, bluish oral mucosa; and urine output < 30 ml/hour. • Assess hemodynamic parameters and laboratory results, including cardiac index, every 2 hours and as needed. Notify doctor of abnormal findings. • Monitor heart rate, ECG, and arterial blood pressure continuously. Notify doctor of new bradycardia or tachycardia, dysrhythmia, or hypotension. • Assist with rapid I.V. fluid administration by a peripheral catheter or a large-bore central catheter. • Administer colloid or crystalloid solutions as prescribed. Consider the use of a rapid-volume infuser, a system that provides for simultaneous rapid volume replacement and fluid warming. • Monitor urine output hourly. • Assess patient for signs of increased bleeding, such as blood seepage from old or current puncture sites, hematuria, excessive bloody chest tube drainage, bloody nasogastric drainage, or increased blood during endotracheal suctioning or mouth care.
Altered tissue perfusion related to malposition of intra-aortic balloon pump (IABP) and occlusion of femoral artery	• No pain or significantly fewer ischemic episodes • Strong, palpable peripheral pulses (2 on a scale of 4) • Urine output > 0.5 ml/kg/hour • Capillary blanch test < 2 seconds on feet or hands • Normal state of consciousness • Warm, dry skin distal to catheter insertion site • Pink sublingual mucous membranes and tongue	• Assess for symptoms of chest pain or altered neurologic status once every hour. • Assess intake and output every 1 to 8 hours. • Monitor quality of peripheral pulses, skin temperature, and color every 1 to 4 hours. • Administer anticoagulants as ordered. • Check patient positioning to avoid more than 30-degree flexion at the hips while IABP is in place.
Altered tissue perfusion related to presence of pressurized tracheal cuff and tracheal edema	• Unimpeded arterial flow in trachea • No tracheal edema	• Maintain minimal leak cuff inflation with cuff pressure < 25 mm Hg. • Use high-volume, low-pressure tracheal cuffs. • Stabilize tube with position changes to keep head aligned with body.
Anxiety, fear, and hopelessness related to life-style changes secondary to disease process and hospitalization	• Decreased anxiety, fear and hopelessness • Restful sleep • Decreased ability to concentrate	• Monitor patient for signs and symptoms of anxiety (voice tremors, insomnia, restlessness, irritability). • Spend 10 to 15 minutes with patient at least twice per shift. Convey a willingness to listen.

(continued)

Cardiopulmonary care plans *(continued)*

Nursing diagnosis	Expected outcomes	Nursing interventions
Anxiety, fear, and hopelessness related to life-style changes secondary to disease process and hospitalization *(continued)*		• Encourage verbalization of emotions and concerns. • Help patient identify sources of anxiety. • Help patient participate in activities of daily living to the degree possible.
Decreased cardiac output related to diminished venous return secondary to increased intrapulmonary pressure possibly caused by positive pressure ventilation, positive end-expiratory pressure (PEEP), pneumothorax, and extremely large tidal volume	• Normal state of consciousness • Urine output > 0.5 ml/kg/hour • Specific gravity 1.010 to 1.015 • Warm, dry skin • Systolic arterial pressure of 90 mm Hg and mean arterial pressure of 65 to 70 mm Hg • Pulmonary capillary wedge pressure (PCWP) 10 to 12 mm Hg • Cardiac output 4 to 8 liters/minute • Cardiac index 2.5 to 3.5 liters/m²/minute • Venous oxygen saturation (SvO_2) within 60% to 80% • Body temperature 98.6° F (37° C) • Arterial blood gas (ABG) levels within normal limits	• Assess for signs of decreased cardiac output, such as hypoxia, clammy skin, weak pulse, changes in level of consciousness and behavior, decreased urine output, and oliguria. • Monitor vital signs. • Administer appropriate I.V. fluids and inotropic agents, as needed. • Manually ventilate or medicate as needed to prevent asynchronous breathing, which causes an increased intrathoracic pressure and further decreases venous return. Assess adequacy of ventilatory support if patient has asynchronous breathing. • Assess for trapping of air secondary to increased thoracic resistance or shortened expiratory time (due to a high ventilatory rate). Check ventilator for increased static pressure and peak inspiratory pressure (PIP). As necessary, adjust ventilator, shorten inspiratory time or increase peak flow rate, decrease minute ventilation to minimal level at which an acceptable pH is maintained, institute intermittent mandatory ventilation, or correct cause of increased respiratory rate (fever, agitation, or metabolic acidosis). • Add or increase PEEP in increments of 3 to 5 cm H_2O while monitoring for signs and symptoms of decreased cardiac output. Check ABG levels 20 minutes after setting change; assess changes in SvO_2 and ear oximetry. • Assess oxygen-carrying capacity by monitoring hemoglobin, cardiac output, SvO_2, and partial pressure of oxygen in arterial blood (PaO_2).
Decreased cardiac output related to dysrhythmias or ventricular failure	• No cardiac dysrhythmias • Cardiac output 4 to 8 liters/minute • Serum potassium > 4 mEq/liter (4 mmol/liter) • PCWP 10 to 12 mm Hg • Hemoglobin within normal limits • Absence of chest pain • SvO_2 within 60% to 80% • PaO_2 > 60 mm Hg when chronic lung disease is absent • Partial pressure of carbon dioxide in arterial blood ($PaCO_2$) 35 to 45 mm Hg • Normal level of consciousness	• Monitor vital signs and hemodynamic parameters for evidence of atrial or ventricular dysfunction, such as decreased blood pressure, decreased cardiac output and index, increased PCWP, increased pulmonary artery pressure, and increased right atrial pressure. Keep in mind that in myocardial infarction or necrosis, higher ventricular filling pressures are necessary to maintain cardiac output. • Assess peripheral perfusion, including pulse checks, skin color, sensation, and movement every 4 hours and as needed. • Observe ECG for atrial or ventricular dysrhythmias. If present, note frequency. Maintain oxygenation to prevent myocardial ischemia and resulting increased irritability. Administer appropriate medications to suppress dysrhythmias. Monitor serum potassium levels because hypokalemia can cause ventricular ectopy. • Administer oxygen to ensure optimal tissue oxygenation. • Schedule activities to allow for rest periods to minimize energy requirements and oxygen consumption, thereby decreasing strain on impaired ventricular function.

Cardiopulmonary care plans *(continued)*

Nursing diagnosis	Expected outcomes	Nursing interventions
Decreased cardiac output related to dysrhythmias or ventricular failure *(continued)*		• Suction as needed, using hyperoxygenation before and after each suction if necessary. In a large pulmonary shunt, a closed tracheal suction system may be preferred. If negative airway pressure is created, a decrease in lung volume can occur, causing alveolar collapse and arterial desaturation. • Observe for bradycardia secondary to hyperinflation and vagal nerve stimulation by suction catheter in tracheobronchial tree above the carina. If present, temporarily discontinue suction catheter. • Observe for Valsalva's maneuver secondary to increased intrathoracic pressure, coughing, gagging, lifting, and defecating. Valsalva's maneuver leads to changes in preload and increased afterload and bradycardia.
Decreased cardiac output related to left ventricular dysfunction	• Normal state of consciousness • Respiratory rate, rhythm, and effort within normal limits • Urine output > 0.5 ml/kg/hour • Specific gravity 1.010 to 1.015 • Warm, dry skin • Systolic arterial pressure of 90 mm Hg and mean arterial pressure of 65 to 70 mm Hg • PCWP 10 to 12 mm Hg • Cardiac output 4 to 8 liters/minute • Cardiac index 2.5 to 3.5 liters/m²/minute • SvO$_2$ within 60% to 80% • Body temperature 98.6° F (37° C) • ABG levels within normal limits	• Assess for dyspnea. • Monitor hemodynamic values every 30 minutes while pulmonary artery (PA) catheter is in place. • Monitor heart rate, blood pressure, and respiratory rate every 15 to 60 minutes as situation warrants. • Administer digitalis, amrinone, nitroprusside, and dopamine as prescribed. Titrate dopamine to achieve systolic blood pressure as ordered or 90 to 100 mm Hg. • Administer oxygen therapy as ordered. • Auscultate heart sounds every 1 to 2 hours as warranted. • Evaluate respiratory status every 1 to 2 hours as indicated. • Maintain patient in semi-Fowler's position. • Measure intake and output every 1 to 8 hours. • Assess for signs and symptoms of decreased cardiac output (jugular vein distention, edema, hepatojugular reflux, pulsus alternans, and abnormal skin color, capillary refill, or pulse quality) every 1 to 4 hours. • While patient is on IABP, assess balloon timing every hour.
Fluid volume excess related to sodium and water retention by the hypoperfused kidney	• Urine output > 0.5 ml/kg/hour • Specific gravity 1.010 to 1.015 • Warm, dry skin • Systolic arterial pressure of 90 mm Hg and mean arterial pressure of 65 to 70 mm Hg • PCWP 10 to 12 mm Hg • Cardiac output 4 to 8 liters/minute • Clear lungs on auscultation	• Assess hemodynamic values every 30 to 60 minutes while PA catheter is in place. • Auscultate breath sounds every 1 to 2 hours as indicated. • Auscultate heart sounds every 1 to 2 hours as needed. • Monitor intake and output every 4 to 8 hours. • Weigh the patient daily. • Restrict fluid intake as ordered. • Administer prescribed medications. • Assess for edema every 1 to 4 hours. Check for hepatomegaly, jugular vein distention, and hepatojugular reflux. • Administer oxygen as ordered.
Impaired gas exchange related to altered oxygen supply secondary to cardiopulmonary arrest	• Bilateral, equal breath sounds on auscultation • pH 7.35 to 7.45 • PacO$_2$ 35 to 45 mm Hg • PaO$_2$ 75 to 100 mm Hg	• Provide artificial ventilation using appropriate technique (mouth-mouth, mouth-nose, mouth-mask, or bag-valve-mask). • Continually assess respiratory status. • Monitor ABG levels.

(continued)

Cardiopulmonary care plans (continued)

Nursing diagnosis	Expected outcomes	Nursing interventions
Impaired gas exchange related to atelectasis	• Unlabored, vesicular breath sounds • $Paco_2$ 35 to 45 mm Hg • Pao_2 > 60 mm Hg	• Assess breath sounds every 1 to 2 hours. • Monitor vital signs every hour, and note low-grade temperature elevation. • Monitor ABG levels for decreased oxygen levels or saturation. • Maintain alveolar ventilation by proper patient positioning and by encouraging deep breathing and intermittent sighing. • Apply suction as needed to prevent mucus plugging. Be sure to appropriately hyperinflate and hyperoxygenate (using 100% fraction of inspired oxygen [FIO_2]) before and after suctioning. • If chest wall trauma exists, cautiously administer appropriate analgesic to reduce chest wall splinting.
Impaired gas exchange related to barotrauma secondary to mechanical ventilation	• Restoration of normal negative pressure in the lungs • Equal bilateral lung expansion	• Assess for signs and symptoms of pneumothorax, such as decreased breath sounds, subcutaneous emphysema, and dyspnea. • Monitor ventilator pressure readings for increased PIP and increased static compliance. • Avoid high-volume or high-pressure settings in high-risk patients. • Use PEEP at lowest optimal levels.
Impaired gas exchange related to hypoxemia secondary to disease process, pulmonary interstitial edema, or reduced lung compliance	• Respiratory rate < 20 breaths/minute • No labored respirations • No adventitious breath sounds • pH 7.35 to 7.45 • $Paco_2$ 35 to 45 mm Hg • Pao_2 > 60 mm Hg • Sao_2 > 90%	• Monitor vital signs and assess respiratory status every hour, including rate and rhythm; presence of crackles, wheezes, bronchial breath sounds, diminished or absent breath sounds; central cyanosis and hypoxia (as evidenced by restlessness, forgetfulness, lethargy, tachycardia, and tachypnea); and use of accessory muscles. For the ventilated patient, also monitor hemodynamic parameters. • Assess ventilatory support if appropriate, including tidal volume, ventilator rate versus patient rate, and FIO_2. • Administer supplemental oxygen, as ordered, during rest and patient activity. • Maintain patent airway, using chest physiotherapy (CPT), suctioning, and position changes. • Avoid placing affected lung in a dependent position because increased blood flow to the dependent, poorly oxygenated lung will increase ventilation-perfusion mismatch. • Monitor ABG levels as needed and 20 minutes after each ventilator change or treatment, such as CPT. • Use sedation and analgesics cautiously to avoid depressing ventilation. • To decrease oxygen need and consumption, schedule patient activities and tests to allow appropriate rest periods.
Impaired gas exchange related to positive water balance	• No adventitious breath sounds • Urine output > 0.5 ml/kg/ hour • Balanced intake and output • Pink, moist mucous membranes • PCWP 10 to 12 mm Hg	• Monitor vital signs, mucous membrane and skin turgor, and accurate intake and output. • Administer crystalloids, colloids, and blood products, as ordered. • Monitor for signs and symptoms of fluid overload, such as PCWP > 18 mm Hg, crackles on auscultation, weight gain, intake greater than output, and edema.

Cardiopulmonary care plans *(continued)*

Nursing diagnosis	Expected outcomes	Nursing interventions
Impaired gas exchange related to positive water balance *(continued)*	• Hematocrit 42% to 52% (0.42 to 0.52) in males and 37% to 47% (0.37 to 0.47) in females	• Assess breath sounds for adventitious sounds, especially crackles in dependent portion of lung fields. Increased blood flow to dependent lung areas causes extravasation of fluid into the alveoli and, thus, increased crackles. • Reposition patient as tolerated, elevating head of bed to maintain gravity effect on fluid.
Impaired gas exchange related to right mainstem bronchus intubation	• Tip of artificial airway 4 to 6 cm above carina, as seen on chest X-ray • No adventitious breath sounds	• Assess for bilateral breath sounds immediately after intubation. • Have doctor review chest X-ray for correct placement. • Check level markings of oral endotracheal tube. Maintain markings at the same level. • After patient or tube position change, monitor for signs of right mainstem bronchus intubation, such as wheezing, respiratory distress, and absence of left side breath sounds.
Ineffective airway clearance related to altered airway protective reflex mechanisms or disease condition	• An intact gag reflex • Vesicular breath sounds • No adventitious breath sounds • Clear, patent airway	• Assess respiratory rate, rhythm, and depth of adventitious breath sounds, use of accessory muscles, stridor, restlessness, and confusion. • Position patient so that airway is open (head midline, slightly hyperextended, if appropriate), and promote optimal lung expansion. • Reposition patient every 2 hours. • Encourage two to three breaths before coughing. • Assess patient's ability to cough effectively. Teach patient an effective coughing technique if necessary. • Use CPT, when tolerated, to loosen secretions. • Suction large airways after coughing to remove any secretions. Be sure to hyperinflate or hyperoxygenate with an FIO_2 of 100% before and after suctioning. • Maintain adequate fluid intake to help keep secretions mobile.
Ineffective breathing pattern related to acute respiratory failure	• Effective breathing pattern restored; rate and depth returned to baseline • $Paco_2$ within normal limits • pH within normal limits • No labored breathing or use of accessory muscles • Dyspnea and anxiety relieved	• Assess rate, depth, and pattern of respirations. • Auscultate for decreased breath sounds. • Position patient for optimal chest expansion as tolerated. • If patient is lethargic, maintain head in midline position to help ensure patent airway. • Encourage patient to deep-breathe and cough once or twice every 5 to 10 minutes. • Instruct and encourage patient to use an effective breathing pattern, such as slow and deep or pursed-lip breathing. • Monitor the work of breathing. • Help patient avoid activities that will increase oxygen consumption. • Avoid medications that depress respirations.
Ineffective breathing pattern related to asynchronous ventilation (fighting the ventilator)	• Synchronous ventilator and spontaneous breaths	• Assess respiratory rate and rhythm, and chest excursion. • Evaluate for signs and symptoms of increased anxiety, fear, pain, hypoxia, hypercarbia, acidemia, and central nervous system (CNS) malfunction, which can cause asynchronous breathing. • Increase peak flow rate if set too low, or decrease inspiratory time if prolonged.

(continued)

Cardiopulmonary care plans *(continued)*

Nursing diagnosis	Expected outcomes	Nursing interventions
Ineffective breathing pattern related to asynchronous ventilation (fighting the ventilator) *(continued)*		• Monitor for altered PIP and static pressure to evaluate compliance and to distinguish airway disease from parenchymal disease. • Sedation and pharmacologic paralysis may be considered if cause of asynchronous ventilation is increased PIP. Control mode ventilation must be used when pharmacologic paralysis is used.
Ineffective breathing pattern related to hyperventilation or respiratory alkalosis	• pH 7.35 to 7.45 • $PaCO_2$ 35 to 45 mm Hg • PaO_2 > 60 mm Hg • SaO_2 > 90%	• Assess for increased respiratory rate accompanied by anxiety, restlessness, discomfort, pain, hypoxemia, CNS malfunction, metabolic acidosis, and dyspnea. • Evaluate for appropriateness of respiratory rate (ventilator breaths at 8 to 12 per minute), tidal volume (should be set at 10 to 15 ml/kg; 10 ml/kg in chronic lung disease), inspiratory-expiratory (I:E) ratio, and peak flow rate. Consider ventilator mode change if breathing pattern continues to be ineffective. • Check PaO_2, and optimize oxygenation by secretion control and comfort measures. • Treat metabolic disturbances. • Increase dead space by adding up to, but no more than, 50 cc of tubing between the Y-piece of the ventilator circuit and the patient's artificial airway. • Maintain sensitivity dial at the level to achieve a negative pressure 2 cm H_2O below the level at the end of expiration. With PEEP therapy, set pressure at 2 cm H_2O below the level of PEEP; for example, if PEEP is at 5 cm H_2O pressure, set pressure level at 3 cm H_2O. • Check ABG levels and breath sounds 20 minutes after every ventilator change. • Monitor for cardiac dysrhythmias, tetany, and seizures secondary to alkalotic electrolyte imbalances.
Ineffective breathing pattern related to hypoventilation or respiratory acidosis	• pH 7.35 to 7.45 • $PaCO_2$ 35 to 45 mm Hg • PaO_2 > 60 mm Hg • SaO_2 > 90%	• Observe for symptoms of hypercarbia, including changes in vital signs, lethargy, drowsiness, and coma. • Check ventilator settings and increase tidal volume or respiratory rate, and decrease dead space. • Evaluate nutritional support because excessive carbohydrates cause surplus glucose to be converted to fat, resulting in increased production of carbon dioxide and increased oxygen consumption. • Monitor minute ventilation, respiratory rate, oxygen concentration, carbon dioxide production and ABG levels. • Observe for increased ventilation-perfusion mismatch secondary to increased airway resistance or decreased compliance. The I:E ratio should be at least 1:2 in adults. Increase end-expiratory pause for optimal diffusion to take place. • If patient has a chest tube, check for bronchopleural air leak (bubbling in water seal chamber of chest tube drainage). If present, decrease loss of tidal volume by decreasing ventilator breaths to lowest level with acceptable ABG values; decrease tidal volume to 10 ml/kg; avoid inflation holds, expiratory retard, PEEP, and continuous positive airway pressure; and explore effect of position changes on decreasing peak flow.

Cardiopulmonary care plans *(continued)*

Nursing diagnosis	Expected outcomes	Nursing interventions
Ineffective individual and family coping related to hospitalization secondary to inability to communicate, anxiety, fear, loneliness, and powerlessness	• Effective system of communication established • Patient and family participation in plan of care • Patient's uninterrupted sleep period at least 4 hours • Family's concerns addressed; fewer than three calls to check on patient's status	• Identify acceptable method of communication, and communicate on nursing care plan. • Place call light within patient's reach at all times. • If necessary, phrase questions so that they require a simple "yes" or "no" answer. • Schedule rest periods to decrease fatigue with communication efforts. • Monitor for signs of distress, such as increased crying, anxiety, restlessness, irritability, aggressiveness, changes in sleep pattern, or nightmares. • Observe for expression of fear (facial expressions and gestures), lack of communication with others, and signs of discomfort, such as increased respiratory rate. • Involve patient's family in care; contact a designated person and set up a regular calling time to give status report. • Encourage expression of feelings by patient and family, and refer them to appropriate resources. • Provide comfort measures, such as touch, analgesia, and distraction. • Provide simple explanations of all procedures and activities, and allow patient to make decisions as able. • Provide emotional support and reassurance. • Provide for familiarity in surroundings by allowing frequent visitors, significant personal belongings, a clock, a calendar, pictures, a television, and consistency of personnel. • Provide for patient's privacy during bathing, procedures, and family visits by closing curtains, using individual cubicles, or providing a screen. • Refer unusual patient or family problems to a clinical nurse specialist, chaplain, or social worker. Include such consultants in planning and implementing care. • If patient's hospitalization is trauma-related, reorient patient to date, time, place, and person every 8 hours and as needed. Explain what happened during the accident and the reason for hospital admission. Notify patient of family's location and times for visitation. • Discuss with significant others and doctor which details to tell patient about the accident, such as who was at fault, who else was injured, and outcome of other passengers' injuries, if pertinent.
Knowledge deficit related to health problems, medical procedures, and self-care responsibilities	Patient able to verbalize understanding of health problems and to demonstrate self-care skills and procedures	• Provide instruction regarding disease process and medical procedures. • Provide opportunity and appropriate environment for discussion and feedback. • Evaluate patient's knowledge level, and develop a new teaching plan to meet any unmet needs.
Pain related to myocardial ischemia	• Patient verbalizes that he is pain-free • Vital signs within patient's normal limits • Patient able to rest	• Assess patient's physical symptoms of pain (type, location and duration, skin color, and temperature). • Monitor vital signs as needed. • Administer oxygen as ordered (usually 4 to 5 liters/minute). • Administer medications as ordered. Evaluate their effectiveness.

(continued)

Cardiopulmonary care plans *(continued)*

Nursing diagnosis	Expected outcomes	Nursing interventions
Pain related to myocardial ischemia *(continued)*		• Obtain a stat ECG according to hospital policy if pain persists. • Keep patient in supine, semi-Fowler's position. • Limit patient's physical activity as necessary. • Provide a calm, quiet environment.
Potential for infection related to altered immunologic or nutritional status, excessive fluid in the alveoli, or disrupted cough reflex	• Temperature within normal limits • White blood cell (WBC) count 5,000 to 10,000/mm³ (5 to 10 × 10⁹/liter) • No local inflammation • No pain	• Check temperature every 4 hours. • Monitor for signs of infection, noting amount, color, and consistency of pulmonary secretions; assess all catheter insertion sites for signs and symptoms of infection. • Mobilize pulmonary secretions. Maintain proper humidification and hydration status. Implement sterile suctioning technique as needed. • Perform CPT every 4 hours as tolerated. • Change patient's position every 1 to 2 hours to help mobilize secretions. • Use proper hand-washing technique to prevent auto- and cross-contamination. • Monitor laboratory data, including WBC count and culture and sensitivity tests. • Maintain skin integrity as barrier to infection. • Clean areas around invasive lines meticulously.
Potential for injury related to dysrhythmias secondary to myocardial ischemia	• Monitor showing normal sinus rhythm or a controlled dysrhythmia with a ventricular rate of 60 to 100 beats/minute • Peripheral pulses will be strong and equal bilaterally • Hemodynamic values within normal limits • Clear breath sounds	• Attach patient to a cardiac monitor and observe for dysrhythmias: ventricular dysrhythmias, such as accelerated ventricular rhythm, premature ventricular contractions (PVCs), ventricular tachycardia, ventricular fibrillation; and supraventricular dysrhythmias, such as premature atrial and junctional contractions, atrial tachycardia, atrial fibrillation, atrial flutter, and supraventricular tachycardia. • Treat symptomatic dysrhythmias as ordered: lidocaine for PVCs greater than 6 per minute, sequential or multifocal PVCs, PVCs close to the T wave, ventricular tachycardia, or ventricular fibrillation. • Have code cart readily available.
Potential for suffocation related to loss of tidal volume secondary to increased airway pressure resulting from biting or kinking of artificial airway, decreased compliance, coughing, or copious secretions	• Peak airway pressure at a level allowing delivery of full tidal volume • Tidal volume at approximately 10 to 15 ml/kg	• Check ventilator settings at least once every 2 hours and with any sudden onset of respiratory insufficiency or low pressure alarm. • If low pressure alarm occurs, evaluate ventilator and its circuitry for an air leak. Check that all connections, humidification jar, and temperature sensing device are intact. To confirm a hole in the tubing, place area where air movement is felt under water to check for bubbling. Check for ventilator power failure or loss of compressed air source. If unable to identify cause of low pressure alarm within 10 to 15 seconds, remove patient from ventilator and provide manual ventilatory support. Make sure ventilator is checked before returning patient to ventilator. • Assess ventilator's ability to operate at prescribed settings. A potential for loss of volume can occur from a combination of high tidal volume, respiratory rate, and peak flow settings that exceed the inherent capabilities of the ventilator. The problem may be corrected by decreasing the peak flow rate,

Cardiopulmonary care plans *(continued)*

Nursing diagnosis	Expected outcomes	Nursing interventions
Potential for suffocation related to loss of tidal volume secondary to increased airway pressure resulting from biting or kinking of artificial airway, decreased compliance, coughing, or copious secretions *(continued)*		lengthening the inspiratory time, decreasing the respiratory rate, or decreasing volume settings. • Prevent occlusion of oral endotracheal airway. Instruct patient not to bite on artificial airway. If necessary, place bite block on oral airway to prevent airway occlusion. • Perform appropriate suctioning to maintain airway patency. • Medicate as needed for wheezing or bronchospasm. • Monitor for increased PIP after position change secondary to poor lung compliance. • Evaluate cause of coughing, such as movement of the tube secondary to poor stabilization; deflated cuff; jarring of the artificial airway secondary to head movement; tube touching the carina; or attempt to talk. If necessary, stabilize tube with tape or ties. Avoid tube movement by supporting the oral endotracheal tube. Evaluate for optimal cuff inflation (higher cuff pressures are needed as PIP increases). Check chest X-ray for proper tube placement. Establish alternate communication method if necessary. • High pressure alarm should be set 10 to 15 cm H_2O above the PIP necessary to ventilate the patient. Consider upward adjustment of the alarm setting as long as the high pressure limit remains at an acceptable level. • Evaluate for proper cuff inflation at least once per shift and as needed. Monitor for insufficient air in cuff, a hole in cuff, leak in air inflation port (one-way valve), or displaced artificial airway by noting movement of air in patient's upper airways or audible vocal sounds. The patient must be reintubated if leak in cuff occurs and placing a syringe or stopcock in the air inflation port does not control it. While waiting for reintubation, increasing the tidal volume may temporarily compensate for leakage of air.

Common bronchodilators

The agents listed here, classified as sympathomimetics and methylxanthines, are the most commonly used bronchodilators.

Sympathomimetics (adrenergics)

albuterol
Proventil, Ventolin

Mechanism of action
Relaxes bronchial smooth muscle by acting on $beta_2$-adrenergic receptors.

Respiratory indications and dosage
• To prevent and treat bronchospasm in patients with reversible obstructive airway disease—
Adults and children over age 13: 1 to 2 inhalations q 4 to 6 hours. Each metered dose delivers 90 mcg of albuterol. More frequent administration or a greater number of inhalations is not recommended. For oral tablets, 2 to 4 mg t.i.d. or q.i.d. Maximum dosage is 8 mg q.i.d.
Children age 6 to 13: 2 mg (1 teaspoonful) t.i.d. or q.i.d.
Children age 2 to 5: 0.1 mg/kg t.i.d., not to exceed 2 mg (1 teaspoonful) t.i.d. or q.i.d.
Adults over age 65: 2 mg t.i.d. or q.i.d.
• To prevent exercise-induced asthma—

Adults: 2 inhalations 15 minutes before exercise.

Adverse reactions
CNS: tremor, nervousness, dizziness, insomnia, headache.
CV: tachycardia, palpitations, hypertension.
EENT: drying and irritation of nose and throat (with inhaled form).
GI: heartburn, nausea, vomiting.
Other: muscle cramps.

Interactions
Propranolol and other beta blockers: blocked bronchodilating effect of albuterol. Monitor patient carefully.

Clinical considerations
• Use cautiously in patients with cardiovascular disorders, including coronary insufficiency and hypertension; in patients with hyperthyroidism or diabetes mellitus; and in patients who are usually responsive to adrenergics. Cardiac arrest can occur.

• Warn patient about the possibility of paradoxical bronchospasm. If this occurs, the drug should be discontinued immediately.
• Patients may use tablets and aerosol concomitantly. Monitor closely for toxicity.
• Albuterol reportedly produces less cardiac stimulation than other sympathomimetics, especially isoproterenol.
• Elderly patients usually require a lower dose.
• Teach patient how to administer metered dose correctly. Have him shake container; exhale through nose; administer aerosol while inhaling deeply on mouthpiece of inhaler; and hold breath for a few seconds, then exhale slowly. Tell him to allow 2 minutes between inhalations.
• Pleasant-tasting syrup may be taken by children as young as age 2. Preparation contains no alcohol or sugar. Store drug in light-resistant container.

epinephrine
Inhalants: Bronkaid Mist, Primatene Mist

epinephrine bitartrate
Adrenalin, Sus-Phrine

Mechanism of action
Stimulates alpha- and beta-adrenergic receptors within the sympathetic nervous system.

Respiratory indications and dosage
• Bronchospasm, hypersensitivity reactions, and anaphylaxis—
Adults: 0.1 to 0.5 ml (1:1,000) S.C. or I.M. Repeat q 10 to 15 minutes, p.r.n. Or 0.1 to 0.25 ml (1:1,000) I.V.
Children: 0.01 ml/kg (1:1,000) S.C. Repeat q 20 minutes to 4 hours, p.r.n. Or 0.005 ml/kg (1:200, Sus-Phrine). Repeat q 8 to 12 hours, p.r.n.
• Acute asthmatic attacks—
Adults and children: 1 or 2 inhalations

of 1:100 or 2.25% racemic q 1 to 5 minutes until relief is obtained; 0.2 mg/dose is usual content.

Adverse reactions
CNS: nervousness, tremor, euphoria, anxiety, cold extremities, vertigo, headache, sweating, cerebral hemorrhage, disorientation, agitation; in patients with Parkinson's disease, the drug increases rigidity and tremor.
CV: palpitations, widened pulse pressure, hypertension, tachycardia, ventricular fibrillation, cerebrovascular accident, anginal pain, ECG changes (including decreased T-wave amplitude).
Metabolic: hyperglycemia, glycosuria.
Other: pulmonary edema, dyspnea, pallor.

Interactions
Tricyclic antidepressants: severe hypertension (hypertensive crisis). Don't give together.
Propranolol: vasoconstriction and reflex bradycardia. Monitor patient carefully.

Clinical considerations
• Drug is contraindicated in patients with narrow-angle glaucoma, shock (except anaphylactic shock), organic brain damage, cardiac dilation, and coronary insufficiency; during general anesthesia with halogenated hydrocarbons or cyclopropane; and in patients in labor (may delay second stage). Use with extreme caution in patients with long-standing bronchial asthma and emphysema who have developed degenerative heart disease. Use with caution in elderly patients and in patients with hyperthyroidism, angina, hypertension, psychoneurosis, or diabetes.
• Don't mix with alkaline solutions. Use dextrose 5% in water (D_5W), normal saline solution, or a combination of D_5W

Common bronchodilators (continued)

Sympathomimetics (adrenergics)

epinephrine
epinephrine bitartrate
(continued)

and normal saline solution. Mix just before use.
• Epinephrine is destroyed rapidly by oxidizing agents, such as iodine, chromates, nitrates, nitrites, oxygen, and salts of easily reducible metals (for example, iron).
• Epinephrine solutions deteriorate after 24 hours. Discard after that time or before if solution is discolored or contains precipitate. Keep solution in light-resis-

tant container and don't remove before use.
• Massage site after injection to counteract possible vasoconstriction. Repeated local injection can cause necrosis at site (from vasoconstriction).
• Avoid I.M. administration of suspension into buttocks. Gas gangrene may occur because epinephrine reduces oxygen tension of the tissues, encouraging growth of contaminating organisms.
• This drug may widen pulse pressure.
• In case of a sharp blood pressure rise, rapid-acting vasodilators, such as nitrites or alpha-adrenergic blocking

agents, can be given to counteract the marked pressor effect of large epinephrine doses.
• Observe patient closely for adverse reactions. If these develop, dosage may need to be adjusted or the drug discontinued.
• If patient has acute hypersensitivity reactions, teach him how to inject epinephrine.
• Epinephrine is the drug of choice in emergency treatment of acute anaphylactic reactions, including anaphylactic shock.

---

isoetharine hydrochloride 1%
Bronkosol

isoetharine mesylate
Bronkometer

Mechanism of action
Relaxes bronchial smooth muscle by acting on beta$_2$-adrenergic receptors.

Respiratory indications and dosage
• Bronchial asthma and reversible bronchospasm that may occur with bronchitis and emphysema—
Adults (hydrochloride): Administered by hand nebulizer, 3 to 7 inhalations (undiluted); by oxygen aerosolization, 0.5 ml, diluted 1:3 in normal saline solution; by intermittent positive-pressure breathing, 0.5 ml, diluted 1:3 in normal saline solution.

Adults (mesylate): 1 to 2 inhalations. Occasionally, more may be required.

Adverse reactions
CNS: tremor, headache, dizziness, excitement.
CV: palpitations, increased heart rate.
GI: nausea, vomiting.

Interactions
Propranolol and other beta blockers: blocked bronchodilating effect of isoetharine. Monitor patient carefully if used together.

Clinical considerations
• Use cautiously in patients with hyperthyroidism, hypertension, or coronary disease, and in those with sensitivity to sympathomimetics.

• Excessive use can lead to decreased effectiveness.
• Monitor for severe paradoxical bronchoconstriction after excessive use. Discontinue immediately if bronchoconstriction occurs.
• Although isoetharine has minimal effects on the heart, it should be used cautiously in patients receiving general anesthetics that sensitize the myocardium to sympathomimetic drugs.
• Instruct patient in the use of aerosol and mouthpiece.
• Because drug oxidizes when diluted with water, pink sputum resembling hemoptysis may appear after inhalation of isoetharine solution. Tell patient not to be concerned.

---

isoproterenol hydrochloride
Isuprel
Inhalants: Norisodrine, Vapo-Iso

isoproterenol sulfate
Medihaler-Iso, Norisodrine

Mechanism of action
Relaxes bronchial smooth muscle by acting on beta$_2$-adrenergic receptors. As a cardiac stimulant, acts on beta$_1$-adrenergic receptors in the heart.

Respiratory indications and dosage
• Bronchial asthma and reversible bronchospasm (hydrochloride)—
Adults: 10 to 20 mg S.L. q 6 to 8 hours.
Children age 6 and over: 5 to 10 mg

S.L. q 6 to 8 hours. Not recommended for children under age 6.
• Bronchospasm (sulfate)—
Adults and children: For acute dyspneic episodes, 1 inhalation initially. May repeat if needed after 2 to 5 minutes. Maintenance dose is 1 to 2 inhalations four to six times a day. May repeat once more 10 minutes after second dose. No more than three doses should be administered for each attack.

Adverse reactions
CNS: headache, mild tremor, weakness, dizziness, anxiety, insomnia.
CV: palpitations, tachycardia, anginal pain; blood pressure may rise and then fall.
GI: nausea, vomiting.

Metabolic: hyperglycemia.
Other: sweating, facial flushing, bronchial edema, inflammation.

Interactions
Propranolol and other beta blockers: blocked bronchodilating effect of isoproterenol. Monitor patient carefully if used together.

Clinical considerations
• Drug is contraindicated in tachycardia caused by digitalis toxicity; in preexisting dysrhythmias, especially tachycardia, because drug's chronotropic effect on the heart may aggravate such disorders; and in recent myocardial infarction. Use cautiously in coronary
(continued)

Common bronchodilators *(continued)*

Sympathomimetics (adrenergics)

isoproterenol hydrochloride
isoproterenol sulfate
(continued)

insufficiency, diabetes, and hyperthyroidism.
• If heart rate exceeds 110 beats/minute, decrease infusion rate or temporarily stop infusion, if ordered. Doses sufficient to increase the heart rate to more than 130 beats/minute may induce ventricular dysrhythmias.
• If precordial distress or anginal pain occurs, stop drug immediately.
• Oral and sublingual tablets are absorbed poorly and erratically.
• Teach patient how to take sublingual tablet properly. Tell him to hold tablet under tongue until it dissolves and is absorbed and not to swallow saliva until

that time. Prolonged use of sublingual tablets can cause tooth decay. Instruct patient to rinse mouth with water between doses; this also helps prevent oropharynx dryness.
• If possible, don't give at bedtime because drug interrupts sleep patterns.
• This drug may cause slight systolic blood pressure rise and slight to marked drop in diastolic blood pressure.
• Use a microdrip or infusion pump to regulate infusion flow rate.
• Observe patient closely for adverse reactions. Dosage may need to be adjusted or the drug discontinued.
• Teach patient to perform oral inhalation correctly. Give the following instructions for using a metered-dose nebulizer:
—Clear nasal passages and throat.

—Breathe out, expelling as much air from lungs as possible.
—Place mouthpiece well into mouth as dose from nebulizer is released, and inhale deeply.
—Hold breath for several seconds, remove mouthpiece, and exhale slowly.
• Instructions for metered powder nebulizer are the same, except that deep inhalation isn't necessary.
• Patient may develop tolerance to this drug. Warn against overuse.
• Warn patient using oral inhalant that drug may turn sputum and saliva pink.
• Drug may aggravate ventilation perfusion abnormalities; although it eases breathing, it may cause arterial oxygen tension to fall paradoxically.
• Discard inhalation solution if it is discolored or contains precipitate.

terbutaline sulfate
Brethaire, Brethine, Bricanyl

Mechanism of action
Relaxes bronchial smooth muscle by acting on beta₂-adrenergic receptors.

Respiratory indications and dosage
• Relief of bronchospasm in patients with reversible obstructive airway disease—
Adults and children over age 11: two inhalations separated by a 60-second interval, repeated q 4 to 6 hours. May also administer 2.5 to 5 mg P.O. q 8 hours or 0.25 mg S.C.

Adverse reactions
CNS: nervousness, tremor, headache, drowsiness, sweating.

CV: palpitations, increased heart rate.
EENT: drying and irritation of nose and throat (with inhaled form).
GI: vomiting, nausea.

Interactions
MAO inhibitors: possible severe hypertension (hypertensive crisis). Don't use together.
Propranolol and other beta blockers: blocked bronchodilating effect of terbutaline.

Clinical considerations
• Use cautiously in patients with diabetes, hypertension, hyperthyroidism, severe cardiac disease, or cardiac dysrhythmias.
• Protect injection from light. Don't use if discolored.

• Make sure patient and his family understand why drug is necessary.
• Give S.C. injections in lateral deltoid area.
• Tolerance may develop with prolonged use.
• Warn patient about the possibility of paradoxical bronchospasm. If this occurs, the drug should be discontinued immediately.
• Patient may use tablets and aerosol concomitantly. Monitor closely for toxicity.
• Teach patient how to administer metered dose correctly. Have him shake container, exhale through nose, administer aerosol while inhaling deeply on mouthpiece of inhaler, hold breath for a few seconds, then exhale slowly.

Methylxanthines

aminophylline (theophylline ethylenediamine)
Aminophyllin, Corophyllin, Phyllocontin, Somophyllin-DF

Mechanism of action
Acts directly on airway smooth muscle to produce bronchodilation.

Respiratory indications and dosage
• Symptomatic relief of bronchospasm—
Patients not currently receiving theoph-

ylline who require rapid relief of symptoms: Loading dose is 6 mg/kg (equivalent to 4.7 mg/kg anhydrous theophylline) I.V. slowly (less than or equal to 25 mg/kg minute), then maintenance infusion.
Adults (nonsmokers): 0.7 mg/kg/hour for 12 hours; then 0.5 mg/kg/hour.
Otherwise healthy adult smokers: 1 mg/kg/hour for 12 hours; then 0.18 mg/kg/hour.
Older patients and adults with cor pul-

monale: 0.6 mg/kg/hour for 12 hours; then 0.3 mg/kg/hour.
Adults with congestive heart failure (CHF) or liver disease: 0.5 mg/kg/hour for 12 hours; then 0.1 to 0.2 mg/kg/hour.
Children age 9 to 16: 1 mg/kg/hour for 12 hours; then 0.8 mg/kg/hour.
Children age 6 months to 9 years: 1.2 mg/kg/hour for 12 hours; then 1 mg/kg/hour.

Common bronchodilators (continued)

Methylxanthines

aminophylline (theophylline ethylenediamine) (continued)

Patients currently receiving theophylline: Aminophylline infusions of 0.63 mg/kg (0.5 mg/kg anhydrous theophylline) will increase plasma levels of theophylline by 1 mcg/ml. Some clinicians recommend a dose of 3.1 mg/kg (2.5 mg/kg anhydrous theophylline) if no obvious signs of theophylline toxicity are present.
• Chronic bronchial asthma—
Adults: 600 to 1,600 mg P.O. daily divided t.i.d. or q.i.d.
Children: 12 mg/kg P.O. daily divided t.i.d. or q.i.d.

Adverse reactions
CNS: restlessness, dizziness, headache, insomnia, light-headedness, convulsions, muscle twitching.
CV: palpitations, sinus tachycardia, extrasystole, flushing, marked hypotension, increased respiratory rate.
GI: nausea, vomiting, anorexia, bitter aftertaste, dyspepsia, heavy feeling in stomach, diarrhea.
Skin: urticaria.
Local: irritation (with rectal suppositories).

Interactions
Alkali-sensitive drugs: reduced activity. Don't add to I.V. fluids containing aminophylline.
Beta-adrenergic blockers: antagonized effects. Propranolol and nadolol, especially, may cause bronchospasm in sensitive patients. Use together cautiously.

Troleandomycin, erythromycin, cimetidine: decreased hepatic clearance of theophylline; elevated theophylline levels. Monitor for signs of toxicity.
Barbiturates, phenytoin: enhanced metabolism and decreased theophylline blood levels. Monitor for decreased aminophylline effect.

Clinical considerations
• Drug is contraindicated in patients with hypersensitivity to xanthine compounds (such as caffeine and theobromine) and in those with preexisting cardiac dysrhythmias, especially tachydysrhythmias. Use cautiously in young children; in elderly patients with CHF or other cardiac or circulatory impairment, cor pulmonale, or hepatic disease; in patients with active peptic ulcer because drug may increase volume and acidity of gastric secretions; and in patients with hyperthyroidism or diabetes mellitus.
• Individuals metabolize xanthines at different rates. Adjust dose by monitoring response, tolerance, pulmonary function, and theophylline blood levels. Therapeutic level is 10 to 20 mcg/ml; toxicity may occur at levels over 20 mcg/ml.
• Plasma clearance may decrease in patients with CHF, hepatic dysfunction, or pulmonary edema. Smokers show accelerated clearance. Dose must be adjusted.
• I.V. administration can cause burning; dilute with dextrose in water solution.
• Monitor vital signs; measure and record intake and output. Expected clini-

cal effects include improved quality of pulse and respiration.
• Warn elderly patients that drug may cause dizziness, a common adverse reaction at the start of therapy.
• GI symptoms may be relieved by taking the oral drug with a full glass of water at meals, although food in the stomach delays absorption. Enteric-coated tablets may also delay and impair absorption. Antacids reportedly do not reduce GI adverse reactions.
• Suppositories are absorbed slowly and erratically; retention enemas may be absorbed more rapidly. Rectally administered preparations can be given if the patient can't take the drug orally. Schedule dose after evacuation, if possible; dose may be retained better if given before a meal. Advise patient to remain recumbent for 15 to 20 minutes after insertion.
• Question patient closely about other drugs used. Warn that over-the-counter remedies may contain ephedrine in combination with theophylline salts; excessive CNS stimulation may result. Tell him to check with doctor or pharmacist before taking any other medications.
• Before giving loading dose, check that patient has not had recent theophylline therapy.
• Teach patient about home care and dosage schedule. Some patients may require a round-the-clock dosage schedule.
• Warn patient with allergies that exposure to allergens may exacerbate bronchospasm.

Selected references

American Heart Association. "Standards and Guidelines for Cardiopulmonary Resuscitation and Emergency Cardiac Care," *Journal of the American Medical Association* 255(21):2842-3044, June 6, 1986.

American Heart Association. *Textbook of Advanced Cardiac Life Support.* Dallas: American Heart Association, 1987.

American Thoracic Society. "Standards for the Diagnosis and Care of Patients with Chronic Obstructive Pulmonary Disease (COPD) and Asthma," *American Review of Respiratory Disease* 136(1):225-44, January 1987.

Anderson, F.D. "Issues in the Postresuscitation Period," *Critical Care Nursing Quarterly* 10(4):51-61, March 1988.

Birdsall, C. "How and When Do You Use Pulse Oximetry?" *American Journal of Nursing* 87(2):158, February 1987.

Bradley, R.D. "Adult Respiratory Distress Syndrome," *Focus on Critical Care* 14(5):48-59, October 1987.

Braunwald, E. *Heart Disease: A Textbook of Cardiovascular Medicine,* 3rd ed. Philadelphia: W.B. Saunders Co., 1988.

Bullas, J.B., and Pfister, S.M. "Variant Angina," *Critical Care Nurse* 7(4):9-12, July-August 1987.

Cardiac Problems. NurseReview Series. Springhouse, Pa.: Springhouse Corp., 1987.

Celentano-Norton, L. "Mechanical Ventilation Strategies in ARDS," *Critical Care Nurse* 6(4):71-74, July-August 1986.

Chalikan, J., and Weaver, T.E. "CE: Mechanical Ventilation: Where It's At, Where It's Going," *American Journal of Nursing* 84(11):1372-79, November 1984.

Cheney, R. "Defibrillation," *Critical Care Nursing Quarterly* 10(4):9-15, March 1988.

Cherniack, R. "Comprehensive Approach to Asthma," *Chest* 87 (1 Suppl):94s-97s, January 1985.

Cohen, S. "Advances in the Diagnosis and Treatment of Asthma," *Chest* 87(1 Suppl):26s-30s, January 1985.

Difilippo, N.M., and Jenkins, A.J. "Pressure Support Ventilation," *American Family Physician* 38(2):147-50, August 1988.

Domigan-Wentz, J. "The CPAP Mask: A Comfortable Approach to ARDS," *American Journal of Nursing* 85(7):813-15, July 1985.

Fishman, A., ed. *Pulmonary Diseases and Disorders.* New York: McGraw Hill Book Co., 1988.

Glauser, F., et al. "Worsening Oxygenation in the Mechanically Ventilated Patient," *American Review of Respiratory Disease* 138(2):458-65, August 1988.

Grossbach, I. "Troubleshooting Ventilator- and Patient-Related Problems, Part I," *Critical Care Nurse* 6(4):58-70, July-August 1986.

Grossbach, I. "Troubleshooting Ventilator- and Patient-Related Problems, Part II," *Critical Care Nurse* 6(5):64-79, September-October 1986.

Gruden, M. "High-Frequency Ventilation: An Overview," *Critical Care Nurse* 5(1):36-40, January-February 1985.

Hess, D. "Bedside Monitoring of the Patient on a Ventilator," *Critical Care Quarterly* 6(2):23-32, September 1983.

Hurst, J.W., ed. *The Heart,* 6th ed. New York: McGraw-Hill Book Co., 1986.

Kenner, C.V., et al. *Critical Care Nursing—Body Mind Spirit,* 2nd ed. Boston: Little Brown & Co., 1985.

Kinney, M., et al. *AACN's Clinical Reference for Critical Care Nursing,* 2nd ed. New York: McGraw-Hill Book Co., 1988.

Kirby, R.R., and Taylor, R.W. *Respiratory Failure.* Chicago: Yearbook Medical Publishers, Inc., 1986.

Lamb, J., and Carlson, V.R. *Handbook of Cardiovascular Nursing.* Philadelphia: J.B. Lippincott Co., 1986.

Lameier, D. "Cardiogenic Shock," in *Difficult Diagnosis in Critical Care Nursing.* Edited by Sommers, M.S. Rockville, Md.: Aspen Systems Corp., 1988.

Lopez, M., and Salvaggio, J. "Bronchial Asthma: Mechanisms and Management of a Complex Obstructive Airway Disease," *Postgraduate Medicine* 82(5):177-90, October 1987.

MacIntyre, N.R., "Respiratory Function During Pressure Support Ventilation," *Chest* 89(5):677-88, May 1986.

Melchior, J.P., et al. "Percutaneous Transluminal Coronary Angioplasty for Chronic Total Coronary Arterial Occlusion," *American Journal of Cardiology* 59(6):535-38, March 1, 1987.

Murray, J.F., et al. "An Expanded Definition of the Adult Respiratory Distress Syndrome," *American Review of Respiratory Disease* 138(3):720-23, September 1988.

O'Mara, R.J. "Ethical Dilemmas with Advance Directives: Living Wills and Do Not Resuscitate Orders," *Critical Care Nursing Quarterly* 10(2):17-28, September 1987.

Selected references *(continued)*

Parchert, M.A., and Simon, J.M. "The Role of Exercise in Cardiac Rehabilitation: A Nursing Perspective," *Rehabilitation Nursing* 13(1):149, January-February 1988.

Persons, C.B. "External Cardiac Pacing in the Emergency Department," *Journal of Emergency Nursing* 12(6):348-53, November-December 1987.

Petty, T.L. "The Use, Abuse, and Mystique of Positive End-Expiratory Pressure," *American Review of Respiratory Disease* 138(2):475-78, August 1988.

Respiratory Care Handbook. Springhouse, Pa.: Springhouse Corp., 1989.

Schroeder, J.S. "Calcium Antagonists for Cardiovascular Emergencies," *Topics in Emergency Medicine* 8(3):37-49, October 1986.

Snyder, D.S. "Digoxin Immune Fab Ovine," *Critical Care Nurse* 8(8):10-11, November-December 1988.

Sommers, M.S., ed. *Difficult Diagnosis in Critical Care Nursing.* Rockville, Md.: Aspen Systems Corp., 1988.

Stone, P.H. "Calcium Antagonists for Prinzmetal's Variant Angina, Unstable Angina, and Silent Myocardial Ischemia," *American Journal of Cardiology* 59(3):101B-115B, January 30, 1987.

Swearingen, P., et al. *Manual of Critical Care: Applying Nursing Diagnoses to Adult Critical Illness.* St. Louis: C.V. Mosby Co., 1988.

Vasbinder-Dillon, D. "Understanding Mechanical Ventilation," *Critical Care Nurse* 8(7):42-56, October 1988.

Weber, K.T., et al. "Pathophysiology of Acute and Chronic Cardiac Failure," *American Journal of Cardiology* 60(5):3C-9C, August 14, 1987.

White, K.M. "Continuous Monitoring of Mixed Venous Oxygen Saturation (SvO$_2$): A New Assessment Tool in Critical Care Nursing—Part I," *Cardiovascular Nursing* 23(1):1-6, January-February 1987.

White, K.M. "Continuous Monitoring of Mixed Venous Oxygen Saturation (SvO$_2$): A New Assessment Tool in Critical Care Nursing—Part 2," *Cardiovascular Nursing* 23(2):7-12, March-April 1987.

Index

i refers to an illustration; t refers to a table

i refers to an illustration; t refers to a table

Sepsis, ARDS and, 219
Shunt studies, ARDS and, 228t, 229
Silent myocardial ischemia, 50
Sinus bradycardia, 24
 AMI and, 123
Sinus dysrhythmias, 24
 AMI and, 123
Sinus tachycardia, 24
 AMI and, 123
Skeletal muscle ventricle, 175
Skin tests, asthma and, 265
Smoking
 angina and, 55
 cardiac arrest and, 6
Sodium bicarbonate, 31, 34, 203, 275
Sodium nitroprusside, 33t
Sorbide TD, 71
Sorbitrate, 71
Sputum changes, ARF and, 191, 209
Stable angina, 47-48
 diagnosis of, 49
 treatment of, 67
Starling's curve, 167i
Static airway pressure, 291
Status asthmaticus, 253
Steroid therapy, 239
Streptase, 111-112t
Streptokinase, 111-112t
Stress test. See Exercise ECG.
Stroke volume, 140, 142-143
Suctioning, 20
 ARDS and, 245, 246i, 247
Sudden cardiac death. See Cardiac arrest.
Supraventricular rhythms, AMI and, 123-124
Surgery as cause of cardiac arrest, 4
Sympathetic activity, increased, as compensatory mechanism, 144
Sympathomimetics, 168t
 as cause of cardiac arrest, 4
Synchronized cardioversion, 26-27
Synchronized intermittent mandatory ventilation, 294t, 296
Systemic congestion, CHF and, 154, 155
Systemic vascular resistance, 161-162
Systolic heart failure, 147
Systolic murmurs, CHF and, 154

T

Technetium pyrophosphate scanning
 AMI and, 103-105, 105t
 comparison of, with thallium scanning, 105t
Tenormin, 72
Tension pneumothorax as complication of mechanical ventilation, 305
Terbutaline, 267, 268, 269
Thallium scanning, 60
 AMI and, 103, 105t
 comparison of, with technetium pyrophosphate scanning, 105t
Theophylline, 267, 269-271, 270t
 clearance of, 272t
Thiazide diuretics, 166, 168
Third-degree AV block, 25
 AMI and, 124
Thrombolytic agents, 110, 111-112t, 113-114
Thrombosis as cause of AMI, 89
Tissue oxygenation, improvement of, in ARDS, 235-237, 242-244
Tissue plasminogen activator, 111t, 113i
Tornalate, 268
Torsades de pointes, 26
T-piece weaning technique, 320
Tracheal intubation, asthma and, 274
Tracheotomy, 18
Transderm-Nitro, 70
Transmural infarcts, 93
 ECG findings in, 101i
Transthoracic pacing, 29
Transtracheal catheter ventilation 18
Transvenous endocardial pacing, 29
Triamcinolone acetonide, 271-273
Tridil, 70
Tube cuff, inflation of, 303

U

Unstable angina, 48
 diagnosis of, 49
 treatment of, 67
Urokinase, 112t

V

Valsalva's maneuver, cardiac arrest and, 5-6
Variant angina, 48-50
 treatment of, 67

Vasodilators, 169-170
Venodilators, 169-170
Venous oxygen saturation, 162
Venous return, diminished, as complication of mechanical ventilation, 304
Ventilation-perfusion mismatch, 183-184
Ventilator alarms, 302
Ventilator dependence
 as complication of mechanical ventilation, 308
 weaning and, 315, 317-321
Ventilators, types of, 288, 288i, 290-292, 290i
Ventilatory failure, 183, 184
 weaning techniques for, 319-320
Ventolin, 268
Ventricular aneurysm as complication of AMI, 131
Ventricular asystole, cardiac arrest and, 8, 9
Ventricular dilation as compensatory mechanism, 142, 143-144
Ventricular dysrhythmias, 26
 AMI and, 122-123
Ventricular ectopy, cardiac arrest and, 5
Ventricular failure, 138, 148
 signs of, 150
Ventricular fibrillation
 AMI and, 123
 cardiac arrest and, 8
Ventricular flutter, 26
Ventricular function curve, 167i
Ventricular hypertrophy, 144
Ventricular tachycardia, 26
 AMI and, 122-123
Ventriculography, 64
Venturi mask, 19, 199i
Verapamil, 33t, 74, 116
Volume-cycled ventilators, 233, 290-292, 290i
V/Q mismatch, 183-184

W

Weakness, CHF and, 152
Weaning from mechanical ventilation, 315, 317-322
 criteria for, 315, 317-318
 failure of, 321
 techniques for, 318-320
Weight gain, CHF and, 151-152

X

Xanthine derivatives, 202-203

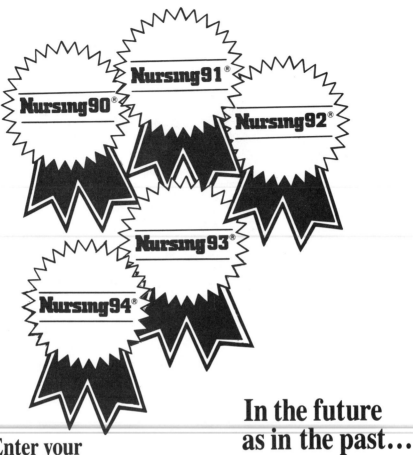

In the future as in the past...

Enter your subscription today

SAVE 38%

You can rely on *Nursing* magazine to keep your skills sharp and your practice current—with award-winning nursing journalism.

Each monthly issue is packed with expert advice on the legal, ethical, and personal issues in nursing, plus up-to-the-minute...

- Drugs—warnings, new uses, and approvals
- Assessment tips
- Emergency and acute care advice
- New treatments, equipment, and disease findings
- Photostories and other skill sharpeners
- AIDS updates
- Career tracks and trends.